HEALTH CARE IN TRANSITION

MEDICAID

POLITICS, POLICY, AND KEY ISSUES

HEALTH CARE IN TRANSITION

Additional books and e-books in this series can be found on Nova's website under the Series tab.

HEALTH CARE IN TRANSITION

MEDICAID

POLITICS, POLICY, AND KEY ISSUES

DANIEL LANFORD, PHD
EDITOR

nova
Medicine & Health
New York

NOTICE TO THE READER

Library of Congress Cataloging-in-Publication Data

Names: Lanford, Daniel, editor.
Title: Medicaid : politics, policy, and key issues / Daniel Lanford.
Description: New York : Nova Science Publishers, [2020] | Series: Health care in transition | Includes bibliographical references and index. |
Identifiers: LCCN 2020027176 (print) | LCCN 2020027177 (ebook) | ISBN 9781536181333 (hardcover) | ISBN 9781536182309 (adobe pdf)
Subjects: LCSH: Medicaid. | Health insurance--United States. | Poor--Medical care--United States.
Classification: LCC RA412.45.U6 M44 2020 (print) | LCC RA412.45.U6 (ebook) | DDC 368.4/200973--dc23
LC record available at https://lccn.loc.gov/2020027176
LC ebook record available at https://lccn.loc.gov/2020027177

Published by Nova Science Publishers, Inc. † New York

CONTENTS

Introduction **ix**
Daniel Lanford

Section I **The Impact of Medicaid in the Age of the Affordable Care Act** **1**

Chapter 1 Personal Narratives from Oregon's Medicaid Expansion **3**
Heidi Allen, Bill J. Wright and Katherine Baicker

Chapter 2 The Impact of the ACA on Insurance Coverage Disparities after Four Years **21**
Charles Courtemanche, Ishtiaque Fazlul, James Marton, Benjamin Ukert, Aaron Yelowitz and Daniela Zapata

Chapter 3 Federally Qualified Health Centers: From the Fringes to the Mainstream **53**
Carolin L. Spice, Bomy Yun, Aaron B. Katz and Paul A. Fishman

Section II	**Challenges in Medicaid Policy and Politics**	**79**
Chapter 4	Administrative Burdens in Medicaid *Pamela Herd and Donald P. Moynihan*	**81**
Chapter 5	The Quiet Politics of Medicaid Work Requirements *Philip Rocco*	**111**
Chapter 6	Medicaid and Racial Restriction: Moving Beyond the Welfare-Entitlement Dichotomy in the Analysis of Income-Targeted Programs *Daniel Lanford*	**141**
Section III	**Challenges Implementing Medicaid**	**179**
Chapter 7	Medicaid Family Planning Expansions: A Case Study of the Implementation of Georgia's Planning for Healthy Babies Program *Sarah C. Blake*	**181**
Chapter 8	Medicaid Coverage across the Income Distribution under the Affordable Care Act *Charles Courtemanche, James Marton and Aaron Yelowitz*	**211**
Section IV	**Program Change**	**259**
Chapter 9	Changes in Medicaid for People with Disability *Madonna Harrington Meyer and J. Dalton Stevens*	**261**

Chapter 10 Medicaid's Consumer Paradox: The Case of Substance Use Disorder **301**
Bikki Tran Smith, Colleen M. Grogan, Christina M. Andrews, Amanda J. Abraham, Melissa A. Westlake and Samantha J. Harris

Chapter 11 Restructuring Medicaid's Long Term Care Benefit: Shifting Services from Institutions to Communities **337**
Jill Quadagno

About the Editor **365**

About the Contributors **367**

Index **377**

INTRODUCTION

Daniel Lanford *
Georgia Health Policy Center
Andrew Young School of Policy Studies
Georgia State University
Atlanta, GA, US

Nearly half of all births in the United States are financed by Medicaid. Over a third of children have health insurance through Medicaid. Over half of all nursing home care is also financed by Medicaid (Paradise, Lyons, and Rowland 2015). Many people have enrolled in Medicaid at some point in their lives, or they are close to somebody who has. Medicaid is the largest single item in most state budgets behind education, and the federal government pays more than the states. Medicaid is often at the heart of U.S. health care politics. Change in the program can be rapid, but it is usually very slow, and it is almost never easy. Recently, despite holding the presidency, the House of Representatives, and the Senate, Republicans in the federal government failed in a years-long effort to make large cuts to the Medicaid program (Quadagno and Lanford 2019).

* Corresponding Author's Email: Daniel Lanford at dlanford1@gsu.edu.

Medicaid is fairly popular among the American people. Americans tend to be more generous in their attitudes toward public benefits in the form of services compared to benefits in the form of cash, and Medicaid is a program that pays for health services. Medicaid is also a major source of income for a large number of health care providers, hospitals, clinics, and managed care organizations. These groups and their representatives can exert effective moral and political pressure when the Medicaid program comes under threat.

Yet while Medicaid is both important and politically resilient, it is not immune to change – sometimes dramatic change. The ACA demonstrated this clearly, placing Medicaid at the center of national politics and reducing the stubborn uninsured rate by 44% in a single fell swoop (Courtmanche et al., Chapter 2 of this volume). The rate most likely would have been reduced further, had the Supreme Court in 2012 not allowed states to opt-out of the ACA-mandated Medicaid expansion, which extended coverage to adults up to 138% of the federal poverty line (a household income of roughly $35,000 for a family of four in 2019 dollars) for states that did not opt-out (Federal Register 2019).

Understanding Medicaid in All Its Complexity

Despite the large changes in Medicaid such as those that came with the ACA, the norm for Medicaid is slow change. A key factor that can impede change is the incredible complexity of the Medicaid program. Within federal guidelines, each states can implement a very different program. This contrasts sharply with Social Security and Medicare, which are operated almost entirely by the federal government. Medicaid is different in that there are effectively as many Medicaid programs as there are states, and they sometimes resemble each other only vaguely.

In recent years, states have in turn ceded much of their own direct control over Medicaid, paying *for*-profit organizations called managed care organizations (MCOs) to administer the programs instead. This complexity, added to an already complex program, can make it difficult for administrative partners to understand Medicaid implementations in a state.

Often, access to data on the program is limited by one of the organizations involved. The difficulty is all the greater when trying to gather program data across fifty states. Understanding Medicaid as a whole is therefore an ongoing challenge for federal administrators, researchers, and policymakers.

Research on Medicaid is important, complex, and often exhausting. Yet it often points the way toward program improvements. For these reasons, it has been an immense honor to work with the scholars whose contributions compose this book. These researchers and practitioners come from a wide variety of academic disciplines and practical backgrounds, and each shines a much-need light into a different corner of this multi-faceted program. My hope is that their efforts help illuminate useful pathways toward the most effective program possible, and toward a better healthcare system in the United States overall – something many of us might agree is sorely needed.

The chapters in this book are arranged into four sections. The first section addresses the impact of Medicaid, especially in the time since the passage of the ACA. This section begins with a chapter giving a very human perspective on Medicaid – a perspective that comes from the people who rely on the program, or who wish they could. Here, Heidi Allen, Bill Wright, and Katherine Baicker take stock of key findings from an important study in Oregon, where lottery access to Medicaid created a natural experiment used to test the effects of Medicaid expansion on those who gained benefits compared to those who did not (Chapter 1). Several interesting findings emerged from the original study. For example, in just two years, Medicaid coverage had improved self-reported health and well-being, but it also increased emergency department usage (Finkelstein et al. 2012; Taubman et al. 2014). Allen and colleagues take a second look at this data from a consumer perspective, reporting on in-depth interviews with Medicaid members. These interviews help explain the earlier findings. For example, while earlier studies showed that emergency room use did not decrease after access to regular primary care was provided, Allen's interviews show that in many cases, individuals had been avoiding emergency care in real emergency situations, only feeling able to go to the emergency room for treatment after knowing that someone (in this case Medicaid) would be able to pay for treatment.

In Chapter 2, Charles Courtemanche and colleagues take a different approach to assessing impact and ask what the ACA and Medicaid expansion did for health insurance coverage across all of the states, with special attention given to the effects that the ACA and its Medicaid expansion had on health insurance coverage disparities between demographic groups. They find, for example, that Medicaid expansion under the ACA reduced the 32.8 percentage-point health insurance coverage gap between the lowest income group (39.5% uninsured) and the highest income group (6.7% uninsured) by 44 percent (14.4 percentage-points). This represents millions of people, many with stories like those related by Allen and colleagues in Chapter 1.

Medicaid doesn't just affect individuals – it also impacts institutions and systems. One key example is the case of America's safety net for individuals seeking primary and preventive care: Federally Qualified Health Centers (FQHS). In Chapter 3, Caroline Spice and colleagues provide a brief history of the relationship between FQHCs and Medicaid, and they bring us up to date on interrelated changes in these programs since the passage of the ACA. Two key developments are, first, the emergence of payment models that in some ways reflect those used in private health care and, second, emerging leadership from FQHCs in the area of integrated health information systems.

Challenges in Medicaid Policy and Politics

The second section of this book addresses key political challenges in Medicaid today. In Chapter 4, Pamela Herd and Donald Moynihan address one of the foremost of these: administrative burden. Some of the most important social and political battles in health care today are fought over the administrative burdens imposed on potential Medicaid beneficiaries. For eligible individuals, obtaining Medicaid benefits can be very easy or very hard. The relevant policies, which vary over time and place and can be quite intentional, play a major role in the number of people who do, and do not, get covered by health insurance. Herd and Moynihan show that the status quo for engaging with the system presents many barriers for potential beneficiaries, and there are many opportunities to improve access to care by lessening administrative burden, even without major policy changes. We might think that folks would be sympathetic to the burdens of dealing with health insurance companies, given that many people have trouble dealing with their insurers whether they use public health insurance *or* private health insurance. However, in the case of Medicaid, the current trend is toward increasing administrative burden. While some administrative burden is no doubt unintentional, this trend is largely born of political choice.

In Chapter 5, Phil Rocco takes another deep dive into political choices around Medicaid. In a chapter that is also highly relevant to administrative burden, he looks at the process by which states have recently implemented new work requirements for Medicaid beneficiaries. These work requirements can be found in a number of recent state waiver applications, and they receive some support from the public. However, this support tends to wane when community health advocates are given the chance to organize and point out the practical consequences of work requirements. For example, most Medicaid people work anyway, and the work requirements end up creating administrative burdens that result in perfectly eligible people being dumped from the program. Those policymakers interested foremost in reducing the number of beneficiaries have therefore minimized the public comment periods required before a work requirement can be enacted, in order to limit their political liabilities. Rocco examines the effects of these constricted public comment periods and finds that community advocates have largely been successful in overcoming the 'mobilization of bias' against the public comment periods. The exception is where the work requirements target only non-parent, non-elderly adults. In such cases, states have effectively reduced public comments.

A related key factor in American politics is that white Americans tend to view low-income people with at least some sympathy, especially when social programs provide services rather than cash benefits. However, that sympathy quickly erodes when the program is believed to primarily benefit minorities (Gilens 1999). Accordingly, two key question are whether white Americans view Medicaid as primarily benefitting minorities and whether Medicaid generosity varies across states according to the racial sympathies and antipathies of the white public. I personally address these questions in Chapter 6, finding that Medicaid is more heavily racialized than its sister program, Medicare, which provides health insurance for the elderly whether they have low-incomes or not. This chapter also shows that in states with more anti-Black racial attitudes, Medicaid eligibility has historically been lower. This is the case net of attitudes toward bigger or smaller government. Accordingly, states with more restrictive Medicaid programs (such as those which have not expanded Medicaid under the ACA with the accompanying very-large federal subsidies) should consider implementing more generous programs as a matter of justice and racial equity.

Challenges Implementing Medicaid

The third section of this book directly addresses issues and challenges with implementing Medicaid *after* the program is already sent down a given course by policy. In Chapter 7, Sarah Blake takes a deep dive into the implementation of a program in Georgia called Planning for Healthy Babies. While the program was by nature at the cutting edge of Medicaid policy, a series of unfortunate circumstances and implementation decisions led to an extremely rough first year of implementation. Everything from decisions about naming the program, to confusion over leadership, to basic complexity stemming from implementation across multiple organizations and agencies, combined together in a disorienting swirl that limited uptake to only a small fraction of the eligible population. Blake shows that the starting point—in this case the noncommittal support from several parts of the state government and insufficient incorporation of community input—plays an important role in later activities. Yet while some problems are easier to prevent than to overcome, constraints are sometimes unavoidable. This case takes a deeper look at communication, showing how communication could have been, and can be, brought to bear in key problem areas to avoid and mitigate problems inevitably encountered with complex health insurance programs like Medicaid.

In Chapter 8, Charles Courtemanche is back with colleagues James Marton and Aaron Yelowitz, this time examining variations in ACA Medicaid expansion implementations across states and across income groups. One findings is that, while access remains a problem for many, some states may have enrolled Medicaid participants with incomes *over* the income-eligibility limits. As in prior chapters, this variation can be explained in part with reference to policy differences across states.

PROGRAM CHANGE

The fourth and final section of this book addresses evolution and change in Medicaid over time. In Chapter 9, Madonna Harrington Meyer and Dalton Stevens highlight changes for people with disabilities. They find that as disability rates in the U.S. have increased, Medicaid disability benefits and eligibility have expanded. However, some states are doing far better than others. Echoing Chapter 4 and foreshadowing Chapter 10, Meyer and Stevens find that obtaining disability-related benefits can be bewilderingly difficult due to a maze of eligibility requirements and administrative red tape. There are policy proposals currently under consideration that will facilitate enrollment as well as proposals that will make it more difficult. An example of the of the latter is the current movement toward work requirements which, despite the fact that they often exclude people with disabilities, will nevertheless affect people with disabilities through a number of pathways, for example by creating additional red tape. Meyer and Stevens also report on the state of managed care for Medicaid members with disabilities, reviewing recent research on the effectiveness of this approach and pointing out reasons for both optimism and skepticism.

In Chapter 10, Bikki Tran Smith and colleagues take a deep dive into the challenges consumers face as they attempt to find information on benefits. They specifically examine the case of Medicaid benefits for substance use disorder (SUD) treatment by exploring the process of finding SUD treatment information on the websites of all 50 states and all 281 Medicaid managed care organizations. While SUD treatment benefits expanded greatly with the ACA, these benefits remain unattainable for many due to informational barriers. Smith and colleagues reveal what they call Medicaid's *consumer paradox*: while the dominant discourse around benefit enrollment puts the burden of finding program information on consumers, Medicaid program administrators and managed care organizations often *do not* provide the means by which the necessary information can be found. This chapter concludes with suggestions for improving program accessibility. Some of these suggestions are likely to be relevant well beyond the realm of SUD treatment.

While most chapters in the fourth section of the book emphasize significant changes in Medicaid, especially since the passage of the Affordable Care Act, Chapter 11 has a slightly different tone. Here, Jill Quadagno demonstrates that some things do not change as much as we might have expected. Quadagno takes a deep historical look at Medicaid Long Term Care (LTC) and finds that despite broad support, efforts to use Medicaid to shift LTC toward home-and-community-based services (HCBS) have met with limited success. Key barriers include the federal-state structure of Medicaid, a shortage of necessary community infrastructure, LTC policy legacies, and the complexity of the HCBS delivery system. Quadagno identifies a number of factors that would need to change in order for there to be a broader transition to home and community care.

USING THIS BOOK

The complex world of Medicaid is swirling with questions. What does Medicaid do for people? Why do people tend to support or oppose Medicaid politically? What is it like to be a Medicaid beneficiary? Where does the program reach, and where does it not reach? Will social divisions or administrative red tape eventually sink the program? Or parts of it? How will benefits be defined in the coming years? What barriers are there to implementing policy once it has already been legislated?

While these questions may seem daunting at first, this book serves as an excellent source for answering them. Each of the chapters in this book has insights that will be useful to practitioners and researchers alike. Not only do these chapters serve as an introduction to key issues in Medicaid, they take deep dives into many of the most important nooks and crannies of the program. There is something for beginners as well as specialists.

My hope is that this book also raises *new* questions. For addressing those new questions, the following chapters offer a wide range investigative techniques that future Medicaid researchers could employ. The task will not be easy. Medicaid is complex and constantly changing. Yet whether readers want to understand the ongoing changes in the Medicaid program or perhaps create changes of their own, they are likely to find much of the information they need in the chapters that follow.

REFERENCES

Finkelstein A, Taubman S, Wright B, Bernstein M, Gruber J, Newhouse J, et al. 2012. "The Oregon Health Insurance Experiment: Evidence from the First Year." *Quarterly Journal of Economics* 127(3):1057-106.

Gilens, Martin. 1999. *Why Americans Hate Welfare: Race, Media, and the Politics of Antipoverty Policy*. University of Chicago Press.

Quadagno, Jill and Daniel Lanford. 2019. "The Obama Health Care Legacy: The Origins, Implementation, and Effort to Repeal the Affordable Care Act of 2010." In *Looking Back on President Barack Obama's Legacy: Hope and Change*, ed. Wilber C. Rich. Cham, Switzerland, Palgrave Macmillan.

Taubman SL, Allen HL, Wright BJ, Baicker K, and Finkelstein AN. 2014. Medicaid Increases Emergency-Department Use: Evidence from Oregon's Health Insurance Experiment. *Science*.

Section I: The Impact of Medicaid in the Age of the Affordable Care Act

In: Medicaid: Politics, Policy, and Key Issues ISBN: 978-1-53618-133-3
Editor: Daniel Lanford

Chapter 1

PERSONAL NARRATIVES FROM OREGON'S MEDICAID EXPANSION

Heidi Allen[1,*], Bill J. Wright[2] and Katherine Baicker[3]
[1]School of Social Work, Columbia University, New York, NY, US
[2]Providence Health and Services, Portland, OR, US
[3]Harris School of Public Policy, Chicago, IL, US

ABSTRACT

Research from the Oregon Health Insurance Experiment, a randomized evaluation of the impact of insuring low-income adults through the Medicaid program, demonstrated that Medicaid increased access to health care, improved overall health and mental health, and had a positive impact on individual finances. In this chapter, we provide illustrative examples of these research findings in the words of real study participants. These narratives add nuance to our understanding on the interplay between Medicaid coverage and well-being for families experiencing poverty.

* Corresponding Author's Email: ha2332@columbia.edu.

Keywords: Oregon Health Insurance Experiment, Medicaid, poverty, health insurance

Introduction

Medicaid coverage can affect enrollees in many different ways. The Oregon Health Insurance Experiment, a randomized evaluation of the impact of covering low income uninsured adults with Medicaid, provided empirical evidence of some of the ways that Medicaid coverage affects the lives of previously-uninsured, low income adults. The results indicated that, in the first one to two years, Medicaid coverage increased access to and use of health care services, reduced financial strain, reduced depression, and improved self-reported health and well-being (Taubman et al. 2014; Baicker et al. 2013; Finkelstein et al. 2012; Finkelstein et al. 2016; Baicker et al. 2018). Medicaid also had a short-lived impact on increasing voter turnout (Baicker and Finkelstein 2019). There was no evidence, however, of measurable improvements in physical health or changes in labor market activity over this period (Baicker et al. 2013; Baicker et al. 2014).

Many of the findings were surprising to policy-makers and analysts. Why does Medicaid increase emergency department use? Why didn't the health care safety net protect the uninsured from financial hardship? How did Medicaid reduce depression? To provide some additional context for these empirical findings, in 2011, we undertook a series of almost 600 in-depth, open-ended interviews with low-income adults who participated in the 2008 Medicaid lottery in Oregon. These narratives give a window into the lives of both the newly insured and the uninsured, providing detail on their health and health care experiences and how those experiences affected their well-being (Allen et al. 2014a; Allen et al. 2010). With many states considering or in the process of expanding Medicaid coverage to low-income adults, these stories complement the previous empirical results from the Oregon Health Insurance Experiment and help illustrate how expanded insurance coverage played out in a population with ongoing health needs and multiple sources of economic strain.

STUDY DESIGN

Background on the Oregon Health Insurance Experiment

In 2008, Oregon opened a waiting list for its previously-closed Medicaid program for low-income adults, Oregon Health Plan (OHP) Standard, and drew names from the list by lottery to allocate a limited number of new slots available in the program. Individuals selected in the lottery were provided with an application; those who completed the application and were deemed eligible were enrolled in OHP Standard. The lottery provided an opportunity to study the effects of Medicaid using a randomized controlled design. We conducted mail surveys and in-person interviews, collected biometric measurements, and compiled administrative data from sources including hospitals, emergency departments, earnings records, and credit reports. The study population was broadly representative of low-income uninsured adults who may be eligible for expanded Medicaid coverage (Finkelstein et al. 2012; Finkelstein et al. 2010). The design of and results from the Oregon Health Insurance Experiment are described in substantial detail elsewhere (Finkelstein et al. 2012; Finkelstein et al. 2010).

The primary findings to date demonstrate that Medicaid coverage (a) increased health care use across a range of settings, including physician visits, prescription drugs, hospitalizations, and emergency department visits (Taubman et al. 2014; Baicker et al. 2013; Finkelstein et al. 2012; Finkelstein et al. 2016; Baicker et al. 2017); (b) improved financial circumstances, including reducing the probability of having medical bills sent to collection agencies and virtually eliminating catastrophic out of pocket medical expenditures, but did not produce statistically significant changes in employment or earnings (Baicker et al. 2013; Finkelstein et al. 2012, Baicker et al. 2014); and (c) lowered rates of depression and improved self-reported health, but did not produce a statistically significant improvement in blood pressure, cholesterol, or diabetic blood sugar control (although it did increase diagnosis of and medication for diabetes) (Baicker et al. 2013). These causal estimates provide important evidence of the impact of expanding Medicaid on this population. Importantly, benefits accrued to both urban and rural populations in Oregon (Allen, Wright, and Broffman 2018). In order to provide further context for these results, this study follows-up on the experiences of that population through the use of free-form narrative interviews to shed additional light on some of the stories behind the numbers. Specifically, for each major study finding (e.g., Medicaid increases emergency department use) we provide real case examples that illustrate this from the patient perspective.

Qualitative Interviews

In 2011, we conducted follow up interviews with a sub-sample of Portland-area individuals who signed up for the 2008 Medicaid lottery and who had completed our in-person survey in 2009-2010. We randomly selected 790 people to recruit for open-ended interviews. We completed 574 face-to-face interviews for a response rate of 74%, after excluding people who had moved out of the area, died, or did not speak English or Spanish (n = 14). Unlike previous data collection efforts, this sample and these interviews were not designed to generate causal estimates of the effects of insurance. Rather, they help provide a more complete picture of the experiences of both the uninsured and the newly insured.

The qualitative interviews, conducted May through September 2011, were designed to elicit nuanced context not easily captured through structured surveys or administrative data (Allen et al. 2014b). We drew on the information collected in the quantitative structured in-person interviews to help guide a discussion of the care participants used, their health and financial situations, and the role of insurance or being uninsured in various aspects of their lives. Interviews took place in a clinic or at the participants' homes and lasted about an hour. Written informed consent was obtained, and human subject protocols were approved by the Institutional Review Board at Providence Health & Services.

Interviews were conducted in English and Spanish by 12 interviewers trained in qualitative data collection methods, audio-taped, and transcribed for textual analysis. The interviews were coded by two independent analysts using ATLAS.ti and an iterative coding dictionary that was updated three times during the study; results were adjudicated by a trained qualitative analyst using the final version of the coding dictionary. Codes were designed to capture subjects' comments about their perception of the relationship between coverage and outcomes such as use of care, experiences with the health care system, changes in financial circumstances, and physical and mental well-being.

For this chapter, we relied on our coding schema to select interview narratives that were illustrative of the main empirical findings of the Oregon Health Insurance Experiment studies. Our purpose was to "give voice" to patient experiences as they relate to the often-cited study findings. The quotes are thus not intended to be representative of the full set of comments made by interviewees. These narratives instead deepen our understanding of the causal impacts of Medicaid we observed in prior analyses by showcasing illustrative, and contrasting, examples of individuals who obtained Medicaid through the lottery versus those who remained uninsured.[1]

EXPERIENCES OF MEDICAID ENROLLEES AND THE UNINSURED

Health Care Use

Primary Care and Prescription Medication

The Oregon Health Insurance Experiment demonstrated that Medicaid increased health care use across a range of settings. Medicaid increased primary and preventive care in the first 2 years, including a 50% increase in the number of outpatient visits, a 50% increase in the probability of having a cholesterol check, and a doubling of the probability that woman had a

---

[1] We focus here on illustrating the statistically significant findings from the Oregon Health Insurance Experiment. As noted above, we found no statistically significant effect of Medicaid on several of the outcomes we studied – including specific physical health measures and labor market activities; in such cases, illustrative anecdotes are likely to be less illuminating.

mammogram (Baicker et al. 2013). Medicaid increased the number of prescription medications taken by more than 33% (Baicker et al. 2017), and increased the use of diabetes medications in particular by more than 80%. Medicaid also increased the probability of having a usual place of clinic-based care by 50% (Baicker et al. 2013).

These increases in primary care access and use were reflected in the stories told by participants. Carmela (all names have been changed) was a 47 year-old woman who was uninsured for a long time before receiving Medicaid and had avoided using care because of the cost. She said, "As soon as I found out that yes, I was covered, I started making phone calls and I got an appointment for primary care, and then I had a couple of references for [redacted women's clinic]. It's an excellent place." After an estimated ten years without coverage, Carmela subsequently went to get a physical and see an OB-GYN because a long time had passed since she had received routine health screenings.

> The first thing I did, well, I went and saw my primary care [provider] for my first visit. I have really bad allergies and I was having pains in my muscle, and so basically it was just a physical. He was absolutely wonderful. He really honestly kind of went through and checked everything, my muscles from head to toe. If I had any questions, he answered all my questions. I [went to an OB-GYN] and got caught up on my Pap and everything. I had my very first mammogram and everything was okay. They have midwives up there. The lady that I picked, she's just absolutely wonderful. She's very informative. I mean, just a great lady, very thorough in anything and everything and very personable.

Richard was a 48 year-old stay-at-home dad with diabetes who gained insurance, like Carmela, through the lottery. While uninsured he accrued significant medical debt with a local hospital. He tried to negotiate a payment plan with the billing representative:

> I tried to explain to them. I'm a stay-at-home dad and my wife works at [redacted retail store]. She goes, 'well, what can you afford to give us?' [I said] 'let me talk to the wife, I'll see what we could do.' So I called her

> up a couple of days later and I said, 'like $20 a month. I'll pay it faithfully until it's paid off.' She goes, 'oh, that's not enough, not for the amount [owed]'… I was willing to do anything. I even jokingly said 'I'm out of work; if you guys got any job openings then you [would] know where the money is coming from anyway'. She didn't find it funny… It's like what can you do? I try to make amends. Here, give me a job and you just take it right out of my check. You just take it until I'm done.

The thought of adding to the family debt led Richard to avoid further care: "I have four children, three of them still living at home. They need and they need. There's hardly ever enough money as it is. If you got to spend money to go to a doctor or medications or whatever - I will be dumbfounded if I was doing insulin and stuff for my diabetes and not have insurance." Once he got insurance, he saw health care providers who put him on insulin and helped him modify his diet.

> The first thing I did when I walked in the doctor's office was [say] I really need to be checked for diabetes…. Since I've been on insulin within the first couple of weeks, it was like a turn-on switch. I mean things were different. I didn't stress out about all the stupid little crap anymore. I didn't get agitated so much, which is a really good thing because there for a while my wife was going 'Your attitude sucks. If you don't change, maybe we should just split up for a while.' I never realized that that's what it was from, just because I eat what I want. I was eating a lot of junk food.

In contrast to Richard and Carmela, Tyrone was 63 years old and uninsured at the time of the interview. He retired at age 50 to care for his ailing mother and hadn't had insurance since. Once a year he paid out-of-pocket to see a doctor and have his prescription for high blood pressure medication refilled. He describes the limitations of out-of-pocket primary care:

> So much worries. It's always on the back of your mind. Am I going to cut myself? Am I going to break a bone? Am I going to do this, am I going to do that? It's still in my mind….Anytime I have a headache, is it a brain tumor or what? You can't go to the doctor. I can't go to the doctor for a

> simple – for anything because it's – my doctor don't like me too much probably because I only see him once a year because it's $150 or $150 per office visit. And what do I do? I walk in and go, 'how are you doing Dr. [redacted]?' He goes, 'hi.' He signs my blood pressure forms. He goes 'Well, I want to give you a test for rectal cancer, colon cancer and all the things.' – He's trying to do his job but I can't afford to have the tests done. He wants to give me a blood test. I go, 'why give me a blood test? So I can find out that this is wrong or that's wrong?' I go, 'if it is wrong or that's wrong, what am I going to do about it? I can't do anything about it.' So he keeps my blood pressure in check anyway, but it's just a nightmare. It really is.

He went on to say:

> Yeah, I've got buddies that ran in to their doctors, of course, they've got health insurance and they have all these tests and cameras running. I mean, it's nothing pleasurable I'm sure but at least they know that they're cancer free or whatever and no polyps in their intestines or whatever and things that can cause problems and I can't have any of those testing. I can't afford them right now. I'll have them done when I'm 65, if I make it.

Another example was Aisha, a 33 year-old uninsured single mother who works as a Certified Nursing Assistant. She won the 2008 lottery and had OHP for two years before she moved from part-time to full time in her job. The increased income put her slightly over OHP eligibility but she couldn't afford coverage through her employer so she had been uninsured for about a year. She had recently cut herself fairly badly but feared an emergency department bill would cost thousands of dollars so she treated it herself; she felt it was healing slowly. She also suffered from depression and asthma.

> Sometimes I've needed an inhaler and I've actually used one of my kids' inhalers. Like I get two for them always, one for at home and one for at school, and yes, I mean it's come to the point that when I felt I needed one, I just used one of theirs, which I know I shouldn't have but I mean I can't afford to go to the doctor.

Hospitalizations

The empirical results from the Oregon Health Insurance Experiment also showed that Medicaid increased the probability of being hospitalized by 30%, concentrated primarily among those stays not originating in the emergency department (Finkelstein et al. 2012). Qualitative interviewees told of their experiences in the acute care setting.

Theresa was a 51 year-old woman who was the caretaker for her husband, who suffered from dementia. She said, "I didn't have insurance [for 5 years] and you couldn't go see a doctor unless you had money. So I just – I know that's one of the reasons why my health went down, because I couldn't be monitored or checked for anything. I mean, I was probably a diabetic for a long time and didn't know it." She had recently been reminded of the consequences of not taking care of herself when her best friend died of cancer. "She was a caregiver for her entire family and she didn't – she was so busy taking care of other people that she didn't take care of herself." After obtaining coverage, Theresa started actively managing a variety of chronic health concerns. She was hospitalized to have double-bypass surgery and started going to cardiac rehabilitation three times weekly.

> Oh, [my health]'s a lot better than it was, just energy level is a lot higher. Tolerating [my husband] is a lot easier. I mean, it's hard because when someone has dementia, it takes a lot out of you physically and emotionally, and it's been a lot easier since my surgery. He has fears because he always thinks he is going to lose me. Well, I'm a lot better than I was.

In contrast, Jose, age 38 and uninsured, reported having a rare untreated illness that he understood would eventually be fatal. He received limited care through safety-net services but was not receiving the specialty care he was told he needed. This affected not just him, but his family.

> Sometimes it is also hard for my family. There are times when my son goes online and, when I ask him what he is doing, he replies he is searching about my disease to see how it can be cured or what doctors say. It hurts me a lot to see that my children are so young and are worried about me.

> My girl is 8 and my other son is 6 years old. Right now, it is time for them to play and enjoy life, not to be thinking about diseases. I think this is destiny. I tell them not to think about it, since we are all going to die in this life; some people die earlier and some others die when they are old people. That is something we can´t control. Sometimes my wife cries, though I tell her not to think about it because everything will be okay. Although I know that, if I don´t see a doctor, it will get worse instead of getting better.

Emergency Department Visits

The Oregon Health Insurance Experiment also found that Medicaid coverage increased emergency department (ED) use (Taubman et al. 2014). Medicaid increased the number of ED visits overall by about 40%, particularly visits for conditions that fall outside the category of emergencies that are only addressable in the emergency department setting. The increase in emergency department use persisted over the two years of the study with no evidence that primary care visits were a replacement for ED use or vice versa (Finkelstein et al. 2016). Debbie, age 41, enrolled in Medicaid after the lottery. Prior to that, she had been uninsured for 8 years and mostly avoided seeking care. Once insured, she found a primary care physician and was diagnosed with type 2 diabetes. Working with her doctor, she experienced some notable improvements in her general health. She used the ED occasionally when the pain from her gout became unbearable; she appreciated having this option when she felt she needed it:

> [Gout] hurts like nothing else. One night I came home and I was kind of limping and then my toe had hurt. When I woke up in the morning it was on fire and I couldn't walk, you know, barely. I didn't know what it was but having diabetes I was kind of concerned and so I thought I'd better get that checked out. I went to the ED. It was nice to have insurance because otherwise I don't know what I would have done. You know, you just can't go to the emergency room anytime you want to [when you are uninsured].

In contrast, James was a 45 year-old man who had gone most of his life without insurance. He worked full time as a gas station attendant and took on as many side jobs (like laying concrete and installing floors) as he could to make ends meet. He avoided care, especially the emergency room, because of cost.

> Lately, I've had a lot of chest – not chest pains but it's kind of internal breathing and it feels like – I get these kind of like butterflies in my chest. I could still breathe and everything but it feels like something tight there, kind of like a pneumonia, maybe something there. I've worked at night, at nighttime when it's cold and wet, so I might have pneumonia and not really know it. Of course, I don't have the money to go to the doctors and have it checked out or go to the emergency room because I can't afford that. So I just kind of wait it out and hopefully it gets better. I drink lots of fluids and try to take care of myself. I [can't] just go to the emergency room, it's like $200 or $300 just to be seen. And then that's not including the tests they got to run over everything else and you go in to $3,000 or $4,000. No way I got that kind of money because I got to pay rent and bills and everything else.

Felicia, a 59 year-old woman described two different situations that occurred in the previous two years. In 2009, while uninsured, she fell and broke her wrist:

> I didn't have a doctor to go to. I couldn't afford to pay him. I probably should've gone somewhere but – it was stupid. I was running on the sidewalk and I didn't see [mimes falling] there was a driveway and so the pavement was a little bit uneven and I was sprawling half on the street and half on the sidewalk. People were [asking] 'Are you okay? Are you okay?' 'Yes, I'm okay'. [Interviewer: Did you ever think about going to the doctor or seeing someone?]. I thought about it but then how could I pay him? But then when I think about it now, I should have gone to the hospital ER or something.

In 2010, after she had gained insurance, she thought she was having a heart attack:

> I was sitting at the computer and I noticed for the past couple of hours, I was having trouble breathing. It would hurt when I take a deep breath and I thought, geez, what's going on here. And then when I laid down, it got worse; oh geez, this isn't good. So after about a day or so…about two in the morning or three, because I couldn't lay down…I hadn't slept the whole night because if I laid down, it would kill me, so I went to the ER. They hooked me up and my [heart] was fine. They gave me a stool softener [laughs].

Financial Security

Information about the effect of Medicaid on financial strain was gathered in the Oregon Health Insurance Experiment from credit reports and from self-reports. Medicaid reduced the probability of having an unpaid medical bill sent to collection by 25%, reduced the probability of having to borrow money or skip paying other bills because of medical expenses by 40%, and virtually eliminated having out-of-pocket medical expenses that exceeded 30% of income (Baicker et al. 2013; Finkelstein et al. 2012).

Qualitative interviewees described the change in their financial circumstances as well as the associated stress. Ashley was a 28-year old mother who also ran a daycare. She had churned on and off OHP several times in the last three years because of fluctuations in her income. She had recently reenrolled in OHP, and described the difference in security compared to when she was not covered:

> I think having health insurance means that there's a lot less burden, not only on me as a person because I know that I can get the healthcare that I need, but on me as a mom because I can take care of myself and be there for my kids and just have a better opportunity to be healthy, and I think that's extremely important. And so it's a huge burden that is lifted off our shoulders when we do have it; and when we don't, it is an insane amount of stress and financial as well as mental and physical and everything else, so it's a big deal. I know that when I don't have insurance, I am constantly worrying about whether something else will come up like an emergency room visit, even having to go to the urgent care can cost you $200 to $300

> now, and worrying about having to cover that cost. Also, the worry when you don't have insurance, of knowing that you really can't properly take care of yourself, it is very stressful.

People were particularly concerned that their unmet health care needs would result in an emergency situation where they would accumulate medical debt and worsen an already precarious financial situation. Audre was age 48 and uninsured. Prior to the study she had had health insurance for one year through her employer, a time when she said she was happy and confident and had a healthy social life. After her hours were cut at work she no longer qualified for insurance, and her reduced income required her to downsize to a basement apartment she described as "a jail." She reported that her mental health was severely affected by combined lack of income and lack of health insurance; she worried about what she would do if anything happened to her, because she couldn't afford care. She occasionally received care at a free clinic, but didn't think the care was comprehensive or of high quality.

> My injury was 19 years ago in a car, my pelvis here was broken. The doctor said there's a possibility that I'm going to have arthritis right now. I'm not going to have medical insurance very soon. I feel like I have nothing again. Anything could happen. How am I going to be able to pay all those bills to the doctors? How? It's right here all the time in my mind because I know I have to pay because I don't have health insurance right now.

Health Outcomes

The Oregon Health Insurance Experiment also examined the impact of Medicaid on mental health, self-reported health, a depression screen, and physical health measures. It found that Medicaid improved mental health, reducing the prevalence of depression by 30 percent (Baicker et al. 2013; Baicker et al. 2018). Medicaid also improved self-reported measures of overall health such as the likelihood that respondents felt their health was stable or improving, or that they would rate their health as good, very good, or excellent, rather than fair or poor (Baicker et al. 2013; Finkelstein et al. 2012).

Interviewees talked about their mental health and overall well-being. Timothy, age 49, was a father of two who discovered that one of his children had been sexually abused. Along with his children, who were also covered by OHP, Timothy attended therapy covered by their insurance.

> OHP saved all of us. I can't stress that enough. If we didn't have health coverage, we would be completely lost. Because we have health coverage and we could seek services and kind of figure out with the help of an advocate what we actually needed, it made all the difference…it's a complete 180-turn-around from where we were a year ago. Now, we're a real family. We're functioning and all the bills are paid and kids are in school passing all of their classes. We're doing really well.

Jade, age 33 and uninsured, had frequent headaches and suffered from depression. She was raising four children and was a caregiver for three more. She felt like going without care hurt her ability to be a good parent or a good partner.

> There are days when I want to cry for everything and there are days when I would like to leave. I don't know, it is difficult because I have four children at home and I need to hold back a lot so as not to explode…It is difficult because when I feel bad, I don't want them to yell or to hear any noise, so I find it hard to hold myself; I ask them not to yell or I tell them to go and play outside until I feel better. It is really difficult.

Kamala was a 52 year-old woman who had not been insured for at least seven years. She generally worked as a waitress or a bartender. She was currently unemployed but felt the restaurant and bar industry provided little security even when she was working because she was often laid-off and was rarely offered benefits such as health insurance. Overall she felt healthy, but not having coverage was a constant struggle:

> I've been feeling really tired. There's a cost of not having insurance. The money layout, the financial piece, and then there's the emotional piece from the little decisions saying, okay, I got cut, I need stitches. But I don't want to go to the emergency [room]. I don't have insurance; it's going to cost me $1,000. I'm just going to wrap my finger and hope for the best. We're juggling medications. There have been times where even that $4 [prescription cost] I'm juggling and didn't have enough, so I went a week without my blood pressure medicine. Did that impact me? Yeah. There's a financial cost and then there's that emotional cost. There are just so many little things to that emotional cost.

DISCUSSION

The narratives reported here illuminate what insurance coverage means to the low-income adults in the Oregon Health Insurance Experiment. A pattern that emerged in story after story was the interplay between access to care, financial security, stress, and overall well-being. The low-income people we interviewed lived with little room for uncertainty. One set-back often cascaded into many others. The safety net provided by insurance translated to improved financial circumstances and enormous reductions in stress.

Some respondents described the relief of learning from a provider that the symptoms they were experiencing were not indicative of a serious health condition – improving their self-perceived health. Many reported improved security in the knowledge that they could seek care if they needed to. As Celia, a 56-year-old insured participant, put it:

> You remember that all-American Express credit card 'don't leave home without it'? That's the way I feel about my Oregon Health Plan because I know that at any given time I don't have that added stress of [knowing that] I don't have any insurance, I can't go to the doctor, or if I go to the doctor, I'm going to get another bill, another medical bill that I can't pay. Having the Oregon Health Plan relieves a lot of pressure.

Beyond the anecdotes that shed light on particular quantitative findings, the stories of the interviewees pointed to an overall general sense of relief from insurance coverage. Most insured interviewees still struggled with poor health and financial difficulties, but they reported that insurance lightened the load and allowed them a bit of grace. Those with coverage almost always identified that coverage in their inventory of blessings, regardless of how much care they used. As one study participant put it: "I love [having the Oregon Health Plan]. It's wonderful. I feel like it's given me some of my dignity back in that, you know, I don't have to be standing on the sidelines of society. I can actually participate in my life and the choices I have over my own health. It's wonderful. It's empowering to have that choice." Another concluded his interview with: "So yes: no insurance horrible, insurance good. Like they needed a study to figure this one out."

ACKNOWLEDGMENTS

This work was Supported by grants from the Office of the Assistant Secretary for Planning and Evaluation, Department of Health and Human Services; the California HealthCare Foundation; the National Institute on Aging (P30AG012810, RC2AGO36631, and R01AG0345151); the Robert Wood Johnson Foundation; the Alfred P. Sloan Foundation; the Smith Richardson Foundation; and the Social Security Administration (5 R RC 08098400-03-00, to the National Bureau of Economic Research as part of the Retirement Research Consortium of the Social Security Administration); and by the Centers for Medicare and Medicaid Services.

REFERENCES

Allen H, Wright BJ, Harding K, Broffman L. The role of stigma in access to health care for the poor. *Milbank Q*. 2014a;92(2):289-318.

Allen H, Wright BJ, Baicker K. New Medicaid Enrollees In Oregon Report Health Care Successes and Challenges. *Health Affairs.* 2014b;33(2): 292-9.

Allen H, Baicker K, Finkelstein A, Taubman S, Wright BJ, Group OHS. What The Oregon Health Study Can Tell Us About Expanding Medicaid. *Health Affairs.* 2010;29(8):1498-506.

Allen H, Wright B, Broffman L. The impacts of Medicaid expansion on rural low-income adults: Lessons from the Oregon Health Insurance Experiment. *Medical Care Research and Review.* 2018;75(3):354-83.

Baicker K, Allen HL, Wright BJ, Finkelstein AN. The effect of Medicaid on medication use among poor adults: Evidence from Oregon. *Health Affairs* (Millwood). 2017;36(12):2110-4.

Baicker K, Taubman S, Allen H, Bernstein M, Gruber J, Newhouse J, et al. The Oregon Experiment - Effects of Medicaid on Clinical Outcomes. *New England Journal of Medicine.* 2013;368(18):1713-22.

Baicker K, Allen HL, Wright BJ, Taubman SL, Finkelstein AN. The effect of Medicaid on management of depression: evidence from the Oregon Health Insurance Experiment. *The Milbank Quarterly.* 2018;96(1):29-56.

Baicker K, Finkelstein A, Song J, Taubman S. The Impact of Medicaid on Labor Market Activity and Program Participation: Evidence from the Oregon Health Insurance Experiment. *American Economic Review: Papers and Proceedings.* 2014;104(5):322-8.

Baicker K, Allen HL, Wright BJ, Taubman SL, Finkelstein AN. The effect of Medicaid on dental care of poor adults: Evidence from the Oregon Health Insurance Experiment. *Health Services Research.* 2017;53(4):2147-64.

Taubman SL, Allen HL, Wright BJ, Baicker K, Finkelstein AN. Medicaid Increases Emergency-Department Use: Evidence from Oregon's Health Insurance Experiment. *Science.* 2014.

In: Medicaid: Politics, Policy, and Key Issues ISBN: 978-1-53618-133-3
Editor: Daniel Lanford

Chapter 2

THE IMPACT OF THE ACA ON INSURANCE COVERAGE DISPARITIES AFTER FOUR YEARS

Charles Courtemanche[1,2], Ishtiaque Fazlul[3], James Marton[3], Benjamin Ukert[4], Aaron Yelowitz[1,*] and Daniela Zapata[5]

[1]Department of Economics, University of Kentucky, Lexington, KY, US
[2]National Bureau of Economic Research, Institute of Labor Economics (IZA)
[3]Department of Economics Andrew Young School of Policy Studies, Georgia State University, Atlanta, GA, US
[4]Department of Health Policy and Management, Texas A&M University, College Station, TX, US
[5]Impaq International, Washington, DC, US

---

[*] Corresponding Author's Email : aaron@uky.edu.

Abstract

In this chapter we estimate the impact of the major components of the ACA (Medicaid expansion, subsidized Marketplace plans, and insurance market reforms) on disparities in insurance coverage after four years. We use data from the 2011–2017 waves of the American Community Survey (ACS), with the sample restricted to nonelderly adults. Our methods feature a difference-in-difference-in-differences model, developed in the recent ACA literature, which separately identifies the effects of the nationwide and Medicaid expansion portions of the law. The differences in this model come from time, state Medicaid expansion status, and local area pre-ACA uninsured rate. We stratify our sample separately by income, race/ethnicity, marital status, age, and gender, in order to examine access disparities. After four years, the fully implemented ACA (i.e., the national components of the ACA combined with the Medicaid expansion) eliminated 44 percent of the coverage gap across income groups, with the Medicaid expansion accounting for this entire reduction. The fully implemented ACA also reduced coverage disparities across racial groups by 26.7 percent, across marital status by 45 percent, and across age groups by 44 percent, with these changes being partly attributable to both the Medicaid expansion and nationwide components of the law.

Keywords: Medicaid, Affordable Care Act, health care finance, disparities in insurance coverage

Introduction

Prior to the main implementation of the Affordable Care Act (ACA) in 2014, there were well documented disparities in insurance coverage along multiple dimensions, such as age, race, and income (Courtemanche, Marton, and Yelowitz, 2016; Yelowitz, 2016; Courtemanche et al., 2019b). The central pieces of the ACA, including the individual mandate, subsidized Marketplace coverage, and state Medicaid expansions, were designed to reduce health insurance coverage disparities by moving the U.S. closer to universal coverage (Obama, 2016; Gruber and Sommers, 2019). The purpose of this book chapter is to examine the extent to which the ACA reduced disparities in coverage after four years (2014-2017).

As will be discussed further below, we measure and report the impact of the ACA on coverage disparities in multiple ways. First, we measure the joint impact of the national components of the ACA (i.e., subsidized Marketplace coverage and the individual mandate) alone. Second, we measure the impact of the Medicaid expansion component of the ACA alone. Third, we combine these first two measures to report the impact of the "fully implemented" ACA in Medicaid expansion states. In other words, the first effect represents what we see in a non-Medicaid expansion state, since individuals in those states were only exposed to the national components of the ACA. The effect in a Medicaid expansion state is given by the sum of effect one and effect two, since individuals in those states were exposed to both the national components of the ACA and their state's own Medicaid expansion. We refer to this sum as the impact of the "fully implemented" ACA.

While gains in insurance coverage after the ACA have been well documented, relatively few papers in this literature examine how the ACA affected coverage disparities and none use data from 2017. Courtemanche et al. (2017) estimate the first-year impact of the ACA on coverage using difference-in-difference-in-differences (DDD) models where the differences come from time, state Medicaid expansion decisions, and pre-ACA local area uninsured rate. Similarly to the approach taken by Finkelstein (2007) and Miller (2012) to study other coverage expansions, this strategy leverages the propensity for universal coverage initiatives to provide the most intense "treatment" in local areas with the highest pre-reform uninsured rates. Using data from the American Community Survey (ACS), Courtemanche et al. (2017) find that the ACA increased coverage by an average of 5.9 percentage points in Medicaid expansion states (i.e., states whose citizens were exposed to the fully implemented ACA, which consists of both the national components of the ACA, such as subsidized Marketplace coverage, and their own state's Medicaid expansion) compared to 2.8 percentage points in non-expansion states (i.e., states whose citizens were only exposed to the national components of the ACA) in 2014. In subsample analyses, the authors show that the fully implemented ACA reduced but did not eliminate the coverage disparities based on education, race, age, and marital status after one year.

Courtemanche et al. (2018a) use the same research strategy and data from the Behavioral Risk Factor Surveillance System (BRFSS), finding that the fully implemented ACA reduced but did not eliminate the coverage disparity between those with incomes above versus below the median after two years (2014-2015). Frean et al. (2017) also use data through 2015 and a DDD approach to find that coverage gains from the Medicaid expansion and Marketplace premium subsidies are larger among childless adult couples than among single adults or adults with children, but the increase from the individual mandate is largest among singles. Courtemanche et al. (2019b) use three years of post-ACA data (2014-2016) from the ACS and find that the ACA Medicaid expansion eliminated 43 percent of the coverage gap across income groups. In addition, the authors find that the fully implemented ACA reduced but did not eliminate coverage disparities across racial groups, age groups, and marital status. These reductions were partly attributable to both the Medicaid expansion and nationwide components of the law.

Other studies in the literature focus solely on the ACA's Medicaid expansion, using difference-in-differences (DD) models to compare changes in coverage over time between Medicaid expansion and non-expansion states. Wehby and Lyu (2018) include two years of post-ACA data (2014-2015) from the ACS and show that the Medicaid expansion reduced but did not eliminate the coverage disparity across age and racial groups. Conversely, Yue et al. (2019) find that the ACA Medicaid expansion led to smaller gains among low-income Hispanics than other low-income individuals, implying a widened disparity. Kaestner et al. (2017) and Wherry and Miller (2016) provide evidence that the ACA Medicaid expansion increased insurance coverage among those with low incomes or levels of education, implying reduced socioeconomic disparities in coverage. Benitez et al. (2018) focuses on Kentucky, finding that much of the reduction in the uninsured rate is due to large coverage gains from areas with higher concentrations of poverty.

We contribute to this literature by using the DDD method described above and elsewhere (Courtemanche et al., 2018b) to uncover the causal impact of the 2014 ACA provisions, both with and without the Medicaid expansion, on coverage disparities after four years. To the best of our knowledge we are the first to include data from 2017 in such an analysis. Given the uncertainty surrounding the future of the ACA, new evidence regarding the impact of the ACA provided by each new year of survey data is extremely valuable to researchers and policy makers. As in Courtemanche et al. (2019b), we evaluate changes in coverage disparities by stratifying our sample by income, race/ethnicity, marital status, age, and gender. We use data from the American Community Survey (ACS) between 2011 and 2017. The ACS is commonly used in the literature because it includes multiple categories of insurance coverage, allowing us to evaluate how the ACA affected coverage disparities via changes to both private (Marketplace) and public (Medicaid) coverage. The ACS includes approximately 3,000,000 observations per year and relatively narrow geographic identifiers, allowing us to precisely estimate the effects for states and many local areas. A final benefit is that the mandatory nature of the ACS reduces concerns about sample selection amongst respondents.

After four years, our results suggest that the fully implemented ACA eliminated 44 percent of the coverage gap across income groups in Medicaid expansion states, with the Medicaid expansion accounting for this entire reduction. The fully implemented ACA also reduced coverage disparities across racial groups by 26.7 percent, across marital status by 45 percent, and across age groups by 44 percent, with these changes being partly attributable to both the Medicaid expansion and nationwide components of the law.

DATA

We use individual level micro-data from the American Community Survey's (ACS) 2011 through 2017 survey waves. The ACS is a nationwide mandatory random survey across all 50 states and the District of Columbia that samples about one percent of the U.S. population annually. Each year of the survey results in about 3,000,000 individual responses per year.[1] The mandatory feature of the survey reduces concerns about sample selection amongst respondents. For this study, we restrict the ACS sample to individual respondents aged 19 to 64 because the ACA was not intended to affect the health coverage of children or those older than 64. We limit the first sample year to 2011 to only isolate the effects of the 2014 provisions of the ACA, and thereby avoid capturing the effect of earlier changes in the insurance market, such as the 2010 dependent coverage mandate that allowed dependents to remain on their parent's insurance plan until their 26th birthday.

The ACS includes geographic identifiers for each survey respondent. In addition to state identifiers, the ACS identifies smaller geographic areas called Public Use Microdata Areas (PUMAs), which represent approximately 2,300 areas of at least 100,000 people nested entirely within a state.[2] The granularity of the PUMA identifier is important for our study since a PUMA can better represent local characteristics than a state identifier.

To detect a causal impact of the ACA marketplace component of the ACA, we utilize local within-state variation in uninsured rates in 2013. Ideally, we would use the PUMA level information associated with each individual in our sample to measure local area uninsured rates, however, the PUMA definitions changed, new boundaries were introduced in the 2010 Census, and the new boundaries were applied to the 2013 ACS wave and later. This complicates our analysis as we cannot identify the same geographic region across time before and after the 2014 ACA components. We address this problem by following Courtemanche et al. (2017) and identifying core-based statistical areas (CBSAs) using the old and new PUMA classification systems. Some CBSAs span multiple states and we isolate the portion of the CBSA in each state as separate local areas. In other cases, CBSAs do not cover all areas within a state, and we create additional

[1] The survey can be completed online or by mailing in a paper questionnaire. In-person interviews are done with respondents in group quarters. See https://www.census.gov/content/dam/Census/programs-surveys/acs/about/ACS_Information_Guide.pdf.

[2] For more information, see: https://www.census.gov/geo/reference/puma.html.

local areas for the non-CBSA portion in each state. These adjustments avoid dropping respondents from the sample living in multistate CBSAs or areas that are not part of a CBSA. Our dataset includes 630 local CBSA and non-CBSA areas that each contain between 356 and 78,781 ACS respondents in 2013, with a median of 1,020 and a mean of 2,811 respondents. This implies that our pre-ACA uninsured rates are computed from a reasonably large sample in each local area. To be clear, individuals in our sample that reside in the same CBSA are assigned that CBSA's uninsured rate.

The ACS collects a large number of socio-demographic characteristics relevant to execute our study and it includes a question on health insurance coverage that allows us to evaluate how the ACA affected both private and public coverage. The ACS asks each individual "Is this person CURRENTLY covered by any of the following types of health insurance or health coverage plans?" and respondents select from eight types of health insurance categories; "insurance through a current or former employer or union", "insurance purchased directly from an insurance company", "Medicare", "Medicaid, Medical Assistance, or any kind of government-assistance plan for those with low incomes or a disability", "TRICARE or other military health care", "VA (including those who have ever used or enrolled for VA health care)", "Indian Health Service", and "any other type of health insurance or health coverage plan."[3] Respondents can choose more than one type of insurance coverage and we classify only those answering "no" to all eight categories as uninsured. We create six binary outcome variables based on the ACS insurance coverage question: any insurance, any private insurance (either employer sponsored or directly purchased), employer-sponsored insurance, directly purchased insurance, Medicaid, and any other coverage (defined as coverage as neither private nor Medicaid coverage). These categories are not mutually exclusive due to the possibility of multiple sources of coverage. The purpose of sub-dividing the private insurance category into employer sponsored and directly purchased is because we expect the ACA to have an impact on directly purchased coverage, but not employer sponsored coverage. Because individuals may

---

[3] See, for example, http://www2.census.gov/programs-surveys/acs/methodology/questionnaires/2014/quest14.pdf.

mistakenly classify their source of private coverage, we also analyze the broader private coverage category as well.

Additionally, the ACS collects information on age, gender, race/ethnicity, origin, family structure, education, labor force participation, and household income. We use this information to create a large number of control variables. Specifically, we create dummy variables for the age of the respondent (binary indicators for each year from 19 to 64), female, race/ethnicity (non-Hispanic white, non-Hispanic black, Hispanic, and other race/ethnicity), foreign born, and U.S. citizenship status. We generate from the family structure responses a binary variable indicating whether the individual is married and separate indicators counting the number of children under the age of 18 living in the household (one, two, three, four, and five or more). We create separate binary indicators for the highest level of completed education (less than a high school degree, high school degree, some college, and college graduate), and we measure labor force outcomes with binary variable indicating whether the individual is a student or not, whether the individual is unemployed or not, and with the continuous Bureau of Labor Statistics' annual state unemployment rate. Lastly, we measure household income by first transforming the income information into percentages relative to the Federal Poverty Limit (FPL), and then create 50 dummies measuring the separate impact for each 10-point increment of income as a percentage of the FPL (with the highest category including everyone over 500 percent).

We add to our ACS individual level micro-dataset state-level ACA variables from the Kaiser Family Foundation. Specifically, we include binary variables on whether a state implemented a Medicaid expansion via the ACA. The majority of states expanded Medicaid effective January 1, 2014, but several states expanded at a later time. At the end of 2017, 32 states expanded their Medicaid program and 25 states expanded Medicaid as of January 1, 2014. Seven states expanded at a later time - Michigan (expansion effective date 4/1/2014), New Hampshire (8/15/2014), Pennsylvania (1/1/2015), Indiana (2/1/2015), Alaska (9/1/2015), Montana (1/1/2016), and Louisiana (7/1/2016).

Finally, we also collect information from the Kaiser Family Foundation regarding the functionality of the 2014 ACA insurance marketplaces. We include dummy variables indicating whether a state set up their own private insurance exchange (as opposed to using the federal exchange) and whether the exchange experienced glitches. These variables speak to aspects that may be related to frictions in outreach and sign-up of the uninsured to Marketplace insurance plans, as well as concerns that these decisions may be correlated with the decision to expand Medicaid coverage.

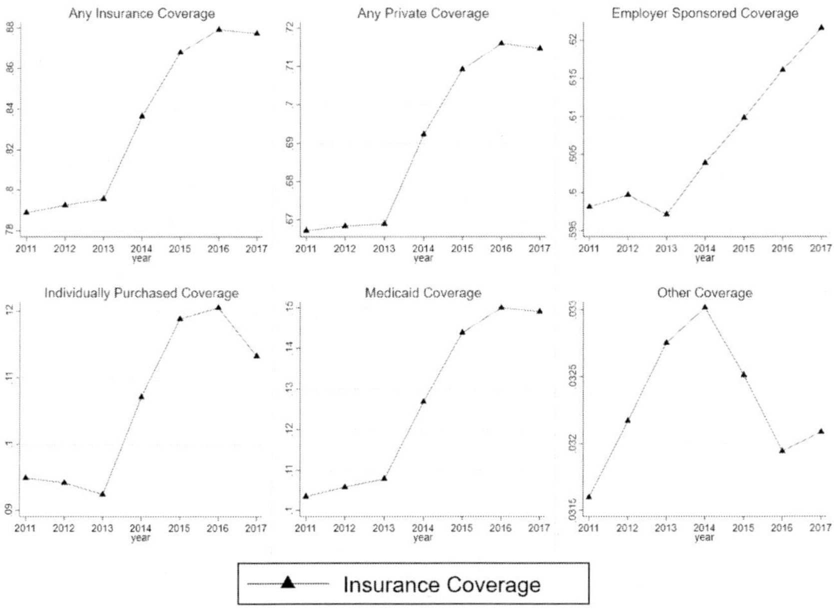

Figure 1. Changes in insurance coverage over time.

Figure 1 simply plots changes in insurance coverage over time for our sample, split by type of coverage. We see sharp increases in the likelihood of having any coverage, any private coverage (both individually purchased and employer sponsored coverage), and Medicaid coverage in 2014. Our DDD model described in the next section will isolate how much of these coverage gains were due to the national components of the ACA and the Medicaid expansion and allow us to examine the extent to which these gains reduced disparities in coverage.

Table 1. Descriptive statistics for insurance coverage

	Full sample	Medicaid expansion; at or above median baseline uninsured	Medicaid expansion; below median baseline uninsured	Non-expansion; at or above median baseline uninsured	Non-expansion; below median baseline uninsured
Any insurance coverage	0.792 (0.406)	0.748 (0.434)	0.849 (0.358)	0.727 (0.446)	0.829 (0.376)
Any private	0.668 (0.471)	0.618 (0.486)	0.721 (0.449)	0.609 (0.488)	0.717 (0.450)
Employer-sponsored	0.598 (0.490)	0.545 (0.498)	0.651 (0.477)	0.542 (0.498)	0.644 (0.479)
Individually purchased	0.094 (0.292)	0.095 (0.293)	0.094 (0.292)	0.089 (0.285)	0.100 (0.299)
Medicaid	0.106 (0.307)	0.114 (0.318)	0.121 (0.325)	0.089 (0.285)	0.080 (0.271)
Other	0.032 (0.176)	0.030 (0.172)	0.024 (0.152)	0.041 (0.198)	0.043 (0.203)

Notes: Standard deviations are in parentheses.

Table 1 provides pretreatment means and standard deviations for the insurance coverage outcomes of interest, while Table A1 does the same for the controls. We also stratify the sample into four groups based on whether the respondent's state expanded Medicaid and whether the local area's pretreatment uninsured rate was above or below the sample median. Table 1 shows that in the baseline year of 2013 79 percent of the sample was enrolled in some type of coverage, including 11 percent with Medicaid and 60 percent with employer-provided coverage. For both the high-uninsured (columns 2 and 4) and low-uninsured (columns 3 and 5) rate subgroups, individuals in Medicaid expansion states were slightly more likely to be covered in 2013 than those in non-expansion states, with the differences being driven entirely by Medicaid coverage. Our DDD model described in the next section will account for such baseline differences. Figure 2 presents changes in our coverage measures between 2011 and 2017, stratified into the same four groups. With six coverage outcomes and four groups, there are a total of 24 lines given in Figure 1. In general, the pre-ACA trends in the figure do not appear to differ meaningfully by state Medicaid expansion status or local area pre-ACA uninsured rate category. This provides preliminary justification for our use of the pre-ACA uninsured rate and Medicaid expansion variables as sources of identification in our analysis. Figure 2 shows that the probabilities of having any coverage, privately purchased coverage, any private coverage, and Medicaid increased in 2014 and generally continued to grow over time. One exception is the dip in individually purchased coverage observed in 2017.

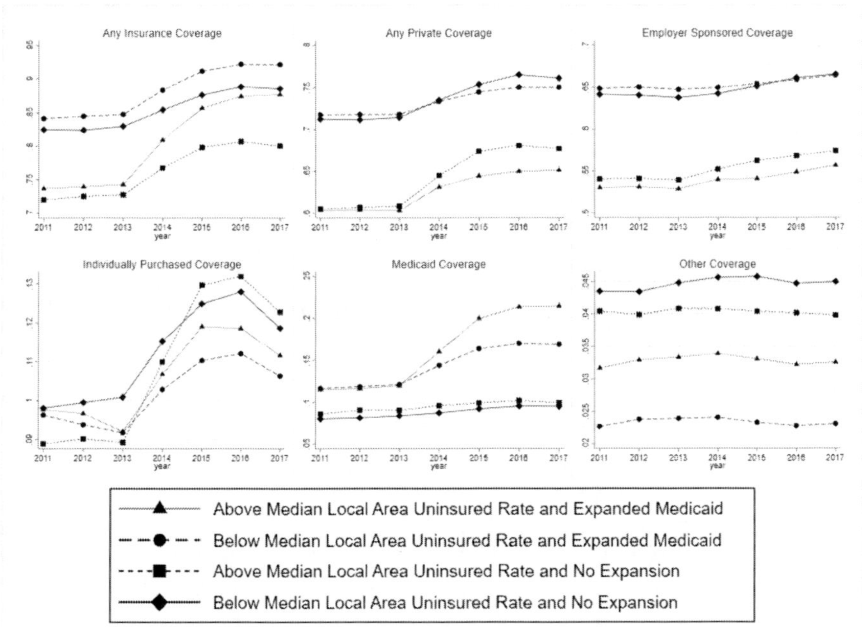

Figure 2. Changes in insurance coverage over time by Medicaid expansion status and local area uninsured rate.

METHODS

Our empirical methodology follows several prior studies that aimed to separately identify the impacts of both the Medicaid and national components of the ACA (Courtemanche et al., 2017; 2018a; 2018b; 2019a; 2019b; 2019c). Specifically, we estimate DDD models where the three "differences" are: (i) before versus after the ACA's implementation, (ii) whether or not the state participated in the ACA's Medicaid expansion, and (iii) the "dose" or "intensity" of the treatment, as measured by the local area's pre-ACA uninsured rate.

We use this strategy because identifying the causal effect of the provisions of the ACA that took effect nationally (i.e., everything but the Medicaid expansion) is challenging due to the lack of a control group. One cannot simply assume that any changes from before to after the ACA represents the law's causal impact, because other factors that influence coverage could have changed at the same time (one of many possible examples is the underlying trend in health care spending that might influence employer plan offerings). The DDD strategy allows us to disentangle the causal effect from these other factors by, in essence, considering areas with high proportion of insured population prior to the ACA to be a control group. If everyone in a local area was already insured before the ACA, then the ACA should have had no impact on the coverage status of individuals in that area. Conversely, if no one in a local area had insurance, then we would expect the ACA to have the maximum impact.

The characteristic feature of a DDD model is the full interaction of the three "difference" variables. This means the interaction of the three variables is included, along with the three possible two-variable interaction terms and each variable separately. In other words, each of the three variables is allowed to modify the influence of both of the others, or the product of both of the others. In our case, that translates to a model of the form:

$$\begin{aligned} I_{iast} = \beta_0 + \beta_1 UNINSURED_{as} + \beta_2 POST_t + \beta_3 MEDICAID_s \\ + \beta_4 (UNINSURED_{as} * POST_t) + \beta_5 (UNINSURED_{as} \\ * MEDICAID_s) + \beta_6 (MEDICAID_s * POST_t) + \\ \beta_7 (UNINSURED_{as} * MEDICAID_s * POST_t) + \beta_8 \boldsymbol{X}_{iast} + \varepsilon_{iast}. \end{aligned} \quad (1)$$

Where,

I_{iast} is a binary variable for whether individual *i* living in local area *a* within state *s* has insurance coverage in year *t*.

$UNINSURED_{as}$ is the 2013 baseline (pre-ACA) uninsured rate in local area *a* in state *s*

$MEDICAID_s$ is an indicator variable for whether state *s* participated in the ACA's Medicaid expansion

$POST_t$ is an indicator variable for whether or not year *t* is after the ACA's implementation (2014 or later)[4]

$\boldsymbol{X}_{iast}$ is a vector of the aforementioned control variables, and

ε_{iast} is the error term.

The covariate-adjusted change in I_{iast} at the time the ACA was implemented is obtained by differentiating with respect to $POST_t$, which yields $\beta_2 + \beta_4 * UNINSURED_{as} + \beta_6 * MEDICAID_s + \beta_7 * UNINSURED_{as} * MEDICAID_s$. The assumption that enables causal inference is that the ACA does not have any effect in a (hypothetical) location with a 0 percent uninsured rate. This means that $\beta_2 + \beta_6 * MEDICAID_s$ represents changes due to factors besides the ACA (and allows them to differ in Medicaid expansion vs. non-expansion states), while the causal effect of the ACA is $\beta_4 * UNINSURED_{as} + \beta_7 * UNINSURED_{as} * MEDICAID_s$.

The effect of the national (non-Medicaid) portion of the ACA is obtained by setting $MEDICAID_s = 0$, yielding $\beta_4 * UNINSURED_{as}$. Note that this is the combined effect of all the national components of the ACA, including the regulations, subsidies, creation of the Marketplace, and individual mandate; the ACS does not have sufficient information to disentangle their separate effects. The impact of the ACA in Medicaid expansion states is obtained by setting $MEDICAID_s = 1$ to yield $\beta_4 * UNINSURED_{as} + \beta_7 * UNINSURED_{as}$. The effect of the Medicaid expansion alone is the difference between these, which is $\beta_7 * UNINSURED_{as}$.

The predicted effects of the ACA therefore vary linearly with an area's baseline uninsured rate. For ease of interpretation, we will focus on the predicted or "implied" effects of the ACA at the sample mean baseline uninsured rate, which is 20.3 percent. When we conduct subsample analyses,

---

[4] For states that expanded Medicaid later than 2014, we adjust the timing of the "post" period in the $MEDICAID_s * POST_t$ and $UNINSURED_{as} * MEDICAID_s * POST_t$ interactions accordingly.

the baseline uninsured rate for each subsample is re-computed using only respondents in that particular subsample. For example, when we estimate separate effects for the married vs. unmarried subsamples, we use pre-ACA uninsured rate for married individuals (14.1 percent) to estimate the average effects on the married and the pre-ACA uninsured rate for unmarried individuals (27.2 percent) to estimate the average effects on the unmarried.

It is worth noting that our assumption that areas with no uninsured people prior to the ACA would not be affected could, if anything, make our estimates conservative. Conceivably, in such an area the ACA could still prevent individuals from *becoming* uninsured over time.

Finally, note that the model we estimate in this chapter is a more complicated version of equation (1) in which we also include year fixed effects, which subsume $POST_t$, and local area fixed effects, which subsume $MEDICAID_s$ and $UNINSURED_{as} * MEDICAID_s$. This approach allows for greater flexibility in measuring confounders, but the intuition and interpretation are the same as in equation (1).

Results

The top panel of Table 2 presents the coefficient estimates for the treatment variables from our DDD model with the full sample. The bottom panel reports the implied effects based on these coefficient estimates for a non-Medicaid expansion state (treated by only the national components of the ACA) and the implied effects for a Medicaid expansion state (treated by both the national components of the ACA and the Medicaid expansion, which we refer to as the fully implemented or full ACA) at the sample mean pre-ACA uninsured rate of 20.3 percent.

Focusing on the top panel first, we see that the coefficient estimate $(\widehat{\beta_4})$ associated with the term $(UNINSURED_{as} * POST_t)$ in equation (1) is a statically significant 0.178. In addition, the coefficient estimate $(\widehat{\beta_7})$ associated with the term $(UNINSURED_{as} * MEDICAID_s * POST_t)$ is a statistically significant 0.252. Taking these coefficient estimates as inputs, the first column of the bottom panel reports that the implied effect of the

ACA on any coverage in a non-expansion state is $\widehat{\beta_4} * \overline{UNINSURED_{as}} = 0.178 * 0.203 = 0.036$. The implied effect of the ACA on any coverage in an expansion state is $\widehat{\beta_4} * \overline{UNINSURED_{as}} + \widehat{\beta_7} * \overline{UNINSURED_{as}} = 0.178 * 0.203 + 0.252 * 0.203 = 0.087$.

Table 2. Implied effects of the ACA at mean pre-treatment uninsured rate for full sample

	Any insurance	Any private	Employer-sponsored	Individually purchased	Medicaid	Other
Non-elderly adults aged 19-64 (pre-treatment uninsured rate=0.203, sample size=12,313,971)						
Coefficient estimates of interest						
Uninsured*Post	0.178**	0.017***	0.037	0.130	0.015	-0.002
	(0.054)	(0.044)	(0.027)	(0.067)	(0.022)	(0.004)
Uninsured*Post*Medicaid	0.252***	-0.032	0.050	-0.081	0.292**	0.005
	(0.059)	(0.052)	(0.170)	(0.070)	(0.039)	(0.007)
Non-elderly adults aged 19-64 (pre-treatment uninsured rate=0.203, sample size=12,313,971)						
Implied effects of the ACA at mean pre-treatment uninsured rate						
ACA w/out Medicaid Expansion	0.036**	0.034***	0.007	0.026	0.003	-0.001
	(.011)	(0.009)	(0.006)	(0.014)	(0.004)	(0.001)
Full ACA	0.087***	0.028***	0.018***	0.010**	0.062***	0.000
	(0.006)	(0.006)	(0.005)	(0.003)	(0.007)	(0.001)

Notes: Results are effects of the ACA on the proportion of residents with the specified type of insurance, evaluated at the mean pre-treatment uninsured rate. Standard errors, heteroscedasticity-robust and clustered by state, are in parentheses. *** indicates statistically significant at 0.1% level; ** 1% level; * 5% level. Sampling weights are used. All regressions include area and time fixed effects and the full set of controls.

What do these estimates imply? They imply that in a typical non-expansion state at the mean pre-ACA uninsured rate the national components of the ACA led to a 3.6 percentage point increase in any insurance coverage. In a typical Medicaid expansion state at the mean pre-ACA uninsured rate the national components of the ACA and the Medicaid expansion combined to produce an 8.7 percentage point increase in any insurance coverage. Thus we can attribute the difference between these two implied effects (5.1 percentage points) to the Medicaid expansion. For each estimate, indicators of statistical significance are given at the 0.1 percent, 1 percent, and 5 percent level.

The remaining columns of Table 2 examine sources of coverage, where we consider any source of private coverage, any employer-sponsored (ESI) plan, any individually purchased plan, Medicaid, and any other coverage source. Our results suggest that, in an area with the mean pre-ACA uninsured rate, the fully implemented ACA increases private coverage by 2.8 percentage points. This is driven by increases in both ESI (1.8 percentage points) and individually purchased coverage (1 percentage point). The full ACA increased Medicaid coverage by 6.2 percentage points, most of which comes from the Medicaid expansion component of the law (5.9 percentage points). Though it cannot be observed directly in Table 2, for the full sample, the Medicaid expansion alone statistically significantly affects the probability of having Medicaid coverage. The full ACA, on the other hand, has a statistically significant positive effect on having any private insurance, ESI, as well as individually purchased insurance.

The validity of the identifying assumptions of our baseline DDD model cannot be directly tested. We test the validity of these assumptions indirectly by reporting the pre-ACA coefficients from an event study model where the treatment variables are interacted with the full set of year fixed effects. We report the results from this event study analysis separately in Tables 3 and 4. Table 3 reports only the estimated pre-treatment (2011 and 2012) coefficients from the event study, while Table 4 reports only the post-treatment implied effects (separately for the years 2014, 2015, 2016, and 2017). This split allows us to focus on the indirect test of our identifying assumptions in Table 3 and decomposing the year-by-year effects of the ACA in the post-period in Table 4. With that in mind, we start by examining the results from Table 3. The numbers in table 3 are not implied effects but estimated coefficients taken directly from the event study regressions, similar to the top panel of Table 2. Here we would expect around 5 percent of the pre-treatment coefficients to be significant by chance. A substantially higher percentage of significant results in the pre-period will call our identification strategy into question. That is because this would suggest an "impact" of the ACA in the years prior to the actual implementation of the

ACA. We see that 2 out of 24 coefficients (8.3 percent) are significant in Table 3, which gives us confidence in a casual interpretation of our results.

Table 3. Event study results for full sample – pre-reform coefficients

	Any insurance	Any private	Employer-sponsored	Individually purchased	Medicaid	Other
Non-elderly adults aged 19-64 (pre-treatment uninsured rate=0.203, sample size=12,313,971)						
Coefficient estimates of interest						
Uninsured*	0.030	-0.0187	-0.018	-0.025	0.039	0.005
Post*2011	(0.030)	(0.036)	(0.037)	(0.020)	(0.027)	(0.010)
Uninsured*	-0.021	-0.009	-0.012	-0.008	-0.007	-0.007
Post*2012	(0.039)	(0.034)	(0.028)	(0.026)	(0.015)	(0.005)
Uninsured*2011	0.010	0.031	0.008	0.040**	-0.008	-0.005
	(0.023)	(0.032)	(0.032)	(0.014)	(0.016)	(0.008)
Uninsured*2012	0.043	0.037	0.008	0.046***	0.010	0.001
	(0.033)	(0.030)	(0.024)	(0.013)	(0.009)	(0.003)

Notes: Coefficient estimates are shown. Standard errors, heteroscedasticity-robust and clustered by state, are in parentheses. *** indicates statistically significant at 0.1% level; ** 1% level; * 5% level. Sampling weights are used. All regressions include area and time fixed effects, the full set of controls, as well as interactions of the treatment variables with the full set of time fixed effects.

Table 4 reports the implied effect of the ACA at mean pre-reform uninsured rate of 20.3 percent in an event study specification where the treatment variables are interacted with the full set of year fixed effects. As mentioned above, this Table reports only the post-treatment implied effects (for the years 2014, 2015, 2016, and 2017) from the same event study model that generates the results reported in Table 3. The table includes indicators at the 0.1 percent, 1 percent, and 5 percent significance level to show if the estimates are statistically significantly different between the first and last post-years (i.e., 2014 vs. 2017) and between 2016 vs. 2017 as well. Two sets of implied effects are reported in Table 4: the impact of the ACA without the Medicaid expansion in panel I and the impact of the full ACA with the Medicaid expansion in panel II. This table essentially shows how the effect of the ACA changed over time.

Table 4. Event study results for full sample – post-reform implied effects

	Any insurance	Any private	Employer-sponsored	Individually purchased	Medicaid	Other
Non-elderly adults aged 19-64 (pre-treatment uninsured rate=0.203, sample size=12,313,971)						
Implied effects of the ACA at mean pre-treatment uninsured rate						
Panel I: ACA w/out Medicaid Expansion						
2014	0.029***	0.028***	0.011***	0.019	0.002	-0.001
	(0.009)	(0.008)	(0.002)	(0.010)	(0.003)	(0.001)
2015	0.046**	0.045**	0.010	0.036*	0.004	-
	(0.016)	(0.013)	(0.004)	(0.017)	(0.005)	0.0002
						(0.001)
2016	0.048**	0.047**	0.010***	0.038*	0.004	-0.001
	(0.018)	(0.014)	(0.003)	(0.016)	(0.006)	(0.002)
2017	0.036*	0.035*	0.003	0.036*	0.004	-0.001
	(0.017)$^{\gamma\gamma\gamma}$	(0.015) $^{\gamma\gamma\gamma}$	(0.003) †† $^{\gamma\gamma}$	(0.017) ††	(0.004)	(0.002)
Panel II: Full ACA						
2014	0.061***	0.028***	.018***	0.010***	0.035***	-
	(0.004)	(.005)	(.004)	(0.003)	(0.006)	0.0000
						(0.001)
2015	0.093***	.032***	.015**	0.016***	0.066***	-
	(0.006)	(.006)	(.004)	(0.003)	(0.008)	0.0003
						(0.001)
2016	0.107***	.032***	.019**	0.012***	0.079***	0.0001
	(0.005)	(.007)	(.006)	(0.003)	(0.008)	(0.002)
2017	0.106***	.026***	.014	0.012**	0.084***	0.001
	(0.006)†††	(.007)	(.008)	(0.004)	(0.007)†††	(0.001)

Notes: Coefficient estimates are shown. Standard errors, heteroscedasticity-robust and clustered by state, are in parentheses. *** indicates statistically significant at 0.1% level; ** 1% level; * 5% level. Statistically significantly different effect in 2017 relative to 2014 is denoted by ††† at 0.1% level, †† at 1% level and † at 5% level. Statistically significantly different effect in 2017 relative to 2016 is denoted by γγγ at 0.1% level, γγ at 1% level and γ at 5% level. Sampling weights are used. All regressions include area and time fixed effects, the full set of controls, as well as interactions of the treatment variables with the full set of time fixed effects.

The first column in panel I shows that the effect of the ACA in non-expansion states on having any insurance increased year over year in the post-reform period until 2016 and then decreased in 2017. The first column in panel II suggests that the effect of the ACA in expansion states on having any coverage combination also increased year over year until 2016. We then see a plateau in the probability of having any insurance between 2016 and

2017 in expansion states. To give a sense of the magnitude of these changes, the probability of having any insurance due the to the fully implemented ACA increased from 6.1 percentage points in 2014 to 10.7 percentage points in 2016. Instead of growing further in 2017, we see an increase in the probability of having any insurance due to the fully implemented ACA of only 10.6 percentage points in 2017, which is not statistically significantly different than the 2016 estimate.

Looking at the sources of insurance in panel I, we see an increase in any private coverage year over year in non-expansion states due to the ACA until 2016 (2.8, 4.5 and 4.7 percentage points for 2014, 2015 and 2016 respectively compared to pre-ACA coverage) and a decrease in coverage growth in 2017 (only a 3.5 percentage point increase in 2017). This change in any private coverage appears to be driving the overall change in coverage due to the ACA in non-expansion states (which increases by 2.9, 4.6, 4.8, and 3.6 percentage points for 2014, 2015, 2016, and 2017 respectively compared to pre-ACA coverage). As mentioned above, panel II in Table 4 shows that between 2016 and 2017 there was a plateau in the growth in "any insurance" due to the full ACA in expansion states (an increase of 10.7 percentage points in 2016 and 10.6 percentage points in 2017 as compared to the pre-ACA period). From the sources of insurance columns, we see that this was the result of continued increasing growth in Medicaid coverage over each of the post-period years (3.5, 6.6, 7.9 and 8.4 percentage point increase in coverage in 2014, 2015, 2016, and 2017) and growth in private insurance coverage in 2014 and 2015, followed by a plateau and a reduction in the growth of coverage from 2015 to 2017 (2.8, 3.2, 3.2 and 2.6 percentage point increase in coverage in 2014, 2015, 2016, and 2017).

Tables 5, 6, and 7 report the implied effects of the ACA in non-expansion and expansion states for various subsamples of interest at the mean pre-ACA uninsured rates for each of those subsamples. Like the bottom panel of Table 2, these tables report implied effects based on the coefficient estimates from the DDD design in equation (1). The first rows for each subsample show the pre-ACA uninsured rate for that subsample, which we use to calculate the pre-ACA disparities in coverage. The two panels of Table 5 stratify the sample into subsamples by income and race.

Since each subsample must contain enough 2013 respondents to accurately compute local area uninsured rates, we are limited to a maximum of two or three subsamples per stratification, as in Courtemanche et al. (2019b). For income, we consider three categories: those with income under 138 percent of the FPL, those between 138 and 400 percent, and those above 400 percent. The under 138 percent of the FPL group was made eligible for Medicaid in states that expanded their Medicaid programs via the ACA. Additionally, those between 100 and 138 percent of the FPL were eligible for subsidized Marketplace coverage in non-expansion states. Those between 138 and 400 percent of the FPL were made eligible for subsidized Marketplace coverage in all states. The highest income group (above 400 percent of the FPL) was also able to purchase non-subsidized Marketplace coverage in all states. The uninsured rate for those in the highest income group in 2013 was 6.7 percent, while it was 39.5 percent for the lowest income group. This implies a 32.8 percentage point coverage gap between the low and high income group.

According to the first column of Table 5, panel I, the fully implemented ACA, which includes the Medicaid expansion and also influences the coverage of higher income individuals through the national components of the ACA, reduced the 32.8 percentage point low-income coverage gap by 14.4 percentage points (= 17 percentage point reduction for the lowest income group – 2.6 percentage point reduction for the highest income group). This represents a 44 percent reduction in the coverage gap between high and low income groups. In results not reported, we estimate that the Medicaid expansion alone, which focuses on lower income individuals, led to a 53 percent reduction in the income coverage gap. Another chapter in this edited volume, Courtemanche, Marton, and Yelowitz (Chapter 8 of this volume), further examines changes in insurance coverage across the income distribution.

We next examine the race stratification in panel II of Table 5. The racial coverage gap in 2013 was 16.1 percentage points, with Hispanic whites and non-whites having an uninsured rate of 30.6 percent, while non-Hispanic whites had an uninsured rate of 14.5 percent. Our results suggest that in non-expansion states the ACA reduced this coverage gap by 2 percentage points (12 percent), while in expansion states the fully implemented ACA reduced the gap by 4.3 percentage points (26.7 percent). The results for sources of coverage show that the Hispanic whites and non-whites enjoy larger gains across-the-board, i.e., the effects of the full ACA on all types of coverage are larger for Hispanic whites and non-whites compared to non-Hispanic whites.

Table 5. Implied effects of the ACA at mean pre-treatment uninsured rate for income and race subsamples

	Any insurance	Any private	Employer - sponsored	Individuall y purchased	Medicaid	Other
Panel I: Income subsamples						
Under 138% FPL (Pre-Treatment Uninsured Rate = 0.395, sample size = 2,237,808)						
ACA w/out Medicaid	-0.014	0.033**	0.013	0.021	-0.057**	0.003
Expansion	(0.017)	(0.011)	(0.019)	(0.022)	(0.019)	(0.003)
Full ACA	0.170***	0.018	0.017	-0.001	0.153***	0.001
	(0.027)	(0.011)	(0.008)	(0.007)	(0.032)	(0.002)
138%-400% FPL (Pre-Treatment Uninsured Rate = 0.238, sample size = 4,814,696)						
ACA w/out Medicaid	0.050***	0.055***	0.020	0.034	-0.003	-0.001***
Expansion	(0.011)	0.010	(0.011)	(.019)	(0.006)	(0.002)
Full ACA	0.106***	0.062***	0.050***	0.014*	0.047***	0.000
	(0.012)	(0.013)	(0.011)	(0.006)	(0.012)	(0.002)
Over 400% FPL (Pre-Treatment Uninsured Rate = 0.067, sample size = 5,292,346)						
ACA w/out Medicaid	0.016	0.016***	-0.001	0.018*	0.000	0.001
Expansion	(0.002)	(0.002)	(0.007)	(0.007)	(0.001)	(0.001)
Full ACA	0.026***	0.018***	0.009	0.007*	0.007*	0.001
	(0.003)	(0.005)	(0.005)	(0.003)	(0.003)	(0.002)
Panel II: Race/ethnicity subsamples						
Non-Hispanic White (Pre-Treatment Uninsured Rate = 0.145, sample size = 8,336,484)						
ACA w/out Medicaid	0.025***	0.017***	0.001	0.014	0.013***	-0.002
Expansion	(0.003)	(0.003)	(0.007)	(0.007)	(0.002)	(0.001)
Full ACA	0.073***	0.021***	0.012**	0.007*	0.061***	-0.003***
	(0.006)	(0.004)	(0.004)	(0.003)	(0.008)	(0.001)
Hispanic White & Non-White (Pre-Treatment Uninsured Rate = 0.306, sample size = 3,977,487)						
ACA w/out Medicaid	0.045*	0.048*	0.012*	0.036	-0.003	-0.002
Expansion	(0.019)	(0.019)	(0.006)	(0.021)	(0.003)	(0.001)
Full ACA	0.116***	0.036***	0.025**	0.014*	0.078***	0.005**
	(0.011)	(0.009)	(0.009)	(0.005)	(0.013)	(0.002)

Notes: Results are effects of the ACA on the proportion of residents with the specified type of insurance, evaluated at the mean pre-treatment uninsured rate. Standard errors, heteroscedasticity-robust and clustered by state, are in parentheses. *** indicates statistically significant at 0.1% level; ** 1% level; * 5% level. Sampling weights are used. All regressions include area and time fixed effects and the full set of controls.

Table 6. Implied effects of the ACA at mean pre-treatment uninsured rate for marital status and age subsamples

	Any insurance	Any private	Employer-sponsored	Individually purchased	Medicaid	Other
Panel I: Marital status subsamples						
Married (Pre-Treatment Uninsured Rate = 0.141, sample size = 6,977,652)						
ACA w/out	0.029***	0.026***	0.007**	0.019*	0.004	-0.001
Medicaid	(0.008)	(0.006)	(0.003)	(0.008)	(0.003)	(0.001)
Full ACA	0.060***	0.021***	0.010***	0.011***	0.041***	0.001
	(0.004)	(0.003)	(0.003)	(0.003)	(0.004)	(0.001)
Unmarried (Pre-Treatment Uninsured Rate = 0.272, sample size = 5,336,319)						
ACA w/out	0.035*	0.038**	0.008	0.008	-0.002	-0.000
Medicaid	(0.015)	(0.012)	(0.010)	(0.018)	(0.006)	(0.002)
Full ACA	0.119***	0.034***	0.027***	0.008	0.088***	0.002
	(0.009)	(0.009)	(0.006)	(0.004)	(0.011)	(0.001)
Panel II: Age subsamples						
Ages 19-26 (pre-treatment uninsured rate = 0.270, sample size = 1,821,602)						
ACA w/out	0.045**	0.036**	0.011	0.023	0.010*	0.001
Medicaid	(0.014)	(0.012)	(0.007)	(0.012)	0.004	(0.001)
Full ACA	0.123***	0.029**	0.025**	0.006	0.097***	0.003*
	(0.010)	(0.009)	(0.008)	(0.004)	(0.013)	(0.002)
Ages 27-34 (pre-treatment uninsured rate = 0.250, sample size = 1,961,736)						
ACA w/out	0.037***	0.026***	0.008	0.016	0.011	0.001
Medicaid	(0,009)	(0.007)	(0.006)	(0.008)	(0.008)	(0.003)
Full ACA	0.094***	0.020*	0.009	0.009*	0.078***	0.003
	(0.009)	(0.008)	(0.007)	(0.003)	(0.009)	(0.003)
Ages 35-49 (pre-treatment uninsured rate = 0.201, sample size = 3,885,153)						
ACA w/out	0.037***	0.034***	0.012**	0.022	0.004	-0.001
Medicaid	(0.011)	(0.009)	(0.004)	(0.011)	(0.005)	(0.001)
Full ACA	0.074***	0.028***	0.019***	0.009**	0.047***	0.001
	(0.005)	(0.005)	(0.005)	(0.003)	(0.006)	(0.001)
Ages 50-64 (pre-treatment uninsured rate = 0.145, sample size = 4,645,480)						
ACA w/out	0.036***	0.038***	0.006	0.032*	0.000	-0.001
Medicaid	(0.007)	(0.005)	(0.008)	(0.013)	(0.003)	(0.002)
Full ACA	0.068***	0.029***	0.015***	0.013***	0.043***	-0.002
	(0.005)	(0.004)	(0.003)	(0.003)	(0.004)	(0.001)

Notes: Results are effects of the ACA on the proportion of residents with the specified type of insurance, evaluated at the mean pre-treatment uninsured rate. Standard errors, heteroscedasticity-robust and clustered by state, are in parentheses. *** indicates statistically significant at 0.1% level; ** 1% level; * 5% level. Sampling weights are used. All regressions include area and time fixed effects and the full set of controls.

Ideally, we would have liked to have been able to separately examine different groups within the Hispanic white and non-white category (e.g., black, Hispanic, Asian), but this is not practical with our particular empirical strategy. Since we need to re-compute the baseline uninsured rate in each local area for each subsample, the subsamples have to have enough people per local area to reliably compute this rate – and this is not, in our judgment, the case for different categories of racial/ethnic minorities.

Panel I of Table 6 examines disparities of coverage by marital status. In 2013 unmarried individuals had a 27.2 percent uninsured rate, while married individuals had a 14.1 percent uninsured rate giving rise to a 13.1 percentage point coverage gap between the two groups. This unmarried coverage gap was reduced by 0.6 percentage points (4.6 percent) by the ACA in non-expansion states, while the fully implemented ACA reduced this coverage gap by 5.9 percentage points (45 percent) in expansion states. The shrinking gap is attributable to larger gains in ESI and Medicaid coverage among the unmarried.

Panel II of Table 6 splits the sample into four age groups: 19-26 years of age, 27-34 years of age, 35-49 years of age, and 50-64 years of age. The rationale for separating 19-26 year olds from 27-34 year olds is that the former was previously affected by the 2010 dependent coverage mandate. Because of the mandate, it is possible that the effect of the 2014 ACA provisions could be weaker among 19-26 than 27-34 year olds. The data, however, shows that those aged 19-26 years still had the highest uninsured rate (27 percent) among the age groups in 2013, three years after the dependent coverage mandate took effect. Those aged 50-64 had the lowest uninsured rate of 14.5 percent. This implies a young adult coverage gap of 12.5 percentage points. The ACA reduced this coverage gap in non-expansion states by 0.9 percentage points (7.2 percent) and the fully implemented ACA reduced it by 5.5 percentage points (44 percent) in expansion states. In results not reported, we find that the larger gain among 19-26 year olds is driven by a much larger increase in Medicaid coverage (9.7 percentage points compared to 4.3 percentage points among 50-64 year olds due to the full ACA).

Table 7. Implied effects of the ACA at mean pre-treatment uninsured rate for gender subsamples

	Any insurance	Any private	Employer-sponsored	Individually purchased	Medicaid	Other
Gender subsamples						
Women (Pre-Treatment Uninsured Rate = 0.186, sample size = 6,389,974)						
ACA w/out	0.030**	.032***	0.010	0.021	-0.002	0.000
Medicaid Expansion	(0.009)	(0.006)	(0.010)	(0.012)	(0.009)	(0.002)
Full ACA	0.093***	0.030***	0.022***	0.007	0.065***	0.002
	(0.007)	(0.007)	(0.005)	(0.004)	(0.010)	(0.001)
Men (Pre-Treatment Uninsured Rate = 0.223, sample size = 5,954,876)						
ACA w/out	0.041***	0.042***	0.010	0.032	0.000	0.001
Medicaid Expansion	(0.011)	(0.009)	(0.009)	(0.017)	(0.005)	(0.002)
Full ACA	0.095***	0.038***	0.029***	0.012*	0.061***	-0.000
	(0.008)	(0.008)	(0.006)	(0.005)	(0.010)	(0.002)

Notes: Results are effects of the ACA on the proportion of residents with the specified type of insurance, evaluated at the mean pre-treatment uninsured rate. Standard errors, heteroscedasticity-robust and clustered by state, are in parentheses. *** indicates statistically significant at 0.1% level; ** 1% level; * 5% level. Sampling weights are used. All regressions include area and time fixed effects and the full set of controls.

Table 7 stratifies the sample by gender. Prior to the ACA, we observe a relatively small coverage gap of 3.7 percentage point for men (22.3 percent uninsured rate for males vs. 18.6 percent for females). In non-expansion states, the ACA reduced the size of this coverage gap by 29.7 percent. The fully implemented ACA reduced the size of the gender coverage gap by 5.4 percent in expansion states due to a larger effect of the full ACA on private coverage for men as compared to women.

DISCUSSION

Prior to the main implementation of the Affordable Care Act (ACA) in 2014, there were well- documented disparities in insurance coverage along multiple dimensions, such as age, race, and income (Courtemanche, Marton, and Yelowitz, 2016; Yelowitz, 2016; Courtemanche et al., 2019b). In this chapter, we investigate whether newly available calendar year 2017 data from the ACS helps to provide further insights into the ACA's effects on insurance disparities.

There are three main overall findings of our investigation. First, there were further reductions in coverage disparities in 2017. After four years, the fully implemented ACA reduced coverage disparities across income groups by 44 percent, racial groups by 27 percent, and across age groups by 44 percent. These results are larger than the ones estimated by Courtemanche et al., (2019b) using only three years of post-implementation data. In addition, reductions in the size of the gender coverage gap emerged that were not present when using only three years of post-implementation data. This reduction is due to the larger effect of the private components of the ACA expansion on insurance coverage for men than women. Finally, the reductions in coverage disparities across marital status were slightly smaller with four years of post-implementation data than the ones obtained with only three years (44 percent versus 45 percent, respectively).

Second, the gains in insurance coverage growth slowed down in 2017 due to a reduction in the growth of private insurance coverage, most of which is due to a reduction in ESI coverage, but also due to a reduction in the growth of individually purchased coverage. Even though we don't have enough data to understand the mechanisms driving this change, it is possible that the 2016 presidential election had a chilling effect on private insurance. In January 2017, President Trump signed his first executive order directing federal agencies to exercise all authority and discretion available to them to waive, defer, grant exemptions from, or delay the implementation of any provision or requirement of the ACA. Whether this and other actions taken by President Trump had an effect on private insurance coverage is a topic that needs further investigation.

Third, our results show that the reductions in coverage disparities are due to both the Medicaid expansion and to the private components of the ACA. Reductions in the growth of private insurance coverage could dampen the reductions in coverage disparities. For example, the reduction in coverage disparities across income groups was larger using four years of data compared to using three years of data, but only slightly (44 percent versus 43 percent, respectively). Similarly, the slight reduction in the coverage disparity by marital status in 2017 is due to a smaller increase in private insurance coverage – particularly individually purchased insurance – among unmarried individuals.

One limitation of our work is that our disparity analyses assume that the subsamples are exogenously determined. In other words, we are assuming people cannot move from one category into another. Income is one source of stratification where this assumption might not hold, since individuals can (endogenously) adjust their income in response to the 2014 ACA provisions. Kaestner et al. (2017) and Leung and Mas (2018) found little impact of the ACA Medicaid expansions on work effort, implying that the effect on income should be minimal. Gooptu et al. (2016) found no impact of the ACA in part-time versus full-time employment or job reductions in 2014. Duggan et al. (2017), on the other hand, found that while labor market outcomes in the aggregate were not significantly affected by the ACA, labor force participation reductions in areas with higher potential exchange enrollment were offset by increases in labor force participation in areas with higher potential Medicaid enrollment.

Our results are broadly consistent with those reported in the Medicaid expansion literature in that both the Medicaid expansion and the fully implemented ACA generally reduce but do not eliminate coverage disparities. These results imply that full repeal of the ACA would exacerbate these disparities. Additionally, it is possible that changes to the ACA after 2017, including regulatory changes, such as Medicaid work requirements, and the elimination of the individual mandate, would lead to further changes in disparities. For example, our finding that the Medicaid expansion eliminated 53 percent of the coverage gap across income groups may change if Medicaid work requirements are widely implemented and end up reducing enrollment. Thus, more work is needed to examine the impact of the ACA as economic conditions change and the ACA itself changes.

APPENDIX

Table A1. Pre-treatment summary statistics for control variables

	Full Sample	Medicaid Expansion; at or above Median Baseline Uninsured	Medicaid Expansion; below Median Baseline Uninsured	Non-Expansion; at or above Median Baseline Uninsured	Non-Expansion; below Median Baseline Uninsured
Demographic controls					
Age dummies (19-24 is omitted base category)[a]					
Age 25-29	0.110	0.114	0.109	0.108	0.113
	(0.313)	(0.318)	(0.311)	(0.311)	(0.317)
Age 30-34	0.109	0.111	0.106	0.108	0.112
	(0.311)	(0.314)	(0.308)	(0.311)	(0.315)
Age 35-39	0.104	0.105	0.101	0.106	0.103
	(0.305)	(0.307)	(0.301)	(0.308)	(0.304)
Age 40-44	0.111	0.110	0.111	0.113	0.109
	(0.314)	(0.313)	(0.314)	(0.317)	(0.312)
Age 45-49	0.114	0.110	0.116	0.114	0.112
	(0.318)	(0.313)	(0.321)	(0.317)	(0.315)
Age 50-54	0.118	0.114	0.122	0.116	0.118
	(0.323)	(0.318)	(0.328)	(0.321)	(0.322)
Age 55-59	0.109	0.105	0.112	0.107	0.108
	(0.311)	(0.306)	(0.316)	(0.309)	(0.310)
Age 60-64	0.095	0.093	0.098	0.096	0.092
	(0.294)	(0.290)	(0.297)	(0.294)	(0.289)
Female	0.510	0.506	0.509	0.513	0.510
	(0.500)	(0.500)	(0.500)	(0.500)	(0.500)
Race/ethnicity dummies (non-Hispanic white is omitted base category)					
Non-Hispanic black	0.121	0.083	0.105	0.169	0.135
	(0.326)	(0.275)	(0.307)	(0.375)	(0.341)
Hispanic	0.163	0.272	0.107	0.198	0.071
	(0.369)	(0.445)	(0.310)	(0.399)	(0.256)
Other	0.080	0.101	0.095	0.051	0.053
	(0.271)	(0.301)	(0.293)	(0.221)	(0.227)
Foreign born	0.171	0.230	0.168	0.162	0.093
	(0.376)	(0.421)	(0.374)	(0.369)	(0.291)
US citizen	0.904	0.867	0.914	0.900	0.944
	(0.295)	(0.340)	(0.281)	(0.300)	(0.231)
Married	0.520	0.508	0.518	0.521	0.544
	(0.500)	(0.500)	(0.500)	(0.500)	(0.498)

Table A1. (Continued)

	Full Sample	Medicaid Expansion; at or above Median Baseline Uninsured	Medicaid Expansion; below Median Baseline Uninsured	Non-Expansion; at or above Median Baseline Uninsured	Non-Expansion; below Median Baseline Uninsured
Dummies for number of children in home (none is omitted base category)					
One child	0.158	0.162	0.157	0.160	0.155
	(0.365)	(0.368)	(0.364)	(0.366)	(0.362)
Two children	0.133	0.135	0.133	0.130	0.134
	(0.339)	(0.341)	(0.340)	(0.336)	(0.341)
Three children	0.052	0.057	0.049	0.053	0.054
	(0.223)	(0.233)	(0.215)	(0.224)	(0.227)
Four children	0.015	0.017	0.013	0.016	0.018
	(0.123)	(0.131)	(0.115)	(0.124)	(0.132)
Five children or more	0.006	0.007	0.006	0.006	0.007
	(0.077)	(0.083)	(0.075)	(0.075)	(0.082)
Economic controls					
Education dummies (less than high school degree is omitted base category)					
High school degree	0.268	0.259	0.263	0.286	0.263
	(0.443)	(0.438)	(0.440)	(0.452)	(0.440)
Some College	0.329	0.337	0.318	0.333	0.343
	(0.470)	(0.473)	(0.466)	(0.471)	(0.475)
College graduate	0.286	0.253	0.328	0.243	0.306
	(0.452)	(0.435)	(0.469)	(0.429)	(0.461)
Unemployed	0.069	0.077	0.067	0.070	0.057
	(0.253)	(0.270)	(0.250)	(0.255)	(0.232)
State unemployment rate	8.161	9.222	8.040	7.970	7.082
	(1.593)	(1.550)	(1.426)	(1.423)	(1.479)
Student	0.110	0.113	0.109	0.106	0.118
	(0.313)	(0.316)	(0.311)	(0.308)	(0.322)
Income dummies (Relative to the Federal Poverty Line)[a]					
Income <100FPL	0.144	0.160	0.126	0.163	0.131
	(0.351)	(0.367)	(0.331)	(0.369)	(0.337)
100FPL≤ Income<200FPL	0.171	0.193	0.143	0.199	0.158
	(0.376)	(0.395)	(0.350)	(0.400)	(0.364)
200FPL≤ Income<300FPL	0.162	0.167	0.148	0.175	0.166
	(0.368)	(0.373)	(0.356)	(0.380)	(0.372)
300FPL≤ Income<400FPL	0.136	0.131	0.136	0.135	0.146
	(0.343)	(0.337)	(0.343)	(0.342)	(0.353)
400FPL≤ Income<500FPL	0.106	0.098	0.113	0.099	0.115
	(0.308)	(0.297)	(0.317)	(0.299)	(0.319)
Income ≥500FPL	0.282	0.251	0.333	0.229	0.285
	(0.450)	(0.434)	(0.471)	(0.420)	(0.451)

	Full Sample	Medicaid Expansion; at or above Median Baseline Uninsured	Medicaid Expansion; below Median Baseline Uninsured	Non-Expansion; at or above Median Baseline Uninsured	Non-Expansion; below Median Baseline Uninsured
Exchange controls					
State set up own exchange	0.344 (0.475)	0.563 (0.496)	0.566 (0.496)	N/A	N/A
State exchange had glitches	0.084 (0.277)	0.065 (0.246)	0.178 (0.383)	N/A	N/A

Notes: Standard deviations are in parentheses.

[a] Our baseline model includes dummy variables for each year of age as well as dummy variables for each 10-point increment of the FPL (50 total dummies). To conserve space, we present our descriptive statistics for age and income in broader categories in this table.

References

Benitez Joseph A., E. Kathleen Adams, and Eric E. Seiber. 2018. "Did Health Care Reform Help Kentucky Address Disparities in Coverage and Access to Care Among the Poor?" *Health Services Research* 53(3):1387–1406.

Courtemanche, Charles, James Marton, and Aaron Yelowitz. 2016. "Who Gained Insurance Coverage in 2014, the First Year of Full ACA Implementation?" *Health Economics* 25(6):778–84.

Courtemanche, Charles, James Marton, and Aaron Yelowitz. 2019. "Medicaid Coverage Across the Income Distribution under the Affordable Care Act." In *Medicaid: Enrollment, Eligibility, and Key Issues*, edited by Daniel Lanford. New York: Nova Science.

Courtemanche, Charles, James Marton, Benjamin Ukert, Aaron Yelowitz, and Daniela Zapata. 2017. "Impacts of the Affordable Care Act on Health Insurance Coverage in Medicaid Expansion and Non-Expansion States," *Journal of Policy Analysis and Management* 36(1):178–210.

Courtemanche, Charles, James Marton, Benjamin Ukert, Aaron Yelowitz, and Daniela Zapata. 2018a. "Early Effects of the Affordable Care Act on Health Care Access, Risky Health Behaviors, and Self-Assessed Health," *Southern Economic Journal* 84(3):660–691.

Courtemanche, Charles, James Marton, Benjamin Ukert, Aaron Yelowitz, and Daniela Zapata. 2018b. "Effects of the Affordable Care Act on Health Care Access and Self-Assessed Health after 3 Years," *Inquiry: The Journal of Health Care Organization, Provision and Financing* 55:1–10.

Courtemanche, Charles, James Marton, Benjamin Ukert, Aaron Yelowitz, and Daniela Zapata. 2019a. "Effects of the Affordable Care Act on Health Behaviors after 3 Years," *Eastern Economic Journal* 45(1):7–33.

Courtemanche, Charles, James Marton, Benjamin Ukert, Aaron Yelowitz, Daniela Zapata, and Ishtiaque Fazlul. 2019b. "The Three-Year Impact of the Affordable Care Act on Disparities in Insurance Coverage," *Health Services Research*, 54(S1):307–316.

Courtemanche, Charles, Andrew Friedson, Andrew P. Koller, and Daniel I. Rees. 2019c. "The Affordable Care Act and Ambulance Response Times," *Journal of Health Economics*, 67.

Duggan, Mark, Gopi S. Goda, and Emilie Jackson. 2017. *The Effects of the Affordable Car Act on Health Insurance Coverage and Labor Market Outcomes.* National Bureau of Economic Research Working Paper 23607.

Finkelstein, Amy. 2007. "The Aggregate Effects of Health Insurance: Evidence from the Introduction of Medicare," *Quarterly Journal of Economics* 122:1–37.

Frean, Molly, Jonathan Gruber, and Benjamin D. Sommers. 2017. "Premium Subsidies, the Mandate, and Medicaid Expansion: Coverage Effects of the Affordable Care Act," *Journal of Health Economics* 53:72–86.

Gooptu, Angshuman, Asako S. Moriya, Kosali I. Simon, and Benjamin D. Sommers. 2016. "Medicaid Expansion did not Result in Significant Employment changes or Job Reductions in 2014," *Health Affairs* 35(1):111–118.

Gruber, Jonathan and Benjamin D. Sommers. 2019. "The Affordable Care Act's Effects on Patients, Providers and the Economy: What We've Learned so Far." National Bureau of Economic Research Working Paper

25932, National Bureau of Economic Research, June. http://www.nber.org/papers/w25932.

Kaestner, Robert, Bowen Garrett, Jiajia Chen, Anuj Gangopadhyaya, and Caitlyn Fleming. 2017. "Effects of the ACA Medicaid Expansion on Health Insurance Coverage and Labor Supply," *Journal of Policy Analysis and Management* 36(3):608–642.

Leung, Pauline and Alexandre Mas. 2018. "Employment Effects of the Affordable Care Act Medicaid Expansions". *Industrial Relations* 57(2):206– 234.

Miller, Sarah. 2012. "The Effect of Insurance on Emergency Room Visits: An Analysis of the 2006 Massachusetts Health Reform," *Journal of Public Economics* 96:893–908.

Obama, Barack. 2016. "United States Health Reform: Progress to Date and Next Steps," *Journal of the American Medical Association* 316 (5):525–532.

Wehby, George L. and Wei Lyu. 2018. "The Impact of the ACA Medicaid Expansions on Health Insurance Coverage through 2015 and Coverage Disparities by Age, Race/Ethnicity, and Gender," *Health Services Research* 53(2):1248–1271.

Wherry, Laura R. and Sarah Miller. 2016. "Early Coverage, Access, Utilization, and Health Effects Associated with the Affordable Care Act Medicaid Expansions: A Quasi-Experimental Study," *Annals of Internal Medicine* 164(12):795–803.

Yelowitz, Aaron. 2016. "How Did the ACA Affect Health Insurance Coverage in Kentucky?" *Schnatter Institute Working Paper*. John H. Schnatter Institute for the Study of Free Enterprise, University of Kentucky, Accessed September. http://isfe.uky.edu/sites/ISFE/files/research-pdfs/Schnatter.2017.Yelowitz.pdf.

Yue, Dahai, Petra W. Rasmussen, and Ninez A. Ponce. 2018. "Racial/Ethnic Differential Effects of Medicaid Expansion on Health Care Access," *Health Services Research* 53(5):3640–3656.

In: Medicaid: Politics, Policy, and Key Issues ISBN: 978-1-53618-133-3
Editor: Daniel Lanford

Chapter 3

FEDERALLY QUALIFIED HEALTH CENTERS: FROM THE FRINGES TO THE MAINSTREAM

Carolin L. Spice[1,*], Bomy Yun[2], Aaron B. Katz[1] and Paul A. Fishman[1]
[1]Department of Health Services,
University of Washington, Seattle, WA, US
[2]Neighborcare Health, Seattle, WA, US

ABSTRACT

As of 2017, Federally Qualified Health Centers (FQHCs) serve one in 12 Americans in the United States (HRSA 2018a). What started in 1965 as a demonstration project with two centers within President Lyndon B. Johnson's Office of Economic Opportunity (OEO) has grown to over 1,400 centers nationwide that serve nearly 28 million people today (RCHN 2019). Though FQHCs have historically cared for those without insurance, their mix of payers in recent years has expanded to include private insurance, Medicare, and Medicaid. In this chapter, we address the question of how the Affordable Care Act of 2010 (ACA) affected the FQHC system.

---

* Corresponding Author's Email: cspice@uw.edu.

Keywords: federally qualified health centers, Medicare, Medicaid, Affordable Care Act, HITECH Act, uninsured

Introduction

In 1975, with support from Senators Edward Kennedy and Jacob Javits, Congress authorized the Community Health Center program as a permanent program. With this authorization, what began as a demonstration program became an enduring health network under Section 330 of the U.S. Public Health Service Act. The program was placed under the Department of Health and Human Services, and in 1989, Congress established FQHC services as a guaranteed benefit within Medicare and Medicaid, offering cost-based payments for services. In 2001, President George W. Bush's Health Center Growth Initiative called for new health centers, and Congress unanimously reauthorized the Health Center Program in 2002. Through these initiatives, reauthorizations, and expansions, federal funding for community health centers covered 18 million people by 2008 (NACHC 2015a).

The goal of the program is to increase access to comprehensive and affordable healthcare for underserved and vulnerable populations. Today, FQHCs provide a range of services to an equal mix of urban and rural residents. By providing comprehensive and affordable care, the FQHC model also improves communities. Accordingly, both the White House Office of Management and Budget and the Institute of Medicine have hailed the FQHC program as one of the most effective of all federal programs, citing FQHCs as "stellar models" of primary care practice (IOM 2003).

Today, FQHCs rely on Medicaid funding to fulfill their missions. With the passage of the ACA in 2010 and the Medicaid expansion it enabled in 2014, it is important to take stock of FQHC changes in states that did and did *not* expand Medicaid income eligibility under the ACA. To that end, this chapter addresses the question of how FQHCs have developed since the passage of the ACA.

MEDICAID AND FQHCS

As a provider of comprehensive health services for low income individuals and families, FQHCs are a unique type of Medicaid healthcare provider. Though FQHCs provide services to privately insured and uninsured individuals, they rely on public funding to remain in operation (HRSA 2018b). This is essential as it allows FQHCs to overcome economic, geographic, or cultural barriers that limit access to affordable healthcare services for the nation's most vulnerable populations. Section 330 of the Public Health Service Act allows FQHCs to receive federal grant funding administered through the Health Resources and Services Administration (HRSA) Health Center Program. Additionally, FQHCs are qualified for enhanced reimbursement from Medicare and Medicaid. Now, one in six Medicaid enrollees are cared for by an FQHC (NACHC 2019a).

Qualifications and Requirements of FQHCs

Health centers must meet a stringent set of requirements to receive and maintain FQHC status. Several key requirements are listed below:

- Serve a designated medically-underserved area or medically-underserved population
- Deliver high quality, comprehensive primary care and supportive services to all, regardless of patients' ability to pay
- Discount cost of care by offering a sliding fee scale to individuals and families whose annual household incomes are below those set forth in the Federal Poverty Guidelines
- Offer accessible locations and hours of operation, including after-hours coverage
- Have an ongoing quality assurance program
- Be governed by a board of directors composed of 9-25 members of which at least 51% must be patients served by the health center

FQHCs can leverage benefits from a number of other federal programs and gain access to the following:

- Medical malpractice coverage under the Federal Tort Claims Act
- Federal loan guarantees for capital improvements and modernization of health center facilities
- Discounts for pharmaceutical products through the 340B Drug Pricing Program
- Free vaccines for uninsured and underinsured children through the Vaccines For Children program
- Assistance in the recruitment and retention of primary care providers through the National Health Service Corps

FQHC LANDSCAPE PRIOR TO THE PASSAGE OF THE AFFORDABLE CARE ACT

In the 15 years preceding the passage of the Patient Protection and Affordable Care Act (ACA) of 2010, FQHC capacity expanded in response to an increased demand for free or low-cost healthcare. Since the mid-1990s, the number of uninsured Americans had grown faster than the general population, with simultaneously declining willingness on the part of private physicians to provide charity care (Cunningham and May 2006). In addition, the proportion of the U.S. population covered by Medicaid increased from approximately 10 percent in 1999 to 17 percent in 2010 (DeNavas-Walt, Proctor, and Smith 2010). Direct federal funding for FQHCs increased from roughly $750 million in 1996 to $2.2 billion in 2010, helping to increase the number of FQHC organizations nationally from about 700 to 1,100 – with close to 7,000 sites of care (NACHC 2017a). The American Recovery and Reinvestment Act of 2009 added another $2 billion in temporary FQHC funding for capital and service improvements through 2010 (NACHC n.d.).

When state Medicaid programs accelerated their use of managed care arrangements in the 1990s, FQHCs worked with state Medicaid programs to be part of health plans' primary care networks. By 2009, nearly half of all Medicaid beneficiaries were enrolled in comprehensive managed care and this number continued to grow in subsequent years (CMS n.d.).

Despite similar missions and parallel growth since their inception, Medicaid and FQHCs are distinct programs. Thus, it may be useful to compare how the ACA Medicaid provisions impacted FQHCs in states that expanded Medicaid income eligibility (also known as Medicaid expansion) with states that did not.

THE STATE OF FQHCS AFTER THE ACA

As of May 2019, 36 states and the District of Columbia expanded Medicaid eligibility based on the ACA income guideline, while the 14 states shown in Table 1 have not (KFF 2019). Because the ACA does not specify a deadline for when states expand their Medicaid income eligibility, and the Supreme Court ruled that states can opt out of Medicaid expansion, this situation is fluid and will likely change in future years. In addition, in many states, voters can decide to pursue or sunset Medicaid expansion through a ballot initiative.

Table 1. Non-expansion Medicaid states

Alabama	Florida
Georgia	Kansas
Mississippi	Missouri
North Carolina	Oklahoma
South Carolina	South Dakota
Tennessee	Texas
Wisconsin	Wyoming

Source: "Status of State Action on the Medicaid Expansion Decision," KFF State Health Facts, updated November 6, 2019. https://www.kff.org/health-reform/state-indicator/state-activity-around-expanding-medicaid-under-the-affordable-care-act/.

An analysis was performed on aggregated state-level FQHC-Medicaid data from the years 2013, 2015, and 2017, obtained from the National Association of Community Health Centers (NACHC 2013; NACHC 2015b; NACHC 2017b). Between 2013 and 2017, Medicaid enrollments at FQHCs increased by an average of nearly 8 percent in states that expanded Medicaid compared to an average 0.5 percent increase across non-expansion states. These findings are consistent with a 2019 report by the Medicaid and CHIP Payment Access Commission (MACPAC), which showed that Medicaid enrollment in Medicaid expansion states increased by 13.1 million or 34.4 percent between 2013 and 2019. In the same period, uninsured patient volumes decreased by an average of 12 percent in expansion state FQHCs, but only decreased by less than 4 percent in the 14 non-expansion states.

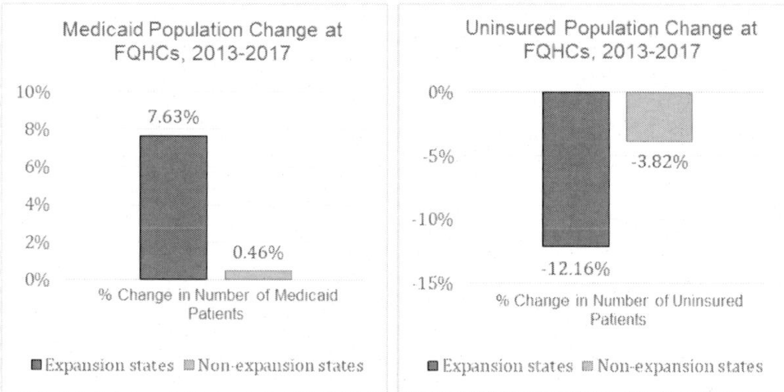

Data Sources: National Association of Community Health Centers. Key Health Center Data by State, Years 2013, 2015, and 2017.

Figure 1. Average percent change in Medicaid and uninsured populations at FQHCs from 2013–2017.

Despite differences in the Medicaid and uninsured populations seen at FQHCs between expansion and non-expansion states, the change in number of visits, employed staff, and number of sites between the two did not differ as appreciably. Encounter volumes at FQHCs increased by an average of 6.9 percentage points and employee full-time equivalent (FTE) by an average of 6.2 percentage points more in expansion states as compared to non-expansion states between 2013 and 2017. A plausible explanation for the greater comparative growth in FQHCs in expansion states is the extra capacity to see more patients and hire more staff allowed by the infusion of capital from Medicaid expansion. Less anticipated was the 1.3 percentage point greater increase in number of sites at FQHCs in non-expansion states compared to expansion states. It is worth noting that a greater number of sites does not necessarily equate to increased access or a greater number of services provided. The national growth of FQHCs is likely due to a multitude of factors, some of which may depend, at the state level, on legislation and characteristics of relationships between state Medicaid agencies, health plans, and FQHCs, but not on the growth of the Medicaid population alone. However, Medicaid expansion has allowed for significantly increased access to healthcare for Medicaid and uninsured populations.

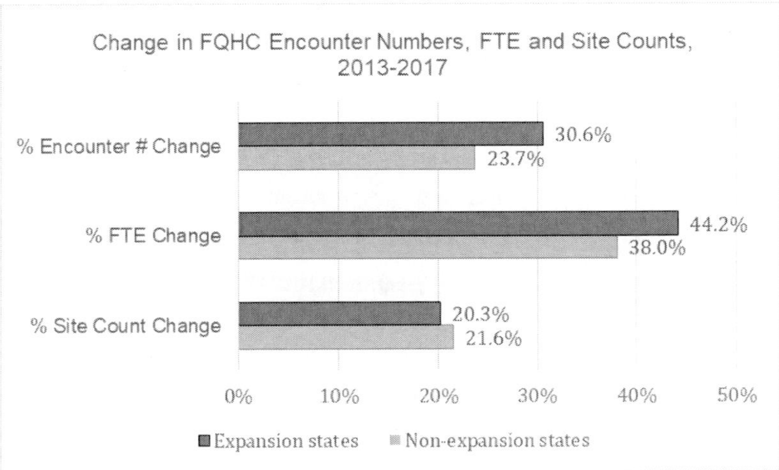

Data Sources: National Association of Community Health Centers. Key Health Center Data by State, Years 2013, 2015, and 2017.

Figure 2. Average percent change of FQHC Encounters, FTEs, and site counts from 2013-2017.

Growth of FQHC Services

What started with two sites in the mid-1960s serving almost 100,000 people grew to 600 sites serving five million people in the mid-1980s, then expanded further by 2010 to almost 7,000 sites serving 20 million people. FQHCs have become an integral part of the United States healthcare system today. As the number of sites have grown, so too have the variety of services that FQHCs provide for their patient populations. Today, FQHCs provide care to one in 12 people nationwide, of which 20 percent are rural residents.

In addition, they serve over 10 percent of the nation's children in traditional ambulatory settings as well as in more than 800,000 school-based health centers.

Grantees, Sites, and Services

As shown in the Figure below, the growth in the number of grantees increased moderately from 2006 to 2017. However, the net increase in sites during this same period grew by almost 5,000, with the largest expansion of 1,291 sites between 2011 and 2012.

In addition to establishing more sites, FQHCs also broadened the number of services provided to their patients during this time. As organizations that have always taken a broader view of health and focused on providing comprehensive care, they responded to the diverse needs of their patient population by incorporating dental, vision, behavioral health, and enabling services (e.g., transportation) to their suite of services. Nationwide, 22 percent of health centers provide all five types of services onsite, while 81 percent of health centers provide dental services and 90 percent of health centers provide behavioral health services onsite (NACHC 2019b).

Between 2010 and 2017, visits for vision services grew by 116 percent, behavioral health service visits grew by 111 percent, and dental visits grew by 70 percent. In addition, enabling services, which are defined as "a wide range of services that support and assist primary care and facilitate patient access to care" (BPHC 2018), grew by 27 percent between 2010 and 2017. Based on research conducted by the Association of Asian Pacific Community Health Organizations, enabling services lead to positive impacts on outcomes, costs, access, and patient satisfaction (AAPCHO 2016). Some examples of enabling services include case management, interpretation services, patient education, outreach, eligibility assistance, and transportation services. For example, some health centers have found effective ways to transport patients to their clinics by utilizing ride-sharing networks and apps (Liu 2018).

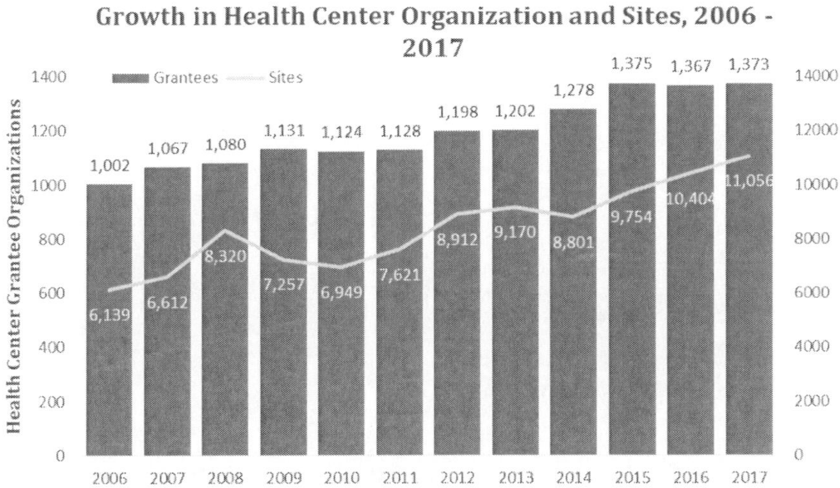

Source: National Association of Community Health Centers. Community Health Center Chartbooks, June 2017 and January 2019.

Figure 3. Growth of FQHC grantees and sites from 2006–2017.

Furthermore, FQHC use of information technology included the implementation of electronic health records (EHRs) resulting in an adoption rate of over 99 percent (HRSA 2017). As of 2017, almost 98 percent of FQHCs send pharmacy prescriptions electronically and over 98 percent use computerized clinical decision support, such as alerts for drug allergies, checks for drug-drug interactions, and reminders for preventive screening tests. Almost 80 percent of FQHCs exchange clinical information electronically with other key providers in health care settings such as hospitals, emergency rooms, or subspecialty clinicians, and over 90 percent engage patients through health IT such as patient portals, kiosks, and secure messaging (i.e., secure e-mail) either through the EHR or through other technologies. Finally, almost 90 percent of health centers use health IT to coordinate or provide enabling services which encompasses outreach, language translation, transportation, case management, or other similar services (HRSA 2017). Some FQHCs have also established partnerships with traditional hospitals within their geographic area such as staffing a hospital's urgent care center after hours, thereby increasing access to specialty care and advanced imaging for their patient population.

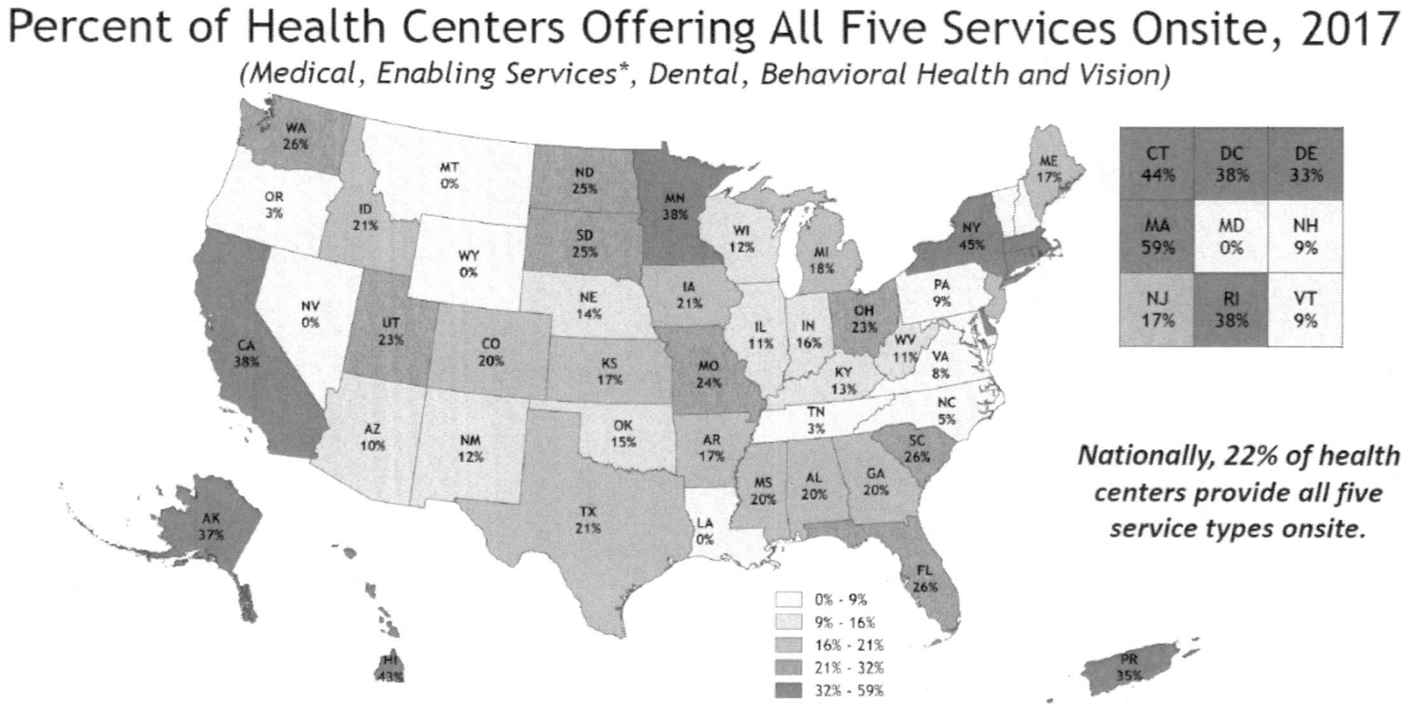

Source: Reprinted with permission from the National Association of Community Health Centers. Community Health Center Chartbook, January 2019.

Figure 4. Percentage of FQHCs offering Medical, Dental, Vision, Behavioral Health, and Enabling Services.

Recent advancements in technology have allowed FQHCs to offer telehealth services to their patients. As of 2017, 44 percent of health centers provide telehealth services, and 52 percent of telehealth programs offer telehealth for behavioral health (NACHC 2019b). Telehealth is "the use of telecommunications and information technologies to share information and provide clinical care, education, public health, and administrative services at a distance" (HRSA 2019c). It applies a variety of technologies, such as videoconferencing, the internet, or store-and-forward of data. Telehealth incorporates telemedicine, which is the remote provision of clinical services. Telehealth is enlisted by FQHCs to provide specialty care, manage chronic conditions, primary care, and oral health, among other services. Adoption of telehealth services by FQHCs stands in contrast to the overall national average wherein 42 percent of hospitals and 15 percent of family physicians in the United States have adopted telehealth (Lin et al. 2018).

Table 2. Percentage of FQHCs with various Electronic Health Record (EHR) functions

EHR Functionalities	Percent of centers
Prescriptions electronically sent to the pharmacy	97.96%
Use of computerized, clinical decision support such as alerts for drug allergies, checks for drug-drug interactions, reminders for preventive screening tests, or other similar functions	98.25%
Electronically exchange clinical information with other key providers/health care settings such as hospitals, emergency rooms, or subspecialty clinicians	79.83%
Patients engaged through health IT components such as patient portals, kiosks, secure messaging (i.e., secure email)	90.17%
Use the EHR or other health IT system to provide patients with electronic summaries of office visits or other clinical information when requested	95.85%
Use health IT to coordinate or to provide enabling services such as outreach, language translation, transportation, case management, or other similar services	79.39%

Source: Health Resources & Services Administration Health Center Program. 2017 National Health Center Data. https://bphc.hrsa.gov/uds2017/datacenter.aspx?year=2017.

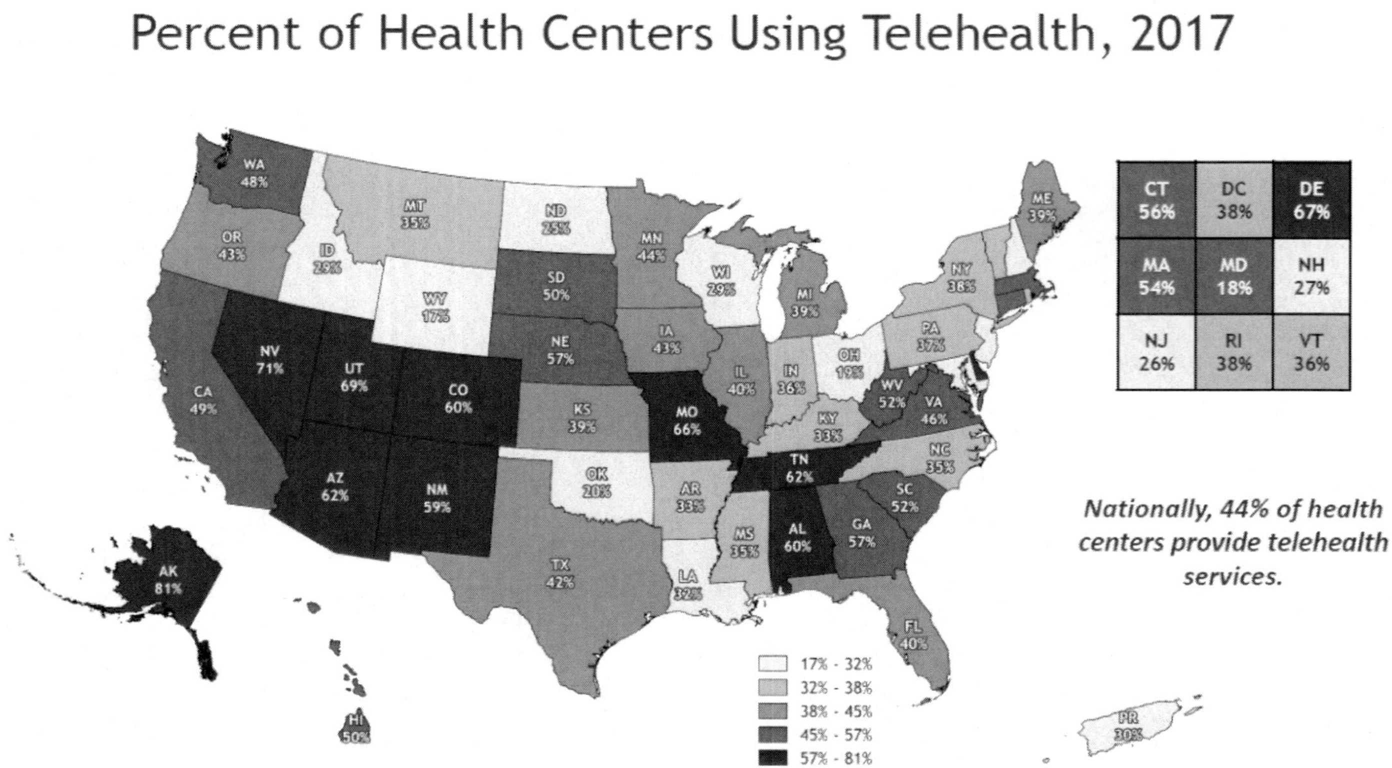

Source: Reprinted with permission from the National Association of Community Health Centers. Community Health Center Chartbook, January 2019.

Figure 5. Percentage of FQHCs using Telehealth.

Quality Focus

Throughout their 50-year history, FQHCs have been recognized for their strong record of implementing innovative models of care and in recent years have incorporated technological advances to extend their models of care. As part of the nation's network of safety net providers, FQHCs have continued to provide a high level of integrated, affordable care to all patients, regardless of their ability to pay.

This focus on quality care has resulted in 75 percent of FQHCs nationwide achieving formal recognition as *Patient Centered Medical Homes* (PCMH) as of July 2018 (NACHC 2019b). In addition, many FQHCs integrate multiple services to address the needs of their patient population (HRSA 2019a). Some clinical quality improvement integration efforts include:

- Behavioral health and primary care
- Hepatitis treatment and primary care
- Oral health and primary care
- Substance use disorders treatment and primary care

Through these quality improvement efforts, FQHCs are able to foster a continuous learning health system in which evidence and experience are used to improve local practices and inform system-wide enhancements. Many of these practices within specific FQHCs have been called out for their "Promising Practices" around care coordination, data and health information technology, diabetes, food security, HIV, substance use disorder, and telehealth (HRSA 2019b). A listing of 21 health centers that have demonstrated promising practices, as determined by experts who conducted 252 operational site visits from January 20, 2018 through June 30, 2018, is shown below (HRSA 2018b).

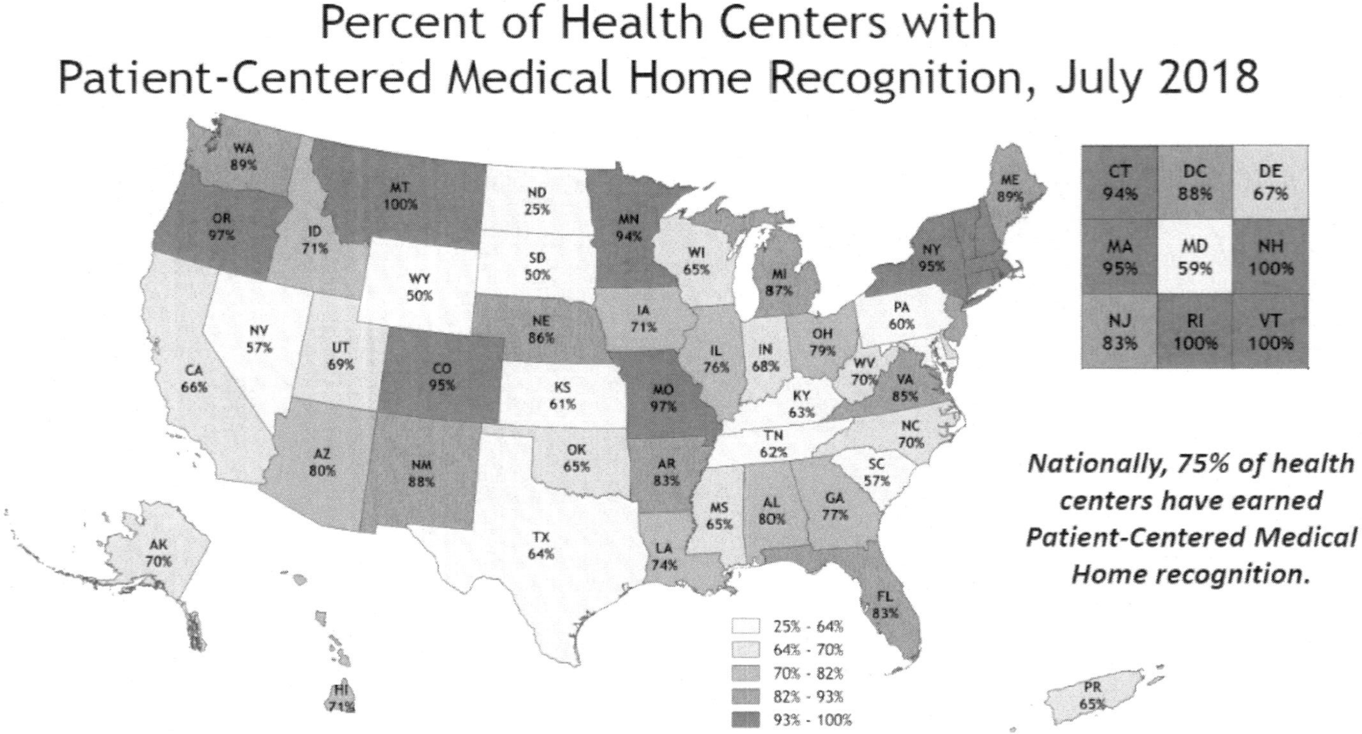

Source: Reprinted with permission from the National Association of Community Health Centers. Community Health Center Chartbook, January 2019.

Figure 6. Percentage of FQHCs with PCMH recognition.

Table 3. Promising Practices

State	Grantee	Type
California	Lifelong Medical Care	Care Transitions
California	Tulare Community Health Clinic	Provider Scans
California	Tulare Community Health Clinic	Substitute for Migratory and Seasonal Agricultural Workers
California	Share Our Selves Corporation	Mailroom for Patients without Addresses
California	Lifelong Medical Care	Patient Scheduling Appointment
California	McCloud Healthcare Clinic, Inc.	Rearranging Health Center Schedules
Colorado	Metro Community Provider Network	Screening, Brief Intervention & Referral to Treatment
Colorado	Metro Community Provider Network	Oral Health
Connecticut	Norwalk Community Health Center, Inc.	Case Management
Florida	Citrus Health Network, Inc.	Chronic Condition Management
Illinois	Erie Family Health Center, Inc.	Clinic Telephones
Maryland	Choptank Community Health System, Inc.	Oral Health
Maryland	Choptank Community Health System, Inc.,	Case Management
Massachusetts	Dothouse Health, Inc.	Hypertension Management
Massachusetts	East Boston Neighborhood Health Center	Project Management
Massachusetts	South End Community Health Center	Chronic Disease Management
Massachusetts	South End Community Health Center	Peer Review
Nebraska	Charles Drew Health Center, Inc.	Health Education
Nebraska	Charles Drew Health Center, Inc.	School-Based Screening
New Jersey	Zufall Health Center, Inc.	Childhood Diabetes
New Jersey	Zufall Health Center, Inc.	Oral Health
New Jersey	North Hudson Community Action Corporation	Diabetes
Ohio	Health Partners of Western Ohio	Pre-Diabetes Screening
Ohio	Signature Health, Inc.	Child Court Drop Area
Oklahoma	Morton Comprehensive Health Services	Transportation Services
Oregon	Lane County	Opioid and Substance
Pennsylvania	Wayne Memorial Community Health Centers	Opioid and Substance

Source: Health Resources & Services Administration Health Center Program. Promising Practices: January 20, 2018 - June 30, 2018. https://www.healthcenterinfo.org/wp-content/uploads/2019/03/PROMISINGPRACTICES-JAN18%E2%80%93JUN18.pdf.

Growth in Staffing and Patient Groups

With the establishment of new sites and ongoing expansion of services, FQHCs have also increased their staffing to provide for these services. Excluding quality improvement and non-clinical facility staff, FQHCs employ 141,478 full-time equivalent clinical staff who engage in over 110 million visits as of 2017 (NACHC 2019b). Sixty-seven percent of these visits were to a medical provider, of which 48 percent were with a nurse practitioner, physician assistant, or certified nurse midwife. In fact, the number of non-physician providers have increased progressively since 2001. Currently, the ratio of physician to non-physician providers at FQHCs is approaching one to one (NACHC 2019b).

In general, FQHCs employ a mix of clinical staff. Other medical staff include laboratory and x-ray personnel. In addition to dentists, dental hygienists and dental therapists provide oral healthcare. FQHCs also employ ophthalmologists and optometrists. The growth of services allowing for integrated healthcare parallels the growth of health center clinical staff since 2008. Such growth has led not only to an increase in the volume of patients, but also the types of patients receiving care at FQHCs. Since 2001, FQHCs have provided care to nearly 17 million additional patients, a 164 percent increase from 2001 to 2017 (HRSA 2018a). As the number of uninsured patients seen within FQHCs decreased from 2013 to 2017, the number of Medicaid patients seen increased during this period. Interestingly, the percentage of patients with private insurance seen at FQHCs also increased, from a little over 3 percent in 2013 to almost 5 percent in 2017 (NACHC 2019b). The payer mix of patients receiving care at FQHCs may be an interesting development to monitor in future years. Given the history of FQHCs in providing cost-effective, high quality care, and their recent expansion of integrated health services enabled with current technologies, FQHCs could become a service provider of choice for private payers as well as public payers as our nation struggles with increasing costs and fragmentation of care.

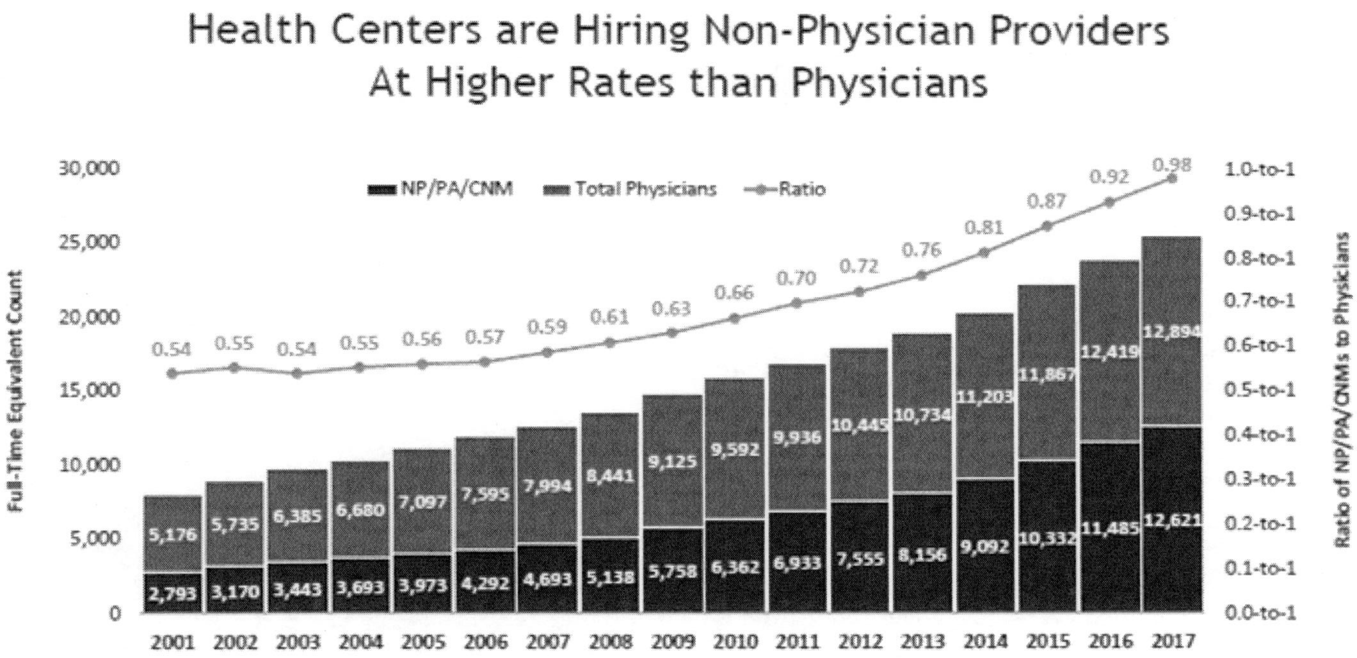

Source: Reprinted with permission from the National Association of Community Health Centers. Community Health Center Chartbook, January 2019.

Figure 7. Ratio of physician to non-physician providers.

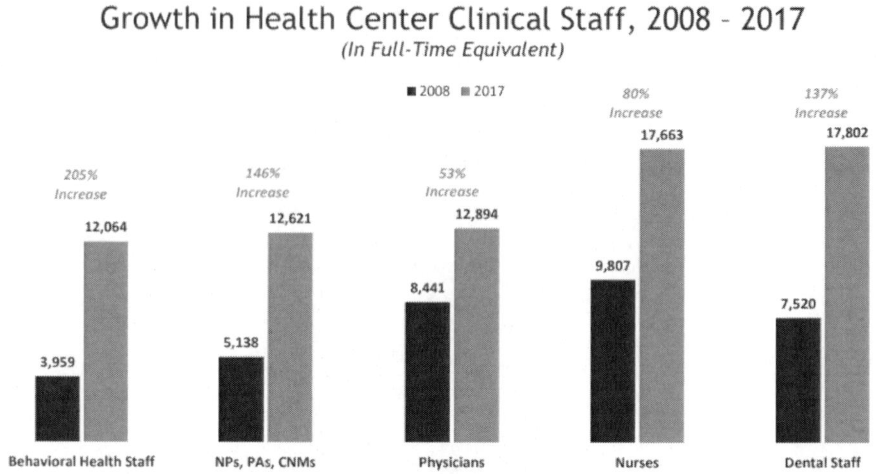

Source: Reprinted with permission from the National Association of Community Health Centers. Community Health Center Chartbook, January 2019.

Note: NP, PA, CNM stand for Nurse Practitioners, Physician Assistants, Certified Nurse Midwives, respectively. Behavioral health staff includes mental health and substance abuse.

2008-2017 Uniform Data System, Bureau of Primary Health Care, HRSA, DHHS.

Figure 8. Growth of FQHC clinical staff from 2008–2017.

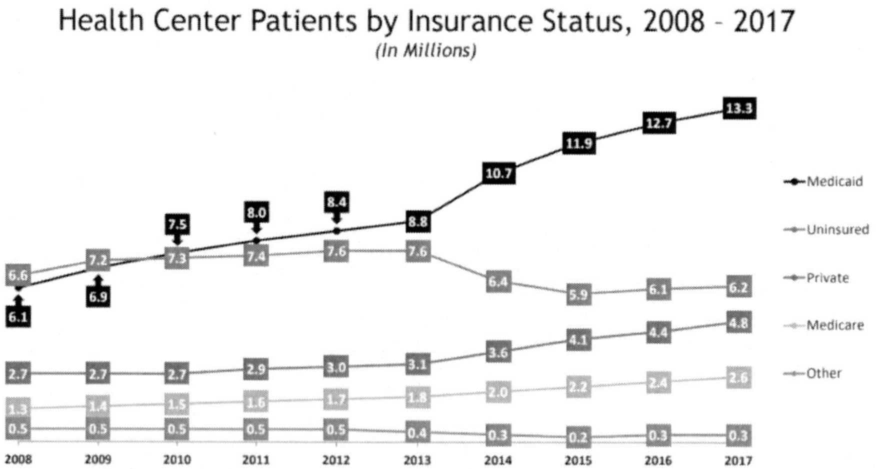

Source: Reprinted with permission from the National Association of Community Health Centers. Community Health Center Chartbook, January 2019.

2008-2017 Uniform Data System, Bureau of Primary Health Care, HRSA, DHHS.

Figure 9. Percentage of FQHC patients by insurance status from 2008-2017.

EHRs and Payment Innovation in FQHCs

EHRs as a Vehicle for Value-Based Care

In 2009, the U.S. Congress passed the Health Information Technology for Economic and Clinical Health (HITECH) Act as part of the American Recovery and Reinvestment Act (ARRA). HITECH provided the U.S. Department of Human and Health Services (HHS) with the authority to establish programs to improve healthcare quality, safety, and efficiency through the promotion of health IT, including EHR and private and secure electronic health information exchange (ARRA 2009). Federal funding provided to community health centers to invest in modernization of health IT infrastructure and participation in EHR incentive payment programs through HITECH has allowed for the widespread implementation and utilization of EHRs at FQHCs.

Since 2008, office-based physician adoption of EHRs has more than doubled nation-wide, from 42% to 86% in 2017 (ONC 2019). Of the nearly 1,400 health centers designated as FQHCs in 2017, 99% had an EHR system installed and in use (HRSA n.d.).

The use of EHRs as a vehicle to standardize care delivery, coupled with the availability of large and specific sets of healthcare data obtained from EHRs, have allowed for the development of new strategies to manage the health of patient populations while improving quality of care and working toward lowering costs of care. Such strategies are consistent with the broader trend in the healthcare industry of shifting from encounter-based or fee-for-service to value-based care in recent years.

Payment Innovation in FQHCs

Healthcare payers across the nation are investing in payment reform methodologies to combat exorbitant healthcare spending and poor health outcomes. In 2016, the federal Centers for Medicare and Medicaid Services

(CMS), the largest healthcare purchaser in the U.S., signaled monumental changes in its payment models to move away from volume-based reimbursement to payments based on value. The Medicare Access and CHIP Reauthorization Act (MACRA) of 2015 created a new framework for payment that rewards healthcare providers with higher reimbursement rates for Medicare beneficiaries for participating in value-based payments or alternative payment models (APMs) beginning in 2019 (CMS 2019a).

Medicaid payment systems are also being transformed alongside Medicare. Medicaid currently covers over 72 million enrollees and represents over $500 billion in government spending annually (CMS 2019b; CMS 2019c). Medicaid is the largest source of revenue for FQHCs, accounting for about 45 percent nationally in 2017 (KFF 2017). In fiscal year 2016, Medicaid spent $4.5 billion for health center services provided to Medicaid beneficiaries (MACPAC 2017). In calendar year 2016, nearly half of FQHC patients – 49.2 percent – had Medicaid as their primary source of insurance (HRSA 2016).

Medicaid payment reform for FQHCs is complicated by the fact that FQHCs are subject to participation in a federal prospective payment system (PPS), which dictates how FQHCs are paid for encounters. However, FQHCs are permitted to work with states to implement an APM that pays the same or more than the federal PPS. Many state Medicaid agencies, managed care organizations (MCOs), and FQHCs are adapting the federal FQHC payment rule in innovative ways to enable payment reform. An example includes fee-for-service alternatives that use value-based payment (VBP) concepts, such as global payment tied to shared savings, in which healthcare providers share in savings accrued through efficiencies, health-related services and supports, and incentives to integrate health and social services (The Commonwealth Fund 2016). Different models of collaborative Medicaid payment reform have arisen around the country. In Washington state, community health centers created their own managed care plan in 1992, called the Community Health Plan of Washington. Some FQHCs have also attempted to become network providers in commercial MCOs to maintain and expand their Medicaid and private insurance market share.

Other established and emerging payment strategies that allow for greater FQHC-VBP integration include pay-for-performance (P4P) and risk-based managed care. In the P4P model, FQHCs are financially rewarded in the form of an incentive payment outside of the PPS rate, typically from health plans, for meeting pre-defined performance benchmarks on various quality measures. While P4P programs still operate within a fee-for-service system, participating in them helps FQHCs move toward value-based care as it ties payment to outcomes driven by metrics, evidence-based best practices, and patient satisfaction, therefore aligning payment with value and quality. In risk-based capitation, FQHCs receive a prospective per member, per month (PMPM) payment to cover a range of services with payment coupled with quality metric performance. As an example, FQHCs throughout California receive sub-capitated payment from health plans or independent physician associations (IPAs), though these arrangements are not always contingent on meeting quality metrics. In evaluating VBP models applicable to FQHCs, a primary benefit of risk-based capitation is suggested to be the development of capacity within FQHCs to manage care and drive outcomes for an attributed population of patients (Howe, McGinnis, and Houston 2019).

Managed care is the predominant delivery system for Medicaid services in most states. States are increasingly focused on implementing APMs and improving quality within MCOs. Among the 39 states with comprehensive risk-based MCOs, 33 states reported that 75% or more of their Medicaid beneficiaries were enrolled in MCOs as of July 2018. Nearly all states have managed care quality initiatives in place, such as P4P or capitation withholds, and an increasing number of states (23 states in fiscal year 2018) are setting a target percentage of MCO provider payments that must be in APMs (Gifford et al. 2018).

CONCLUSION

In conclusion, the history and development of FQHCs throughout the past five decades have helped to establish them as an enduring structure in the fabric of the U.S. healthcare system today. What had been considered marginal providers that provided a safety net to the most vulnerable in society has been woven into the network of healthcare delivery within entire communities. How FQHCs develop in the next 50 years will be of great import as they incorporate the potential range of care transformation and payment innovation that is occurring at present and anticipated to ramp up in the future.

REFERENCES

AAPCHO. 2016. *Enabling Services: Gateways to Better Care*.

American Recovery and Reinvestment Act of 2009. HR 1, 111th Congress, *Congressional Record*. https://www.congress.gov/111/plaws/publ5/PLAW-111publ5.pdf.

BPHC. 2018. 2018 *UDS Reporting Manual*.

CMS. n.d. *Medicaid Managed Care Trends and Snapshots*, 2000-2013.

CMS. 2019a. *CMS' Value-Based Programs*.

CMS. 2019b. *April 2019 Medicaid & CHIP Enrollment Data Highlights*.

CMS. 2019c. *NHE Fact Sheet*.

Cunningham, P. J., and J. H. May. 2006. "A Growing Hole in the Safety Net: Physician Charity Care Declines Again." *Tracking Report* (13):1-4. Center for Studying Health System Change.

DeNavas-Walt, Carmen, Bernadette D. Proctor, and Jessica C. Smith. 2010. "*Income, Poverty, and Health Insurance Coverage in the United States: 2009*." U.S. Census Bureau, Washington, D.C.

Gifford, Kathleen, Ellis, E., Edwards, B. C., Lashbrook, A., Hinton, E., Antonisse, L., and Rudowitz, R. 2018. "*State Focus on Quality and Outcomes Amid Waiver Changes: Results from a 50-State Medicaid Budget Survey for State Fiscal Years 2018 and 2019*." Kaiser Family Foundation.

HHS. 2005. *Using Medicaid to Support Working Age Adults with Serious Mental Illnesses in the Community: A Handbook*, edited by the Department of Health and Human Services.

Howe, Greg, Tricia McGinnis, and Rob Houston. 2019. "*Accelerating Value Based Payment in California's Federally Qualified Health Centers: Options for Medicaid Health Plans*." Centers for Health Care Strategies, Inc. http://www.chcs.org/media/CA-VBP-FQHC-Report_041619.pdf.

HRSA. n.d. *Health Information Technology Capabilities and Quality Recognition*. https://bphc.hrsa.gov/uds/datacenter.aspx?q=tehr&year=2017&state=&fd=.

HRSA. 2016. *2016 Health Center Program Awardee Data*. https://bphc.hrsa.gov/uds/datacenter.aspx?q=tall&year=2016&state=&fd=.

HRSA. 2017. *Health Information Technology Capabilities and Quality Recognition: National Data*.

HRSA. 2018a. *Health Center Program: Impact and Growth*, edited by Bureau of Primary Health Care: Health Resources and Services Administration.

HRSA. 2018b. *Health Center Program Compliance Manual*. https://bphc.hrsa.gov/programrequirements/compliancemanual/index.html.

HRSA. 2018c. *Promising Practices: January 20, 2018 - June 30, 2018*. https://www.healthcenterinfo.org/wp-content/uploads/2019/03/PROMISINGPRACTICES-JAN18%E2%80%93JUN18.pdf.

HRSA. 2019a. "*Clinical Quality Improvement*." https://bphc.hrsa.gov/qualityimprovement/clinicalquality/qualityimprovement.html.

HRSA. 2019b. "*Health Center Promising Practices*." https://bphc.hrsa.gov/qualityimprovement/promising-practices/index.html.

HRSA. 2019c. *Telehealth Programs*.

IOM. 2003. *Fostering Rapid Advances in Health Care: Learning from System Demonstrations*, edited by Janet M. Corrigan, Ann Greiner and Shari M. Erickson. Washington, DC: The National Academies Press.

KFF. 2017. *Community Health Center Revenues by Payer Source*. Kaiser Family Foundation. https://www.kff.org/other/state-indicator/community-health-center-revenues-by-payer-source/?currentTimeframe=0&sortModel=%7B%22colId%22:%22Location%22,%22sort%22:%22asc%22%7D.

KFF. 2019. *Status of State Action on the Medicaid Expansion Decision*. Kaiser Family Foundation. https://www.kff.org/health-reform/state-indicator/state-activity-around-expanding-medicaid-under-the-affordable-care-act/?currentTimeframe=0&sortModel=%7B%22colId%22:%22Location%22,%22sort%22:%22asc%22%7D.

LeBron, L., and M. Lugalia-Hollon. 2014. "*Interview - Category: Volume 6 Jack Geiger, MD, M.Sc., ScD*." http://wearepublichealthproject.org/interview/jack-geiger/.

Lin, C. C., A. Dievler, C. Robbins, A. Sripipatana, M. Quinn, and S. Nair. 2018. "Telehealth In Health Centers: Key Adoption Factors, Barriers, And Opportunities." *Health Affairs (Millwood)* 37 (12):1967-1974. doi: 10.1377/hlthaff.2018.05125.

Liu, A. 2018. *Non-Emergency Medical Transportation (NEMT): Technology Solutions Landscape*.

MACPAC. 2017. *Issue Brief: Advising Congress on Medicaid and CHIP Policy. Medicaid and CHIP Payment and Access Commission*. https://www.macpac.gov/wp-content/uploads/2017/12/Medicaid-Payment-Policy-for-Federally-Qualified-Health-Centers.pdf.

MACPAC. 2019. *Medicaid Enrollment Changes Following the ACA. Medicaid and CHIP Payment and Access Commission*. https://www.macpac.gov/subtopic/medicaid-enrollment-changes-following-the-aca/.

NACHC. n.d. *The American Recovery and Reinvestment Act of 2009 FAQ*. http://www.chcanys.org/clientuploads/Your_CHCANYS/NACHC_ARRA_FAQ_2_17_09.pdf.

NACHC. 2013. *Key Health Center Data by State, 2013*. http://www.nachc.org/wp-content/uploads/2015/06/2013-Key-facts-by-state-data.pdf.

NACHC. 2015a. "*Community Health Center Past Present and Future: Building on 50 Years of Success*." National Association of Community Health Centers. http://www.nachc.org/wp-content/uploads/2016/12/NACHC_50th-Report.pdf.

NACHC. 2015b. *Key Health Center Data by State, 2015*. http://www.nachc.org/wp-content/uploads/2016/10/Key-Health-Center-Data-by-State_2015.pdf.

NACHC. 2017a. "*Community Health Center Chartbook*." http://www.nachc.org/wp-content/uploads/2017/06/Chartbook2017.pdf.

NACHC. 2017b. *Key Health Center Data by State, 2017.* http://www.nachc.org/wp-content/uploads/2018/08/Key-Health-Center-Data-by-State-2018FINAL.pdf.

NACHC. 2019a. "*America's Health Centers.*" http://www.nachc.org/wp-content/uploads/2019/07/Americas-Health-Centers-Final-8.5.19.pdf.

NACHC. 2019b. "*Community Health Center Chartbook.*" http://www.nachc.org/wp-content/uploads/2019/01/Community-Health-Center-Chartbook-FINAL-1.28.19.pdf.

Office of the National Coordinator for Health Information Technology (ONC). 2019. Office-Based Physician Electronic Health Record Adoption. *Health IT Quick-Stat* #50.

Phillips, H. 2014. "The return of the Pholela experiment: Medical history and primary health care in post-Apartheid South Africa." *Am Journal of Public Health* 104 (10):1872-6. doi: 10.2105/AJPH.2014.302136.

RCHN. n.d. (Accessed 6/15/2019). "*Health Centers Then & Now.*" RCHN Community Health Center Foundation. https://www.chcchronicles.org/histories.

RCHN. 2011. Dr. H. Jack Geiger and Dr. John Hatch on the Earliest CHCs. In *Dr. H. Jack Geiger and Dr. John Hatch on the Earliest CHCs.*

SECTION II: CHALLENGES IN MEDICAID POLICY AND POLITICS

In: Medicaid: Politics, Policy, and Key Issues ISBN: 978-1-53618-133-3
Editor: Daniel Lanford

Chapter 4

ADMINISTRATIVE BURDENS IN MEDICAID

Pamela Herd and Donald P. Moynihan*
Georgetown University, Washington, DC, US

ABSTRACT

This chapter presents the concept of administrative burdens and applies it to Medicaid. Administrative burdens are the learning, compliance, and psychological costs people experience in their interactions with the state. Administrative burdens are consequential (they have large effects on program access), distributive (they fall hardest on the most vulnerable groups), and are often a function of political preferences. These points are illustrated through case-based examples of government efforts to minimize and increase burdens for Medicaid recipients. Drawing from a case-study of Wisconsin, we examine how different administrations, both Republican and Democratic, shifted burdens onto the state and away from beneficiaries, thus facilitating access to health insurance. We conclude by detailing how work requirements limit access to Medicaid by increasing burdens. While most of those affected by the requirements are eligible for benefits, the reporting procedures involved are onerous enough that even eligible beneficiaries lose coverage.

* Corresponding Author's Email: Donald.moynihan@georgetown.edu.

Keywords: Medicaid, administrative burdens, learning costs, compliance costs, psychological costs, healthcare access

INTRODUCTION

In this chapter we describe how administrative burdens facilitate or limit access to government benefits and services. Administrative burdens are the frictions of interacting with government, or the experience of policy implementation as onerous (Burden et al. 2012). They arise via three primary mechanisms: the costs that people encounter when they (1) search for information about public services (learning costs), (2) respond to rules and requirements (compliance costs), and (3) experience stress, loss of autonomy, frustration, or stigma during the above activities in the process (psychological costs) (Herd and Moynihan 2018).[1] Table 1 provides more detail.

Table 1. The components of administrative burden

Learning costs	Time and effort expended to learn about the program or service, ascertaining eligibility status, the nature of benefits, conditions that must be satisfied, and how to gain access.
Compliance costs	Provision of information and documentation to demonstrate standing; financial costs to access services (such as fees, legal representation, travel costs); avoiding or responding to discretionary demands made by administrators.
Psychological costs	Stigma arising from applying for and participating in an unpopular program; loss of autonomy that comes from intrusive administrative supervision; frustration at dealing with learning and compliance costs, unjust or unnecessary procedures; stresses that arise from uncertainty about whether citizen can negotiate processes and compliance costs.

Adapted from Herd and Moynihan 2018.

[1] Our focus on government in the definition of administrative burdens is not intended to suggest that such frictions do not occur in the private sector. They certainly do. Rather, the terminology reflects the emergence of the concept from public administration scholarship (for an early example, see Herd, DeLeire, Harvey and Moynihan 2013). An analogous concept that has emerged more frequently is "sludge" – defined as unjustified frictions in either public or private domains (Sunstein 2019).

Cumulatively, these burdens color our experience and perception of government (Michener 2018). They are, to some degree, inevitable, but they are often deployed unnecessarily. In the first part of the chapter we make three basic claims to demonstrate why burdens are relevant to public policies. First, burdens are consequential – they make a difference in our lives. Second, administrative burdens are distributive, some groups, like the poor, are more burdened than others. Third, burdens are a function of political and administrative choices.

To illustrate these points, we trace the evolution of administrative rules and practices in Wisconsin under three different governors. This case shows how political goals shaped the bureaucratic logics that made health insurance more or less accessible to low-income groups over time. The federal government is part of this process, using its Medicaid waiver process power to block or encourage the use of burdens depending upon its political goals. To examine the federal role in more detail, we interweave into the Wisconsin case a discussion of how the Trump administration has used administrative burdens as a tool to limit the effectiveness of a policy it tried, and failed, to eliminate: the Affordable Care Act. The Trump administration has hampered the Act by making it harder to find out about, and apply for, benefits. It has also encouraged states to adopt new barriers, such as co-payments and work requirements. In the final section of the chapter we offer evidence that such work requirements reduce coverage for people who are eligible for Medicaid benefits, but struggle to overcome the new compliance costs they face.

The Relevance of Burdens to Public Policy

In this section we argue that burdens are relevant to understanding public policies for three reasons. First, burdens are consequential – in the area of social programs, they have large effects on whether people are able to gain access to the program. Estimates of Medicaid take-up of program benefits vary a good deal and are confounded by variance in take up across different states, but typically anywhere from 30 to 50 percent of eligible beneficiaries do not access Medicaid (Herd and Moynihan 2018). Among the non-elderly eligible for Medicaid and not receiving other health insurance, seven out of ten participate in the Medicaid program. Take-up rates vary significantly across states, ranging from 48 percent in Texas to 96 percent in the District of Columbia (Kenney et al. 2016). Administrative burdens play a significant role in this variance across states. Program characteristics such as presumptive eligibility improve take up among eligible participants, while burdensome asset tests reduce it (Bansak and Raphael 2006; Wolfe and Scrivner 2005).

Second, administrative burdens are distributive. They affect some groups more than others, and in doing so, tend to reinforce inequalities in society. A classic definition of politics – "who gets what, when, where, and how" – underlines its essentially distributive nature (Lasswell 1936). Administrative burdens play a central role in determining when, how, and where goods, services, and rights are distributed and, in practice, who is likely to receive them. If burdens are the product of governmental rules and procedures, this raises the question of whether they are distributive, i.e., do they help or hurt some groups more than others? If so, who are the winners and losers?

Those who are least advantaged tend to more systematically face burdens, even as they have fewer resources to manage and overcome them. In general, those who lack political power or who are seen as undeserving tend to be less successful in winning benefits from the policy process (Schneider and Ingram 1997), and the same insight applies to administrative burdens: those who are powerless or are categorized as undeserving are more likely to be targeted with burdens. Using Schneider and Ingram's framework, Medicaid beneficiaries traditionally fall into the category of "contenders" – sympathetic but with limited political power. This means they may be more subject to burdens, especially if politicians can shift the framing of beneficiaries from being contenders to "deviants" i.e., those viewed unsympathetically and with little political power. For example, the imposition of work requirements assumes that beneficiaries are so likely to shirk collective responsibilities that they must routinely document their work history.

For many Americans, especially poor Americans, the experience of government is predominantly the experience of burdens. Individuals applying for means-tested programs such as Medicaid are also likely applying for SNAP and possibly the EITC. These same individuals are also less likely to have IDs or live in neighborhoods that provide sufficient polling places, making it harder to access the right to vote. Poor women are disproportionately more likely to have unplanned pregnancies and also to need access to abortion services—which many states are making more difficult to access; shuttered clinics, due to unreasonable and unnecessary regulations, and mandatory waiting periods all increase the already high costs of getting an abortion, further ensuring it's an out-of-reach option for poor women (Herd and Moynihan 2018). In short, it's not just that policies targeted at the poor that are more burdensome; it's that the poor are more likely to experience government as routinely burdensome.

Third, burdens, like public policies themselves, are constructed via administrative and political choices, and are therefore central to policymaking and politics. In some cases, burdens may arise inadvertently, through history, accident, limited administrative capacity, or lack of foresight. In other cases, burdens serve legitimate purposes, such as program integrity. But political ideology or policy preferences also lead politicians to use burdens to make government a source of hindrance rather than help. Policymakers sometimes deliberately construct administrative burdens – as a complement or alternative to traditional forms of policymaking – to achieve their policy goals.

Fights over burdens are fights about political values, such as access or program integrity or the deservingness of recipients. The venues for these fights are often within and between bureaucracies, such as waiver applications in Medicaid, where values are converted into bureaucratic logics. Social policies offer a straightforward illustration of how burdens reflect competing values. As far back as the Nixon administration, social programs have been designed to ensure there are no mistaken payments to ineligible beneficiaries, rather than ensuring that eligible beneficiaries receive needed benefits (Brodkin 1987). Federal quality control guidelines offered states stronger incentives to avoid overpayment rather than to enroll eligible participants (Hanratty 2006). Performance evaluations of welfare programs maintain this tradition by rewarding reductions in fraud, but neglecting beneficiary take-up (Wichowsky and Moynihan 2008). During the George W. Bush administration, the White House used this technique to curb state efforts to expand Medicaid, pressuring state governments to reduce take-up error rates in Medicaid – and consequently increase administrative burden (Thompson 2012). Ultimately, the Obama administration withdrew the policy amidst threats of litigation from states over the failure of the Bush administration to follow the rulemaking process for this relatively dramatic reinterpretation of law.

To provide a granular analysis of how changes in administrative actions are linked to evolving political preferences, this next section tracks changes in administrative burdens in a single state (Wisconsin) in Medicaid over two decades, from 1995-2019.

Medicaid in Wisconsin: The Case of Political Preferences

To demonstrate the political construction of administrative burdens, we show how gubernatorial policy and ideological preferences align with attempts to alter administrative burdens. Two Governors, one Republican and one Democrat, sought to reduce burdens, albeit for different reasons, while one Republican Governor took actions that increased burdens.[2]

---

[2] This chapter is drawn heavily from collaborative work with Hope Harvey and Tom DeLeire. Data for the case study were collected from 24 interviews of state and local elected officials, their staff, administrators, and stakeholders involved in changes in the programs. Unless otherwise cited, quotes in the chapter come from these interviews. Program documentation was also analyzed to establish a timeline of changes and the nature of those changes. These included all state operations memos from 1999 to 2012 that referred to Medicaid, BadgerCare, and BadgerCare Plus eligibility procedures, all available application forms from 1999 to 2011; state eligibility handbooks; Department of Health Services internal documents archived at the Wisconsin Historical Society; state audits and external of the program (Gavin et al. 2003; Sirica 2001; Swart, Troia and Ellegard 2004); and waiver requests submitted to the federal

Governor Thompson: Making Work Pay

Governor Tommy Thompson (1987-2001) was a pioneer in the movement to tie welfare benefits to employment, passing a version of welfare reform that informed later federal policy changes. Welfare reform was a defining political issue for Thompson. He saw changes in public health insurance as inextricably tied to his policy goal of "making work pay": a means of encouraging individuals to move off welfare, as well as a basic matter of fairness, arguing that that those on public assistance should not enjoy better health insurance than the working poor.

The "making work pay" frame shaped how the Thompson administration wanted health insurance to work. Even if the program was technically welfare, those in the Governor's administration saw it differently. One said, "a simple message needs to be marketed—Medicaid and BadgerCare are health insurance for working families." Another noted: "They wanted it not to be an entitlement. They wanted it more like an employer plan, and they really wanted to cover families." That the Governor saw it as a benefit earned, rather than welfare, shaped strategies to limit the administrative burdens that participants faced.

BadgerCare (named after the state symbol) expanded Medicaid to the working poor using a mixture of funds from federal Medicaid and the Children's Health Insurance Program (CHIP). BadgerCare required a waiver from the U.S. Department of Health and Human Services. The waiver process gave the Clinton administration an opportunity to influence the design of the program. President Clinton was troubled by the estimated 1.37 million decline in Medicaid coverage for eligible children across the United States after the 1996 federal welfare reform. The Clinton administration's desire to reduce burdens was reflected in the conditions placed on Wisconsin's waiver request, including the elimination of its asset test, a simplified application form, and a mail-in application process for Medicaid and BadgerCare.

Centers for Medicare and Medicaid Services by the state and federal responses to these waiver requests.

Thompson accepted the conditions, received the waiver, and BadgerCare was implemented in July 1999, covering parents and children below 185 percent of the federal poverty level. Enrollment was restricted to those ineligible for Medicaid funds, but BadgerCare was designed to be integrated with Medicaid for applicants and participants. From the perspective of participants, there was only one program, reducing learning and compliance costs. BadgerCare participants with higher incomes had to pay premiums, but all received the same benefits as other participants in Wisconsin's relatively comprehensive Medicaid program.

Outreach efforts reduced learning and psychological costs. The Wisconsin Department of Health Services sent a direct mailing with information about BadgerCare to 18,000 families who had lost Aid to Families with Dependent Children (AFDC) or Temporary Aid to Needy Family (TANF) benefits, but who might still be eligible for BadgerCare. In Milwaukee, National School Lunch Program applications also contained an additional form for those interested in applying for Medicaid or BadgerCare, resulting in the enrollment of several hundred new families. Advertising campaigns by the state specifically targeted low-income populations with a message meant to reduce the stigma traditionally associated with public health insurance. A television commercial featured Thompson promoting the new program, a "back-to-school" initiative promoted BadgerCare and Medicaid among schoolchildren, and public health officials educated parents whose children were participating in an immunization program.

Department of Health Services operations plans instructed all direct marketing materials to be "written in prose that is easily understandable," and at no higher than a sixth-grade reading level. Department of Health Services also targeted outreach to non-English speakers.

Governor Thompson tapped into active community outreach to increase enrollment. The state benefited from the Robert Wood Johnson Foundation's "Covering Kids Expansion" project in Wisconsin, supplemented by additional funding from the Department of Health Services. Working with community organizations, healthcare providers, and translators, these outreach efforts trained hundreds of workers from schools, public health agencies, dental providers, utility companies, legal service agencies, food pantries, and homeless shelters in BadgerCare and Medicaid eligibility (Swart, Troia and Ellegard 2004).

Outreach matters in three ways. First, the provision of information can reduce the learning costs of finding out about the existence of the program and understanding eligibility. Second, the ability of outreach workers to directly provide a helping hand to individuals completing applications reduces compliance burdens and raises application completion rates. Third, if done well, outreach that utilizes non-profits and healthcare providers who are known to, and trusted by, the target population can reduce psychological costs. Outreach workers are more likely to be recognized as advocates for the individual, and applicants are likely to encounter peers also seeking to receive benefits.

To begin an application, clients had to sign and date the form in the presence of an eligibility worker. To reduce this compliance burden, workers were located at county, tribal, social, and human services departments; state agencies; local community centers, health clinics, and schools; and various outstation sites like federally qualified health centers. Out-stationed eligibility workers had laptop computers with dial-up capacity to link them to state databases. Allowing participants to sign up at out-stationing sites, rather than only welfare offices, was also meant to decrease psychological costs by making BadgerCare look more like private insurance and less like welfare.

A change in state law in 2000 reinforced the notion that the role of eligibility workers was to help clients. Case workers generally have discretion in how they interact with beneficiaries. The state law set an expectation that agency workers should prioritize access over verification. This provided a frame for how agency workers saw applicants and how they used discretion during the application process. If applicants were not able to obtain the required verification on their own, the law stated that "the agency may not deny assistance but shall proceed immediately to verify the data elements." In an internal operations memo, eligibility workers were instructed to "only verify those items required to determine eligibility and benefits," not to over-verify by "requiring excessive pieces of evidence for any one item," or "exclusively require a particular type of verification when various types are possible."

By putting multiple state medical assistance programs and funding sources under the umbrella of a single program, the state was able to streamline the marketing message and make it easier for individuals to understand if they were eligible. The efforts to increase access appear to have been successful. Between its implementation in 1999 and 2008, prior to the implementation of BadgerCare Plus, which is discussed below, enrollment in the program more than doubled from approximately 215,000 to 510,000.

Governor Doyle: All Kids

Unlike Governor Thompson, Democratic Governor Jim Doyle (2003-2011) did not view health insurance as a benefit tied to employment, but as a basic right. Doyle set a goal of 98 percent of citizens having access to health coverage. Doyle pushed his "all kids" goal through policy changes, expanding BadgerCare and consolidating it with Medicaid and Healthy Start effective February 2008, creating BadgerCare Plus. BadgerCare Plus also led to the implementation of several changes to administrative procedures in the program that were intended to reduce administrative burden for recipients and increase enrollment.

Wisconsin again needed a federal waiver to expand BadgerCare to BadgerCare Plus. Winning this waiver required negotiating with the Bush administration, which had become increasingly concerned about the growing size of CHIP and Medicaid. Under President Bush, the federal government pressured states to reduce take-up error rates in Medicaid – and consequently increase administrative burden (Thompson 2012).

In 2005 Congress required Medicaid applicants to provide citizenship documentation. Prior to this point, self-declaration of citizenship status was deemed sufficient unless the claim was questionable, in which case eligibility workers could require documentation. The Wisconsin Department of Health Services sought to buffer the impact of these requirements, creating a series of policy guidelines that gave applicants flexibility in providing information. Further, state workers were instructed to collect the information from other sources if it was possible to do so. The CHIP Reauthorization Act of 2009 maintained these verification requirements, but allowed states to create a data exchange with the Social Security Administration, which in turn reduced the need for states to seek verification from applicants.

Nevertheless, Governor Doyle pursued higher insurance coverage through a reduction of administrative barriers. According to one advocate for low-income families, the Doyle administration "was genuinely committed to coverage for kids and he gave [state employees] the green light. And then they felt they had a license to remove all the barriers they could." These efforts were encouraged by a federal environment that became friendlier to the goals of the Doyle administration after the election of President Obama in 2008, coupled with Democratic control of Congress.

The new Congress quickly passed the CHIP Reauthorization Act in 2009, which put in place a series of financial incentives to increase access. To qualify for federal bonuses, states had to increase enrollment with active outreach programs and implement features explicitly designed to reduce learning and compliance costs, such as: reducing the frequency of renewal of status requirements for children; liberalizing asset requirements; combining Medicaid and CHIP application forms; eliminating in-person interviews; providing presumptive eligibility for children; and utilizing auto- or administrative enrollment. One hundred million dollars was allocated to outreach, with the vast majority provided to state and local governments and community organizations. Error-reporting requirements passed under Bush were restructured to avoid discouraging efforts to increase take-up. These incentives aligned with initiatives that Wisconsin was already pursuing, allowing it to win bonus funds of $23,432,822 in 2010 and $24,541,778 in 2011.

In the month prior to implementation of BadgerCare Plus, the Department of Health Services carried out a one-time auto-enrollment effort of people who state data suggested were eligible. Auto-enrollment is a technique that makes use of information technology and administrative data to more efficiently capture eligible beneficiaries. For example, Massachusetts used it to enroll a pool of uninsured individuals into a state-run insurance program, allowing the state to claim the lowest uninsured rate in the country (Dorn, Hill and Hogan 2009).

The Wisconsin auto-enrollment was not initially planned, but when gearing up for the implementation of BadgerCare Plus, the Department of Health Services reviewed its administrative files and discovered a large group of individuals who were eligible for the program. This included individuals who had been eligible for the original BadgerCare program, as well as individuals those who would be eligible under the new, more generous eligibility guidelines established by BadgerCare Plus. Essentially, the state decided to enroll all citizens as long as it had credible information about their eligibility.

A total of 44,264 people were enrolled as a result of this one-time auto-enrollment (DeLeire and Friedsam 2010). Auto-enrollees looked similar to non-auto-enrollees in terms of income – indeed almost three-quarters were already income-eligible – and stayed enrolled at about the same rates as those not auto-enrolled, suggesting that they valued and needed health insurance as much as other enrollees.

BadgerCare Plus incorporated many different Family Medicaid programs under one program name and with one set of rules, making it easier for people to understand if they were eligible and reducing the need to apply for multiple programs with multiple applications. This reduced learning and compliance costs. The change was a response to the complexity that resulted from decades of adding programs on top of one another – from AFDC to Medicaid to Healthy Start to BadgerCare – "we had this very organic, but very disorganized, chaotic system," according to one state employee. Another employee noted that "we were conscious that the system that had evolved had complexity in it which we wanted to streamline. We weren't deliberately trying to make the system difficult, but as you build system and add pieces, that happens."

Program simplification made the application process easier in tangible ways. Individuals could fill out just one form to apply for multiple programs. The application did become somewhat longer, but was made user-friendly with larger font, clearer formatting, and more space for applicants' responses. Program simplification also allowed the Department of Health Services to simplify its communications with beneficiaries. By simplifying the rules and explanations, Department of Health Services made BadgerCare Plus easier for applicants and enrollees to understand, reducing learning costs.

By putting the many state medical assistance programs and funding sources under the umbrella of a single program, the state was also able to streamline the marketing message around the "all-kids" theme. This mattered in two ways. First, it communicated broad eligibility for the program, reducing learning costs that come from potential beneficiaries trying to figure out which, if any, public programs they are eligible for. Second, the marketing sought to reframe the negative conceptions of welfare, thereby reducing psychological costs. Department of Health Services administrators believed the all-kids frame allowed for broad-based marketing which made it less likely that eligible parents would be confused about their status.

Prior to the passage of BadgerCare Plus, the state sought to significantly streamline the application process via a new website named ACCESS. By making it easier for potential applicants to determine whether they were likely to be eligible and what eligibility information they needed to provide, the website reduced learning costs. By making it easier for outreach workers to enroll applicants and facilitating single applications for multiple programs, ACCESS reduced compliance costs. ACCESS supplemented, but did not replace, notices and other communication with caseworkers, and it allowed users to find the date their benefits began, the date of their next review, information on cost-sharing, reasons for denials of benefits, items needed by their caseworker (such as verification documents), contact information for their case worker, a history of changes in benefits, and answers to frequently asked questions. By 2010, the online system had become the most popular method of applying for the program. Critically, however, this was viewed as a supplement, rather than a replacement, to other application methods. Poor people and older adults—those disproportionately more likely to be applying for Medicaid—are less likely to have access to, and use, the internet.

The lessons of community outreach from BadgerCare Plus point to the importance of utilizing a diverse mix of third-parties who have robust incentives to enroll participants, while still providing strong oversight by the state. The state contracted with county income maintenance or tribal offices to process Medicaid enrollment forms and to help individuals apply for the program. While income maintenance offices continued to play a central role, the state broadened the number of agencies on the ground to help people apply for the program, even allowing them to do presumptive enrollment. Indeed, states that have increased enrollment of Medicaid beneficiaries also engaged in active outreach with partners in the non-profit and health-care community (Kaiser Commission on Medicaid and the Uninsured 2012).

The implementation of BadgerCare Plus built on the Thompson administration's practice of third-party outreach. The state relied heavily on community-based organizations to assist enrollment efforts. In these strategic partnerships, the Department of Health Services provided community organizations with monetary incentives and training, as well as bilingual and culturally-specific marketing materials. The Department of Health Services encouraged cooperation by offering a $50 "finder's fee" for organizations and providers for every person they enrolled in BadgerCare Plus. In addition, it awarded mini-grants of up to $25,000 to 32 organizations to help finance locally-based outreach efforts. Approximately 3,000 people from almost 200 community organizations and healthcare providers were trained by state officials to provide outreach about the new program and to enroll eligible individuals (Hynes and Oliver 2010). These included community groups likely to have direct interaction with eligible applicants, such as groups providing Head Start, and Women, Infant and Children programs, as well as community health clinics, schools, and faith-based groups. One county eligibility expert said of the community partnerships, "I would say that media attention has been good but I don't think that's the most significant factor, I think it's the involvement of so many external partners that has generated a level of buzz that is unprecedented" (Hynes and Oliver 2010).

Governor Walker: Increasing Burdens

The reductions in burden under the Doyle administration increased program enrollment, even among those who were previously eligible before the introduction of BadgerCare Plus (Herd et al. 2013). However, Doyle's successor, Republican Scott Walker (2011-2019), challenged the underlying assumptions of BadgerCare, and especially BadgerCare Plus. The Walker administration saw the program as too large, covering individuals who were not truly poor. By covering children up to 300 percent of the poverty line, around half of state households had become income-eligible under Doyle. The Walker administration also argued that innovations that had reduced administrative burden made the program vulnerable to "all kinds of fraud and abuse." Walker's Department of Health Services sought to reduce the size of the program, partly by using administrative procedures to limit access in the name of curbing fraud.

As one of his first acts as Governor, Walker created a Commission on Waste, Fraud, and Abuse. The commission criticized "an explosion in public assistance spending and program expansions over the last decade with no corresponding investment in program integrity," identifying the efforts of the prior administrations to reduce burden as part of the problem. The Commission argued that ex-post punishments for fraud were ineffective and called for moving the burden of proof back on the citizen at the front-end of the application process, increasing the frequency of program eligibility re-certifications, and requiring face-to-face interviews for eligibility verification when possible. The actual evidence of applicant fraud was largely anecdotal, and there was no discussion of the impact that administrative burden would have on eligible beneficiaries. This willingness to ignore the burdensome effects of proposed requirements may have been linked to Governor Walker's generally skeptical view of government-provided welfare supports and his argument that the program had grown unnecessarily large.

In a waiver application, the state proposed a series of changes that would have increased administrative burdens and beneficiary costs. For example, it proposed redefining household income to require the provision of evidence of income from all residing in the house for more than 60 days (excluding grandparents) including boyfriends, girlfriends, siblings, friends, and other relatives with no legal obligation to support the mother or child actually claiming benefits. Finally, the state sought to require verification of state residency before providing aid, having an effect similar to an identification requirement.

The Obama White House administration largely rejected Walker's proposed changes, consistent with prohibitions on states from making their ACA medical assistance "eligibility standards, methodologies, or procedures" more restrictive. Some proposed waiver changes for adult applicants were allowed. Premiums were increased, and eligibility changed. This altered administrative burden. Increases in premiums in Medicaid and CHIP, even small ones, have been shown to reduce participation, especially among those with the lowest incomes (Artiga, Ubri and Zur 2017). Recipients who failed to pay a premium were required to wait an additional six months to re-enroll. New income reporting requirements were added, with failure to verify these changes resulting in the loss of eligibility. Clients faced a new $60 processing fee to pay for their renewal in the program, which previous evidence suggests will reduce Medicaid take-up among individuals with low incomes (Wright et al. 2005).

Walker's reliance on administrative burdens to reduce access to Medicaid was made less pressing by the 2012 Supreme Court decision in National Federation of Independent Businesses (NFIB) vs. Sibelius, which gave states more discretion in determining eligibility levels than was allowed in the ACA. Rather than adding administrative burdens to restrict access to the program, states could simply alter eligibility criteria to restrict access. Governor Walker rejected new federal funding from the ACA, reducing Medicaid access to citizens above the federal poverty line. The state 2013-15 budget reduced maximum income eligibility levels for BadgerCare Plus from 200 to 100 percent of the federal poverty line for parents (approximately 97,000 parents would lose coverage) and would not expand the Medicaid program to cover childless adults above 100 percent of the FPL, leveraging NFIB vs. Sibelius to contradict the original provisions of the ACA.

A decline in health insurance coverage created a political risk for Walker in the 2014 election year. The creation of a federal health insurance marketplace through the ACA offered an opportunity to offset losses in state-provided insurance. While his predecessors had used outreach to expand BadgerCare and BadgerCare Plus, Walker now used this tool to direct Wisconsinites to the federal marketplace. Walker's Department of Health Services maintained relationships with third-parties who helped individuals gain coverage via the federal marketplace, and ACA Navigators were given support by the federal government for outreach. Walker benefited from existing networks of public and private healthcare providers, local governments, community organizations, tribal representatives, and others. These groups formed regional enrollment networks dedicated to maintaining outreach. The Milwaukee network alone involved 100 public and private organizations. The Department of Health Services disseminated Milwaukee's network as a model for other parts of the state to follow and helped to coordinate other networks.

However, other parts of the Walker administration sometimes worked at cross-purposes with the outreach goal. The Office of Consumer Insurance placed extra requirements on Navigators, increasing learning costs, and publicly stated that it believed that the costs of marketplace plans would soar in the future. While Doyle and Thompson tried to simplify branding and send positive messages about health insurance, the Office of Consumer Insurance described the federal exchange as the provider of "public assistance" products. The different actions by the Department of Health Services and the Office of Consumer Insurance reflected the paradox of Walker's own position: he was both a vocal critic of Obamacare, while also relying on it to maintain health insurance coverage for many in his state.

The election of President Trump offered Governor Walker a federal partner that shared his political views about Medicaid and his fondness for administrative burdens. Even as the Trump administration failed to repeal the Affordable Care Act, the Center for Medicare and Medicaid Services (CMS) vigorously, and effectively, employed administrative burdens to make it less effective. It largely eliminated advertising of the program during the enrollment period and slashed funding for those providing enrollment help from $63 million to $10 million. While under the Obama Administration, the Department of Health and Human Services had tried to reduce learning and psychological costs about the Affordable Care Act. New government promotional materials featured videos of people explaining how the ACA had harmed them (CBPP 2019). They also cut ACA promotional partnerships with organizations that had direct access to potential beneficiaries, such as companies whose low-wage employees might be eligible, faith-based organizations, and medical groups. Finally, HHS ended contracts with private firms that provided in-person assistance for enrollees and cut the Navigator budget by about 40 percent (CBPP 2019). The lack of outreach has increased learning costs and hurt enrollment. A Kaiser Family Foundation poll found that only one in four people who buy their own insurance knew the correct enrollment deadline. Enrollment declined by 4 percent at the end of 2018 relative to the previous year, with a 15 percent drop in first-time enrollees (Goldstein 2018). The drop in first-time enrollees bodes ill for long term enrollment trends.

While Trump's CMS declined to allow Walker's request to be the first state to drug-test Medicaid recipients, it did allow other changes, such as additional premiums of about $8 a month for those with incomes approximately between $6,000 and $12,000 a year. Another change they made were to introduce mandatory health-risk assessments, a requirement that other states have adopted with little benefit. For example, Iowa and Michigan adopted wellness programs where premium payments would be waived for healthy behaviors, such as undertaking a health risk assessment. But such programs can fall short because of the learning and compliance costs involved. A review of Michigan's program found that while many beneficiaries had undertaken a health risk assessment, most were unaware of the connection between it and reduced payments, or that such a benefit even existed, making it unlikely they would take advantage of it (Michigan Health and Human Services 2016). CMS also approved Walker's requests for work requirements, which, as we discuss below, are proving to raise significant costs in the one state in which they have been implemented.

Walker was succeeded by Democrat Tony Evers in 2019. Evers made the expansion of Medicaid an election priority, but was stymied from this goal by a Republican legislature. Further, in a post-election lame duck session, the legislature passed a law that shifted the Governor's powers to submit Medicaid waivers to the state legislature. One of Walker's last significant acts of Governor was to sign this bill, removing a tool from Evers that Walker himself enthusiastically used, as well as breaking with a tradition of legislative deference to the executive branch on Medicaid policy that went back to Thompson.

Medicaid Work Requirements: The Case of Arkansas

While Medicaid work requirements have not yet been implemented in Wisconsin (though they now have permission to do so from CMS), their use in Arkansas provides a telling example of how they dramatically increase administrative burdens. The Trump administration released an executive order on April 10, 2018 that directed agencies to deploy "work requirements when legally permissible" in means-tested social programs. But even before that order, CMS Administrator Seema Verma had already telegraphed her desire to impose work requirements into Medicaid. In late 2017, she told state policymakers: "The thought that a program designed for our most vulnerable citizens should be used as a vehicle to serve working age, able-bodied adults does not make sense…These are individuals who are physically capable of being actively engaged in their communities, whether it be through working, volunteering, going to school or obtaining job training. Let me be clear to everyone in this room, we will approve proposals that promote community engagement activities" (Pear 2017). Ten states, all led by Republican Governors, quickly sought waivers from the Trump administration to impose work requirements. The nature of the work requirements varied, though all are required to exempt people with disabilities, pregnant women, and the elderly. However, individuals exempt from these requirements will often need to document and prove those exemptions, itself a form of administrative burden.

The issue of work requirements is a fascinating example of the slippery nature of espoused political values in justifying burdens, and the role of evidence in rebutting political claims. The primary justification for work requirements is economic: to increase employment by moving people from welfare (that is, health insurance) to work. While increased labor force participation is a valid political goal, the statutory goal of Medicaid is not to increase employment, but to improve access to healthcare. The Medicaid Act seeks to enable each state "to furnish medical assistance" to individuals "whose income and resources are insufficient to meet the costs of necessary medical services" and to provide "rehabilitation and other services to help such families and individuals attain or retain capability for independence or self-care." The law specifies that waivers are only to be provided to the extent that they facilitate the objectives of the Medicaid Act.

The addition of work requirements faced legal challenges because, plaintiffs argued, CMS used the waiver process to undermine the statutory intent of Medicaid. This posed a problem for the Trump administration, so they claimed that the work requirements did not just enhance the economy, they would also improve health outcomes because those who are working tend to enjoy better health. This argument, however, ignores that many people enroll in Medicaid precisely because they are in poor health. Moreover, there is no evidence to suggest that removing health coverage, or other types of welfare, from those who are not working improves health. Instead, the opposite is closer to the truth. A randomized control trial of a Florida program that made benefits conditional on workforce participation found that participants had a 16 percent higher mortality rate 18 years later relative to a control group not subject to such conditionality (Muennig, Rosen and Wilde 2013). Another study found that welfare reform programs that emphasized quick entry into the workforce contributes to depressive symptoms among parents with pre-school age children (Morris 2008). Workfare therefore appears to worsen rather than improve health outcomes. The Trump administration also ignored heterogenous effects in the relationship between work and health. Those working in low-wage jobs are especially likely to have health problems, many of which start in childhood (see for example Marmot et al. 1991). The US labor market is shifting from jobs with stable hours to more precarious forms of employment, and low-wage jobs with uncertain schedules for Medicaid beneficiaries are also associated with psychological distress and poor sleep quality (Schneider and Harknett 2019).

A closer look at the logic behind work requirements illustrates why these burdens create costs with little gain. Almost all non-disabled working-age Medicaid-eligible individuals are already working (Silvestri, Holland and Ross 2018). This means there is not a large population of unemployed claimants ready to move into the workforce. Work requirements therefore cannot solve a problem – low labor-force participation among Medicaid beneficiaries – that does not exist. On the other hand, if most are already working, what is the problem with the requirements? To understand the effects of work requirements in Medicaid we need to properly understand them as *work-reporting requirements,* since it is the reporting part that causes people to lose healthcare.

Reporting work means documenting work activity or exemption from the requirement because of a disability, a pregnancy, or another status. For many working in informal low-income self-employed or service jobs, work documentation may not be straightforward. Work-reporting requirements assume stable work patterns. Arkansas required people to work 80 hours per month. But low-income workers in the service industry have unstable hours, where they may be called in to work for 40 hours one month and 120 hours the next (Schneider and Harknett 2019), meaning they may be locked out of the program because of the shifting commodification of work by employers. The work-reporting requirements also assume it is easy to document work, which is less likely to be the case for more informal work, or self-employed workers. Sarah and Matt Burress offer an example (Goodnough 2018). The Medicaid coverage they gained after Matt started his own lawn care business was crucial: Matt's glaucoma would have led to blindness without treatment. But the informal, irregular and seasonal nature of his work did not align well with new documentation requirements. Sarah noted, "Do his clients have to say, 'Yeah, he mowed my grass this week?' Part of it feels like they're trying to catch you, by burying people in paperwork and making it a huge inconvenience." Their case is not atypical. Bill Wagner, who managed primary care clinics in poorer Kentucky neighborhoods, had been helping people enroll in Medicaid prior to the Trump administration. With the Trump administration, "We're shifting our focus from helping people gain coverage to helping people keep it." (Goodnough 2018).

Work-reporting requirements may pose a difficulty for people because of learning costs. With any new program it takes a great deal of effort and communication to make the public aware. For example, with the creation of Social Security, the federal government undertook a huge informational campaign solely focused on communications and outreach, including an entire organization that directed promotional films (Herd and Moynihan 2018). More recent programs have not invested in the same fashion. For example, even after years of intense debate and campaigning about the Affordable Care Act, more than one-third still did not understand that it was the same policy as "Obamacare." That lack of knowledge was even higher for low-income and younger people most likely to be using the policy (Dropp and Nyhan 2017). The probability that the public will be closely attuned to *administrative changes* in an existing policy is much lower, especially if those changes are poorly advertised. People generally assume that existing policies will continue to work as they have. A qualitative study of Arkansas Medicaid recipients found that two-thirds had not heard about the change (Greene 2018):

> "First time I've ever heard anything [about it]," a 31-year old man, who had started a vocational training program the day we spoke, said. "You'd think it'd be on the news or something. I ain't seen it on the news, and I watch Channel 8 news every night." Others echoed his surprise: "I've never even heard of it" and "I can't believe I ain't heard something about it on the news." (Greene 2018).

The compliance costs of documentation create a new demand on all recipients, but will be especially intense for those with low administrative literacy. In the case of Arkansas, reporting was online-only, but 30 percent of Medicaid adults report they never use a computer, 28 percent say they do not use the internet, and 41 percent do not use email. It is unrealistic to expect that such a population will possess the technological literacy to navigate online documentation processes (Garfield, Rudowitz, Musucemi and Damico 2018).

The Kaiser Family Foundation sought to estimate the effects of work requirements on Medicaid enrollment based on existing studies that had examined the effect of reporting requirements for Medicaid and state waiver estimates of enrollment (Garfield, Rudowirz, Musumeci 2018). Across a variety of assumptions, the vast majority (between 62 and 91 percent) of those who would lose benefits would do so not because they were not satisfying the requirements, but because they would struggle with the administrative burdens involved.

Arkansas was an early adopter, the canary in the coalmine. Almost 17,000 people lost health insurance coverage in just four months. The state did not track these individuals, so it was possible that they had found insurance in the private sector with new jobs. But this proved not to be the case. An analysis in the *New England Journal of Medicine* tracked the effects on 6,000 Medicaid recipients, focusing on 30-49 year-old recipients in Arkansas, but using recipients in Kentucky, Texas and Louisiana as controls (Sommers et al. 2019). The results demonstrated that work requirements did not increase labor market participation, and those who lost insurance had largely not found new coverage.

At the same time, the results validated concerns about significant loss in Medicaid take-up because of reporting requirements. Coverage of the low-income adults surveyed declined from 70.5 percent to 63.7 percent, even though 95 percent of those who lost benefits were actually completing the required work or should have qualified for an exemption. The problem was that they could not overcome the onerous reporting processes. Learning costs played a significant role. One-third of those affected had not heard about the new requirements, and 44 percent were unsure if the requirements applied to them. Compliance costs also played a role: one-third of adult Medicaid recipients in Arkansas lack access to the internet, making the online-only reporting process a major barrier. In short, a policy justified as increasing work not only failed in that goal, but instead caused large numbers of low-income beneficiaries to lose health insurance, for which they were eligible, because of administrative burdens.

CONCLUSION

The conventional wisdom on the politics of government regulation is clear enough: conservatives seek to lift the dead hand of government from individual liberties and free enterprise, while liberals use the tools of government to correct perceived inequalities in society. This image may be accurate for economic and regulatory policies to which businesses are subject, but it is not the case for many other policies like Medicaid. Where partisans oppose a policy, or are unsympathetic to the beneficiaries, they will apply burdens as a tactic to limit access to rights or benefits. Where they support a policy, or see it as conducive to a broader political goal, they will reduce burdens.

The Wisconsin case shows not only that administrative burdens can reduce access to health insurance, but also points to concrete ways that states can reduce burdens on citizens in order to increase enrollment, using means such as auto-enrollment, simpler forms, online information and application systems, and better outreach. By contrast, the use of work requirements demonstrates how governments can put in place processes that will reduce participation in Medicaid.

The cases also illustrate the interactive nature of efforts to reduce burdens. In the Wisconsin example, an online-enrollment tool worked hand-in-hand with aggressive outreach and presumptive eligibility to capture difficult-to-reach citizens. The shifting of burdens onto the state required more government capacity, but led to reduced administrative burden for applicants and beneficiaries. In sum, if states want to maximize enrollment, they need to find ways to shift burdens away from beneficiaries and onto the state. In Arkansas, the new reporting requirements were onerous enough in their own right, but their effects were amplified by requiring beneficiaries to deal with an online-only reporting system.

Any discussion of the politics of administrative burden in an intergovernmental program must also consider the role of the federal government. Federal actors adjudicated waiver requests necessary for significant program reform, sometimes pushing Governors to further reduce burdens or blocking efforts to increase burdens. Presidents and Congress also offered financial incentives that encouraged states to impose or reduce burdens. The creation and expansion of BadgerCare occurred under federal waivers from standard rules. Federal regulators pushed Governor Thompson to reduce burden with the creation of BadgerCare (which the Thompson administration effectively implemented) and were supportive of Governor Doyle's reforms. Governor Walker found himself largely stymied to implement the changes he wanted by the Obama administration, but found gained a more willing partner with the Trump administration. Trump administration efforts to impose burdens has found support in Republican-leaning states, and some resistance in Democrat-leaning states (Nadel 2019).

The generally opaque nature of administrative burdens makes them valuable as a form of 'policymaking by other means.' Where overt changes are unpopular (such as reducing benefits), administrative burdens offer a low-profile alternative. For example, directly changing Medicaid social benefits requires legislative battles. By contrast, constructing complex, confusing, and time-consuming application procedures is a less visible form of policymaking that can effectively thwart an individual from accessing benefits, even if eligible by law. In short, burdens are one of the tactics in contemporary political battles that determine how policies are delivered.

REFERENCES

Artiga, Samantha, Petry Ubri, and Julia Zur. 2017. "The Effects of Premiums and Cost Sharing on Low-Income Populations: Updated Review of Research Findings." *Kaiser Family Foundation.* Accessed July 2, 2019. https://www.kff.org/medicaid/issue-brief/the-effects-of-premiums-and-cost-sharing-on-low-income-populations-updated-review-of-research-findings/.

Bansak, Cynthia, and Steven Raphael. 2007. "The effects of state policy design features on take-up and crowd-out rates for the state children's health insurance program." *Journal of Policy Analysis and Management* 26(1): 149-175.

Brodkin, Evelyn. 1987. "Policy Politics: If We Can't Govern, Can We Manage?" *Political Science Quarterly* 102: 571-587.

Burden, Barry C., David T. Canon, Kenneth R. Mayer, and Donald P. Moynihan. 2012. "The effect of administrative burden on bureaucratic perception of policies: Evidence from election administration." *Public Administration Review* 72: 741-751.

Center for Budget and Policy Priorities. 2019. "*Sabotage Watch*." Accessed July 1, 2019 https://www.cbpp.org/sabotage-watch-tracking-efforts-to-undermine-the-aca.

DeLeire, Thomas, and Donna Friedsam. *Enrollment, Take-Up, Exit, and Churning: Has BadgerCare Plus Improved Access to and Continuity of Coverage? Evaluation of Wisconsin's BadgerCare Plus Healthcare Coverage Program.* Madison, WI: University of Wisconsin Population Health Institute, 2010.

Dropp, Kyle and Brendan Nyhan. 2017. "One third don't know Obamacare and Affordable Care Act are the same." *New York Times* February 7th, Accessed July 1, 2019. https://www.nytimes.com/2017/02/07/upshot/one-third-dont-know-obamacare-and-affordable-care-act-are-the-same.html.

Garfield, Rachel, Robin Rudowitz, MaryBeth Musucemi and Anthony Damico. 2018. "*Implications of Work Requirement in Medicaid: What Does the Data Say*." Kaiser Family Foundation, Accessed July 1, 2019 https://www.kff.org/medicaid/issue-brief/implications-of-work-requirements-in-medicaid-what-does-the-data-say/.

Gavin, N., Nathan David West, Nancy F. Lenfestey, and Jamie Chriqui. "Evaluation of the BadgerCare Medicaid demonstration." *Report. Research Triangle Park, NC: Research Triangle Institute* (2003).

Goldstein, Amy. 2018. Last minute scramble for ACA plans seems unaffected by court rulings. December 19. *Washington Post*. Accessed July 1, 2019. https://www.washingtonpost.com/national/health-science/last-minute-scramble-for-aca-plans-undampened-by-court-ruling/2018/12/19/e1a730aa-03bc-11e9-9122-82e98f91ee6f_story.html?utm_term=.db6b82800d28.

Greene, Jessica. 2018. "*Medicaid Recipients' Early Experience With the Arkansas Medicaid Work Requirement*." Accessed July 2, 2019. https://www.healthaffairs.org/do/10.1377/hblog20180904.979085/full/.

Hanratty, Maria. 2006. "Has the Food Stamp program become more accessible? Impacts of recent changes in reporting requirements and asset eligibility limits." *Journal of Policy Analysis and Management* 25: 603-621.

Herd, Pamela and Donald P. Moynihan. 2018. *Administrative Burden: Policymaking by Other Means*. New York: Russell Sage Foundation.

Herd, Pamela, Thomas DeLeire, Hope Harvey, and Donald P. Moynihan. 2013. "Shifting Administrative Burden to the State: The Case of Medicaid Take-Up." *Public Administration Review*. 73 (s1): S69-S81.

Hynes, Emma, and Thomas Oliver. 2010. *Wisconsin's BadgerCare Plus health coverage program*. Madison, WI: University of Wisconsin Population Health Institute.

Kaiser Commission on Medicaid and the Uninsured. 2010a. *Medicaid: A Primer*. Menlo Park, CA: Kaiser Family Foundation. Available at http://www.kff.org/medicaid/upload/7334-04.pdf.

Marmot, Michael G., Stephen Stansfeld, Chandra Patel, Fiona North, Jenny Head, Ian White, Eric Brunner, Amanda Feeney, and G. Davey Smith. 1991. "Health inequalities among British civil servants: the Whitehall II study." *The Lancet* 337: 1387-1393.

Michener, Jamila. 2018. *Fragmented Democracy: Medicaid, Federalism, and Unequal Politics*. Cambridge University Press, 2018.

Michigan Health and Human Services. 2016. "*Michigan Adult Coverage Demonstration Section 1115 Annual Report*." Access June 22, 2019 https://www.medicaid.gov/Medicaid-CHIP-Program-Information/By-Topics/Waivers/1115/downloads/mi/Healthy-Michigan/mi-healthy-michigan-annual-report-DY6.pdf.

Morris, Pamela A. (2008). "Welfare program implementation and parents' depression." *Social Service Review* 82,: 579-614.

Muennig, Peter, Zohn Rosen and Elizabeth Wilde. 2013. "Welfare Programs That Target Workforce Participation May Negatively Affect Mortality." *Health Affairs*. 32: 1072–1077.

Nadel, Jesse. 2019. *How States are Combating Trump's ACA Sabotage*. August 1. Access September 3, 2019 https://www.americanprogress.org/issues/healthcare/news/2019/08/01/472615/states-combating-trumps-aca-sabotage/.

Pear, Robert. 2017. "Trump administration will support work requirements for Medicaid." *The New York Times,* November 7. Access July 1, 2019. https://www.nytimes.com/2017/11/07/us/politics/trump-work-requirements-medicaid.html.

Schneider, Anne L., and Helen M. Ingram. 1997. *Policy Design for Democracy*. Lawrence, KS: University Press of Kansas.

Schneider, Daniel, and Kristen Harknett. 2019. "Consequences of Routine Work-Schedule Instability for Worker Health and Well-Being." *American Sociological Review* 84: 82-114.

Silvestri, David M., Margaret L. Holland, and Joseph S. Ross. 2018. State-level population estimates of individuals subject to and not meeting proposed Medicaid work requirements." *JAMA internal medicine* 178: 1552-1555.

Sirica, Coimbra. 2001. "The origins and implementation of BadgerCare." *Milbank Memorial Fund*, Report.

Sommers, Benjamin, Anna L. Goldman, Robert J. Blendon, John Orav, and Arnold M. Epstein. 2019. "Medicaid Work Requirements — Results from the First Year in Arkansas." *New England Journal of Medicine.* Accessed June 19, 2019. DOI: 10.1056/NEJMsr1901772.

Sunstein, Cass R. 2019. Sludge and Ordeals. *Duke Law Journal* 68: 1843–83.

Swart, Chris, Nina Troia, and Dorothy Ellegaard. 2004. *BadgerCare Evaluation*. Wisconsin Department of Health and Family Services Office of Strategic Finance Evaluation Section.

Thompson, Frank. 2012. *Medicaid Politics: Federalism, Policy Durability and Health Reform*. Washington DC: Georgetown University Press.

Wichowsky, Amber, and Donald P. Moynihan. 2008. "Measuring how administration shapes citizenship: A policy feedback perspective on performance management." *Public Administration Review* 68: 908-920.

Wolfe, Barbara, and Scott Scrivner. 2005. "The devil may be in the details: How the characteristics of SCHIP programs affect take-up." *Journal of Policy Analysis and Management* 24(3): 499-522.

Wright, Bill J., Matthew J. Carlson, Tina Edlund, Jennifer DeVoe, Charles Gallia, and Jeanene Smith. 2005. "The impact of increased cost sharing on Medicaid enrollees." *Health Affairs* 24: 1106-1116.

In: Medicaid: Politics, Policy, and Key Issues ISBN: 978-1-53618-133-3
Editor: Daniel Lanford

Chapter 5

THE QUIET POLITICS OF MEDICAID WORK REQUIREMENTS

Philip Rocco*
Department of Political Science,
Marquette University, Milwaukee, WI, US

ABSTRACT

In 2018, the Trump administration announced that for the first time, the federal government would allow states to require individuals to work as a condition of eligibility for Medicaid. While there is modest public support for work requirements in many states, they impose significant administrative burdens on Medicaid beneficiaries and have met with strong opposition from beneficiary advocates. Such opposition may drive state officials who wish to institute work requirements to limit public input. This paper investigates the extent to which states minimized opportunities for public input in the development of Section 1115 waivers and the effect such efforts had on public participation. The results suggest that, while some states took steps to minimize public participation, the effect on participation has been mixed. States that imposed work requirements on the Medicaid expansion population alone tended to have less public

* Corresponding Author's Email: philip.rocco@marquette.edu.

participation in the public comment process compared with states that imposed work requirements on traditional Medicaid populations. This suggests that the mobilization of bias was outweighed by the mobilization of Medicaid advocates.

Keywords: Medicaid, work requirements, Section 1115, waivers, intergovernmental relations

INTRODUCTION

State governments have been an engine of change within the Medicaid program since its creation in 1965 (Thompson 2012). Under Section 1115 of the Social Security Act, the Secretary of Health and Human Services can allow states to waive certain requirements to experiment with policies that that are "likely to assist in promoting the objectives" of the Medicaid Act (42 U.S.C. 1315(a)). Beginning in the 1990s, states like Minnesota, New York, and New Jersey used waivers to expand coverage to new populations of low-income Americans and improve the quality of care (Thompson 2012). These changes have helped to transform Medicaid from "welfare medicine" into a broader and more encompassing insurance program with significant benefits for recipients (Ajkay et al. 2018; Ali et al. 2016; Wen et al. 2017).

While federal and state officials have historically used Section 1115 waivers to create new eligibility restrictions in programs such as Temporary Assistance to Needy Families and the Supplemental Nutritional Assistance Program, the same cannot be said for Medicaid (Hahn et al. 2017). Because Section 1115 waivers are supposed to promote the objectives of the original Medicaid law, federal officials have been reluctant to approve state modifications that would deny potential beneficiaries access to medical care (Somodevilla et al. 2019).

Yet beginning in 2018, the Trump administration advised states that it would approve Section 1115 waivers that required individuals to participate in "employment-related activities," including paid employment or job training as well as unpaid volunteer work or community service (CMS 2018). As of 2019, 16 states submitted such waiver applications to the

Centers for Medicare and Medicaid Services (CMS) for review (see Table 1). Waiver policies vary from state ot state. For example, Wisconsin's waiver would penalize enrollees who fail to come into compliance with requirements after 48 months. In Utah, penalties for noncompliance kick in after three months. In states like South Dakota and Alabama, waiver proposals suggest that penalties will kick in after 90 days. Activities qualifying as work range from paid employment to education and volunteering, yet in many state it is not transparent how these requirements will be enforced. Further, waiver exemptions vary. In most states, pregnant women are exempt, and in several states (e.g., Arizona, Virginia), post-partum women are as well (NASHP 2019). Typically, waivers require Medicaid beneficiaries, as a condition of eligibility, to certify 20 hours per week (or 80 hours per month) of participation in paid work or other activities. Ten of these waivers have received CMS approval. Of these, one is currently being implemented, and three have been set aside by federal courts (KFF 2019).

Work requirements impose barriers to accessing social services (Herd and Moynihan 2019). For example, Arkansas' implementation of Medicaid work requirements within Medicaid resulted in statistically significant losses in insurance coverage with no significant change in the levels of employment. Specifically, coverage among the low-income Arkansas adult population ages 30–49 fell from 70.5 percent in 2016 to 63.7 percent following the implementation of work requirements (Sommers et al. 2019). While both CMS guidance and state applications claim that work-requirements will improve health outcomes, higher earnings, and enhanced fiscal stability, little evidence exists—including in the studies these documents cite—to support these claims (Musumeci and Zur 2017; MACPAC 2017; Antonisse and Garfield 2018; Sommers et al. 2019). Perhaps because of these findings, states and the federal government have begun to argue before the courts that the purpose of work-requirements is not to improve health, but to promote Medicaid programs' fiscal sustainability. Thus far, federal courts have not found this argument persuasive (Rosenbaum and Somodevilla 2019).

Table 1. Characteristics of Medicaid Section 1115 waivers containing work requirements

Location	Waiver Status	Traditional Population Affected?	Expansion Population Affected?	Hours Required
Alabama	Pending	Yes	No exp	35/week**
Arizona	Approved	No	Yes	80/month
Arkansas	Blocked by court	No	Yes	80/month
Indiana	Implemented	Yes	Yes	Ramps up to 20/week
Kentucky	Blocked by court	Yes	Yes	80/month
Michigan	Approved	No	Yes	80/month
Mississippi	Pending	Yes	No exp	20/week
New Hampshire	Blocked by court	No	Yes	100/month
Ohio	Approved	No	Yes	80/month
Oklahoma	Pending	Yes	No exp	Ramps up to 20/week
South Carolina	Approved	Yes	No exp	80/month (quarterly average)
South Dakota	Pending	Yes*	No exp	80/month (or monthly milestones)
Tennessee	Pending	Yes	No exp	20/week average
Utah	Approved	Yes	Yes	No hour requirement***
Virginia	Pending	Yes	Yes	Ramps up to 80/month
Wisconsin	Approved	Yes	No exp	80/month

*Limited to two counties.

**20/week for parents or caretakers with a child under age 6).

***Specified job search/training activities required unless working 30/week.

Source: Adapted by author from Kaiser Family Foundation (2019).

Despite recent rulings against work requirements, state governments around the country have continued to submit them, and CMS has continued to approve them. In doing so, they have faced both political opportunities and constraints. On the one hand, opinion polls suggest that a majority of Americans support allowing states to impose work requirements on non-disabled adults (Kirzinger et al. 2017). Yet at the same time, a plurality of Americans believe that states are pursuing work requirements only to limit the number of people on the program (Kirzinger et al. 2018). Moreover, there is strong opposition to work requirements among Medicaid recipients, patient advocates, medical professionals, and other organized groups (Jarlenski et al. 2017). Anecdotal evidence suggests that—when these groups are highly mobilized—they can slow down or even halt states formulation of Medicaid work-requirements (Willard and Gomez 2018).

For opponents of work requirements, administrative procedures created by the Affordable Care Act (ACA) offer one important leverage point. Under the ACA, state governments must publish and circulate notices explaining the goals of their waivers and their potential effects on enrollment. Additionally, states must allow for a 30-day comment period, after which they must respond to comments in writing. Federal officials are required to hold a similar comment period and must also respond to comments. There is some evidence that these new requirements have generated greater participation under Section 1115. In a survey of Medicaid waivers proposed between 2012 and 2015, Jarlenski et al. (2017) identify a surprisingly high level of quality citizen participation in these processes.

The foregoing evidence suggests that states developing Medicaid work requirements have strong incentives to engage in the "mobilization of bias," manipulating institutional procedures or rhetorical frames to prevent opponents of work requirements from expanding the scope of conflict (Schattschneider 1956; Bachrach and Baratz 1962; Crenson 1971). To be sure, a certain level of participatory bias is baked into decisions about work requirements. Technically complex regulatory decisions do not typically invite wide citizen participation (Yackee and Yackee 2006; Golden 1998). Means-tested social policies can also reinforce social ascriptions that delimit political incorporation (Schneider and Ingram 1993; Michener 2018). Even so, as Herd and Moynihan (2019) suggest, policymakers have strong incentives to limit public scrutiny of efforts to create new barriers to accessing these programs.

This paper examines the extent to which state officials have manipulated the process of developing Medicaid work requirements in ways that may limit broad participation in the policy process. To this end, I analyzed actions taken by 16 states in the development of Medicaid waivers. I examined the process states used to develop general policy on Medicaid work requirements, the amount and quality of information states provided to the public about the effects of work requirements, the procedures states used to invite public comment, and the extent to which states responded to public comments. The results suggest that, while states have taken steps to minimize public participation, the effect of these actions on the scope of conflict has been mixed. States that imposed work requirements on the Medicaid expansion population alone tended to have less public participation in the public comment process compared with states that imposed work requirements on traditional Medicaid populations. In the latter cases, it appears that the mobilization of bias was outweighed by the mobilization of Medicaid advocates.

SECTION 1115 WAIVERS: THE POLITICS OF PARTICIPATION

Intergovernmental programs—jointly administered and financed by the federal and state governments—have been a hallmark of American social policy since the early twentieth century. Yet the number and complexity of intergovernmental relationships has long posed challenges for citizen participation in the policymaking process. As early as 1979, the US Advisory Commission on Intergovernmental Relations observed that participatory opportunities in intergovernmental programs failed to engage citizens. Not only were these opportunities provided only at later stages of the decision process (a hearing immediately prior to the finalization of a decision), they were also largely informal and poorly advertised to affected parties (ACIR 1979).

Within Medicaid, there have long been concerns that citizens lacked meaningful opportunities to influence the design of Section 1115 waivers (Grogan and Gusmano 2007). In response to these and other concerns, Congress made several changes to Section 1115 waivers when it passed the Patient Protection and Affordable Care Act (ACA). Specifically, the ACA required that proposed demonstration projects go through notice-and-comment processes at both the state and federal levels that were "sufficient to ensure a meaningful level of public input" (42 USC 1315(d)(2)). Additionally, the ACA required states to make public specific details of their proposed demonstrations, including "expected State and Federal costs and coverage projections" ((42 USC 1315(d)(2)).

In 2012, CMS issued regulations requiring states to hold a 30-day notice-and-comment period prior to submitting demonstration applications or applications to extend existing demonstration projects (42 CFR 431.408). States were required to publish a notice that included information about a variety of features in demonstration programs, including the expected increase and decrease in enrollment and expenditures and hypotheses to be tested in the evaluation. States were also required to publish an abbreviated public notice, either in their state's register/regulatory bulletin or in large-circulation newspapers in all cities with populations over 100,000. Notice processes also had to include at least two hearings and tribal consultation. Finally, states had to respond to comments in writing when submitting applications to CMS. CMS, in turn, was to hold a second 30-day comment period and respond to comments in writing in considering the approval of demonstration projects (42 CFR 431.416).

These new requirements were a significant departure from the pre-ACA status quo. Indeed, as Jarlenski et al. (2017) show, they opened up opportunities for participation in the Medicaid waiver process, not only among organized stakeholders but among low-income participants in the Medicaid program. Nevertheless, the regulations contain ambiguities that enable policy conversion, or the strategic redeployment of rules to pursue alternative policy goals (Mahoney and Thelen 2010). A 2019 report by the Government Accountability Office (GAO) suggested that, among other things, CMS inconsistently applied transparency requirements in approving states' initial waiver applications. State public notice processes deviated from rules requiring information on how waivers would affect coverage and enrollment. Moreover, both CMS and state governments provided inconsistent or inadequate responses to comments raised during the public-notice process. These findings raise important questions about whether states are staking steps to limit public participation in the development of Section 1115 waivers when these programs have adverse consequences for Medicaid beneficiaries. Unpacking the process by which states developed work-requirements waivers can help us gain purchase on this question.

Data and Methods

To examine variation in the development of Medicaid Section 1115 waivers containing work requirements, I first identified all states where such waivers are pending or have been approved by the federal government (see Table 1). I collected each state's initial application, as well as any applications for a waiver amendment (see Appendix A for a list of application documents). I excluded applications for waiver extensions from the list. Drawing on data from these applications, I examined several types of evidence concerning state efforts to expand or minimize conflict over work requirements.

First, I collected data on the process by which states took up the issue of work requirements. The process of initiating intergovernmental policies can have a significant impact on whether they become open to political contestation (Beland et al. 2016; Rocco et al. 2018). I collected several pieces of data on aspects of state public-notice processes that may have contributed to (or detracted from) waiver salience. Given that work-requirements are likely to result in disenrollment from Medicaid, I noted whether states' full-length and abbreviated public notices included projections of how waivers would impact future enrollment, as required by federal regulations (42 CFR 431.408). I collected similar data on a comparison set of public notices for waivers that did not include work requirements (for a list of these waivers see Appendix B).

Federal regulations also give states a choice about how to disseminate information about proposed Section 1115 waivers. I thus considered whether states chose to publish the notices in newspapers and compared this to the number of cities with population over 100,000 and at least one daily newspaper. For states that opted to publish notices via the state register or regulatory bulletin, I additionally collected all stories regarding the waiver during the notice and comment period in the paper with the largest in-state circulation. Similarly, I collected data on public hearings held by the state in conjunction with the waiver. Federal regulations require states to conduct two hearings within the 30-day comment window, but do not specify where these hearings are to take place geographically. I thus noted whether the state held at least one hearing in the capital city and one hearing in the largest city in the state (if not also the capital city).

Beyond the initiation and public-notice processes, the design of waiver provisions may also have a significant effect on waiver salience. As Table 1 shows, 11 of 16 waivers in the data set imposed work requirements on traditional Medicaid populations, at or below 100 percent of the federal poverty level (FPL). Waivers imposing work requirements on the traditional Medicaid population may (perhaps unintentionally) have generated a greater level of salience than those focused exclusively on the expansion population. Poverty and patient advocacy organizations may have been more likely to mobilize around these provisions, since they jeopardized benefits for large existing client population rather than limiting benefits enjoyed by new (or in some cases, prospective) beneficiaries.

To examine whether these elements of state waivers had effects on participation at a sufficiently early stage of the process, I collected data on the volume of comments collected in the state comment process. This comment process occurs prior to the state's submission of the waiver application to the federal government and states must respond to these comments in writing as part of their submission package. I also collected data on the federal comment process in all states where that process had concluded by the time of analysis. This left only one state out of the analysis (South Carolina).

RESULTS

Notifying the Public

A great deal of variation exists in how states interpreted and implemented federal public notice requirements. As the top panel of Table 2 shows, 9 of the 17 applications surveyed (53%) ignored the federal requirement to include projections about waivers' enrollment effects in the full-length public notice. While not required, only one state (Ohio) included enrollment projections in both the full-length and abbreviated public notices. Among those states that included enrollment projections in their full-length public notices, one state (Tennessee) suggested enrollment effects would be "negligible" but failed to provide information on enrollment effects, suggesting that it would not be "possible to reliably project the magnitude of this decrease in enrollment at this time" (TennCare 2018, 5). No such information was provided in Tennessee's abbreviated notices (see Figure 1). Failure to include enrollment projections appears to be distinctive to work-requirements applications. As the bottom panel of Table 2 shows, in a random sample of ten Section 1115 waiver applications that do not include work requirements, only three (30%) failed to provide enrollment projections.

Table 2. Process of initiating Medicaid work-requirements waivers

State	Initiated through
Alabama	Executive-Branch Action
Arizona	Legislation
Arkansas	Legislation
Indiana	Executive-Branch Action
Kentucky	Executive-Branch Action
Michigan	Legislation
Mississippi	Executive-Branch Action
New Hampshire	State Budget
Ohio	State Budget
Oklahoma	Legislation
South Carolina	Executive-Branch Action
South Dakota	Executive-Branch Action
Tennessee	Legislation
Utah (2017)	Executive-Branch Action
Utah (2018)	Legislation
Virginia	State Budget
Wisconsin	State Budget

Source: Author's analysis of Medicaid Section 1115 waiver applications.

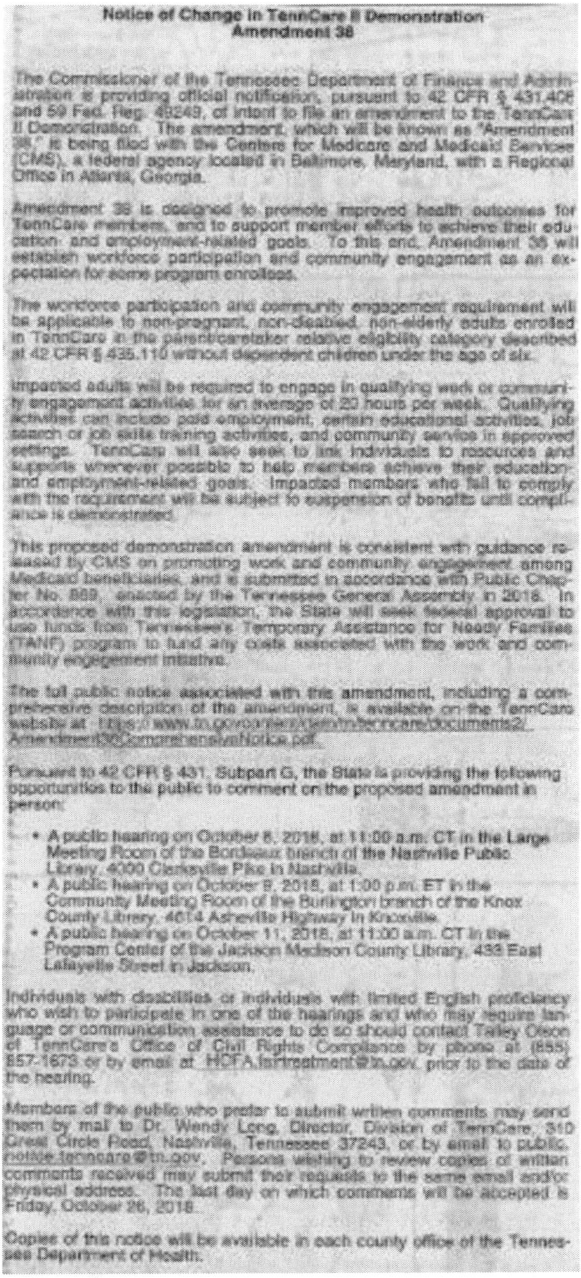

Notice of Change in TennCare II Demonstration
Amendment 38

The Commissioner of the Tennessee Department of Finance and Administration is providing official notification, pursuant to 42 CFR § 431.408 and 59 Fed. Reg. 49249, of intent to file an amendment to the TennCare II Demonstration. The amendment, which will be known as "Amendment 38," is being filed with the Centers for Medicare and Medicaid Services (CMS), a federal agency located in Baltimore, Maryland, with a Regional Office in Atlanta, Georgia.

Amendment 38 is designed to promote improved health outcomes for TennCare members, and to support member efforts to achieve their education- and employment-related goals. To this end, Amendment 38 will establish workforce participation and community engagement as an expectation for some program enrollees.

The workforce participation and community engagement requirement will be applicable to non-pregnant, non-disabled, non-elderly adults enrolled in TennCare in the parent/caretaker relative eligibility category described at 42 CFR § 435.110 without dependent children under the age of six.

Impacted adults will be required to engage in qualifying work or community engagement activities for an average of 20 hours per week. Qualifying activities can include paid employment, certain educational activities, job search or job skills training activities, and community service in approved settings. TennCare will also seek to link individuals to resources and supports whenever possible to help members achieve their education- and employment-related goals. Impacted members who fail to comply with the requirement will be subject to suspension of benefits until compliance is demonstrated.

This proposed demonstration amendment is consistent with guidance released by CMS on promoting work and community engagement among Medicaid beneficiaries, and is submitted in accordance with Public Chapter No. 869, enacted by the Tennessee General Assembly in 2018. In accordance with this legislation, the State will seek federal approval to use funds from Tennessee's Temporary Assistance for Needy Families (TANF) program to fund any costs associated with the work and community engagement initiative.

The full public notice associated with this amendment, including a comprehensive description of the amendment, is available on the TennCare website at https://www.tn.gov/content/dam/tn/tenncare/documents2/Amendment38ComprehensiveNotice.pdf.

Pursuant to 42 CFR § 431, Subpart G, the State is providing the following opportunities to the public to comment on the proposed amendment in person:

- A public hearing on October 8, 2018, at 11:00 a.m. CT in the Large Meeting Room of the Bordeaux branch of the Nashville Public Library, 4000 Clarksville Pike in Nashville.
- A public hearing on October 9, 2018, at 1:00 p.m. ET in the Community Meeting Room of the Burlington branch of the Knox County Library, 4614 Asheville Highway in Knoxville.
- A public hearing on October 11, 2018, at 11:00 a.m. CT in the Program Center of the Jackson Madison County Library, 433 East Lafayette Street in Jackson.

Individuals with disabilities or individuals with limited English proficiency who wish to participate in one of the hearings and who may require language or communication assistance to do so should contact Talley Olson of TennCare's Office of Civil Rights Compliance by phone at (855) 857-1673 or by email at HCFA.fairtreatment@tn.gov, prior to the date of the hearing.

Members of the public who prefer to submit written comments may send them by mail to Dr. Wendy Long, Director, Division of TennCare, 310 Great Circle Road, Nashville, Tennessee 37243, or by email to public.notice.tenncare@tn.gov. Persons wishing to review copies of written comments received may submit their requests to the same email and/or physical address. The last day on which comments will be accepted is Friday, October 26, 2018.

Copies of this notice will be available in each county office of the Tennessee Department of Health.

Source: TennCare (2018).

Figure 1. Example of Abbreviated Public Notice (Tennessee).

Table 3. Description of enrollment impact in state public notices

(a) Work Requirements Waivers

State	Enrollment impact mentioned in state notices?
Alabama	Full-length only
Arizona	No
Arkansas	No
Indiana	Full-length only
Kentucky	Full-length only
Michigan	No
Mississippi	Full-length only
New Hampshire	No
Ohio	Yes
Oklahoma	No
South Carolina	Full-length only
South Dakota	No
Tennessee	No*
Utah (2017)	No
Utah (2018)	No
Virginia	Full-length only
Wisconsin	Full-length only

*Notice states that enrollment impact will be negligible, but fails to provide estimate.
Source: Author's analysis of Medicaid Section 1115 waiver applications (See Appendix A for list).

(b) Comparison Group: 1115 Waivers without Work Requirements

State (Year)	Demonstration	Enrollment impact mentioned in state notices?
Alaska (2018)	Behavioral Health Demonstration Application	Full-length only
Louisiana (2017)	Healthy Louisiana OUD/SUD Demonstration	No
Iowa (2013)	Wellness Plan	Full-length only
Rhode Island (2015)	Comprehensive Demonstration Extension	Full-length only
Massachusetts (2016)	Mass Health Extension	Full-length only
North Carolina (2017)	Medicaid Reform Demonstration	Full-length only
Mississippi (2017)	Family Planning Waiver Extension	Full-length only
New Mexico (2017)	Centennial Care 2.0	Full-length only
Washington (2015)	Medicaid Transformation Project	No
Georgia (2014)	Family Planning Demonstration Extension	No

Source: Author's analysis of Medicaid Section 1115 waiver applications (see Appendix B for list).

Under federal regulations, states can publish notices either in their register or regulatory bulletin, or in newspapers with wide circulation in cities with populations of 100,000 or more. As Table 3 shows, public notices for 13 of 17 waivers were published in newspapers, while four states provided information only in their state register or on public state websites. States also varied in the extent to which they leveraged newspapers to disseminate information. Alabama, for example, published notices about its proposed waiver in four of its five large cities with large-circulation newspapers. By contrast, while Arizona contains six cities with populations over 100,000 and a large-circulation newspaper, Arizona only published notices in the *Arizona Republic*.

Five applications in the data set indicated that states provided newspaper notices but did not provide affidavits of publication or specific information about which papers were notified. In these states, news coverage of the waivers varied substantially. Table 4 presents the number of stories about each waiver published in the state's most widely circulated newspaper in the thirty-day comment window. In both Kentucky and Mississippi, coverage of the waiver was more substantial. During Kentucky's comment window, the Louisville *Courier Journal* published 12 stories on the state's waiver. The Jackson *Clarion-Ledger* published five stories on Mississippi's waiver. By contrast, news coverage of Section 1115 waivers in Michigan, South Carolina, and Utah was sparse.

All states in the data set complied with federal requirements to hold at least two public hearings during the 30-day comment period (see Table 5). Seven of these states held more hearings than required. All but three states (Alabama, Kentucky, and Virginia) held at least one hearing in the state's most populous city. And all but one state (Wisconsin) held at least one hearing in the state's capital city. To be sure, the extent of public participation in these hearings also varied. Mississippi, for example, received a total of four comments across the two public hearings it held in the fall of 2017 (Mississippi Division of Medicaid 2018). Combined attendance at hearings in South Dakota was 32 (South Dakota Division of Social Services 2018).

Table 4. Notice publication method

State	Method	Number of Newspaper Notices	Cities with pop. >100K and newspaper
Alabama	Newspaper	4	5
Arizona	Newspaper	1	6
Arkansas	Newspaper	1	1
Indiana	Register	0	4
Kentucky	Newspaper	n.a.	2
Michigan	Newspaper	n.a.	6
Mississippi	Newspaper	n.a.	1
New Hampshire	Newspaper	1	1
Ohio	Register	0	6
Oklahoma	Newspaper	6	4
South Carolina	Newspaper	n.a.	2
South Dakota	Register	0	1
Tennessee	Newspaper	8	6
Utah (2017)	Newspaper	n.a.	3
Utah (2018)	Newspaper	1	3
Virginia	Register	0	4
Wisconsin	Newspaper	3	4

Register = primary place of notice publication was state register or regulatory bulletin.
n.a. = No data available on number of newspaper publications.

Table 5. News coverage of Medicaid waiver during 30-day comment window in largest newspaper in 5 states

State	Largest newspaper (by circulation)	Waiver Stories during 30-Day Comment Window
Kentucky	Courier Journal	12
South Carolina	Post and Courier	1
Utah (2017)	Deseret News	1
Michigan	Detroit Free Press	0
Mississippi	The Clarion-Ledger	5

Source: Author's analysis.

Evaluating Public Participation

The volume of public comments on Medicaid work-requirements waivers varied widely, both at the state and federal level. As the top panel of Figure 2 shows, the number of state-level comments ranged from 11 in Mississippi to 1,832 in Virginia. States received 566 comments on average, with a standard deviation of 583. A similar pattern can be found in the federal-level comments (see bottom panel of Figure 2). At the low end, CMS received 17 comments on Arkansas' waiver. At the high end, the number of comments on Tennessee's waiver exceeded 13,000. There was a weak negative correlation between the number of comments received at the federal and state level ($r = -0.05$). There was a positive correlation between the logged number of enrollees and comments at the state level ($r = .50$) and federal level ($r = .24$).

Table 6 presents the results of negative binomial regression analyses of the number of state-level comments. The first column presents the results of a reduced model which includes variables associated with a state's process for creating the waiver, including indicators of whether states' notices mentioned enrollment effects of the waiver, whether states published notices in local newspapers, and whether states held more than the required number of hearings.[1] The second model includes an indicator of whether the waiver's work requirements applied to the traditional Medicaid population (i.e., below 100 percent FPL). The third model includes all of these variables. Each model also controls for the logged number of Medicaid enrollees in each state. In both the reduced and full models, variables associated with states' public-notice processes appeared to have no statistically significant effect on the number of comments a state received. By contrast, waivers imposing work requirements on the traditional Medicaid population had a positive and statistically significant relationship with the number of comments a state received (in the full model, $b = 1.55$; $p < .05$).

The results at the federal level were generally similar to those at the state level (see Table 7). In both the reduced and full models, waivers imposing work requirements on the traditional Medicaid population were positively and significantly associated with the number of comments (in the full model, $b = 2.22$, $p < .001$). States which held more than the required number of

[1] Further analysis revealed that there were no statistically significant correlations between any of these process variables.

hearings also invited a significantly higher number of comments at the federal level (in the full model, $b = 1.58$, $p < .01$). States which published newspaper notices also had a significantly higher number of federal-level comments (in the full model, $b = 1.43$, $p < .05$).

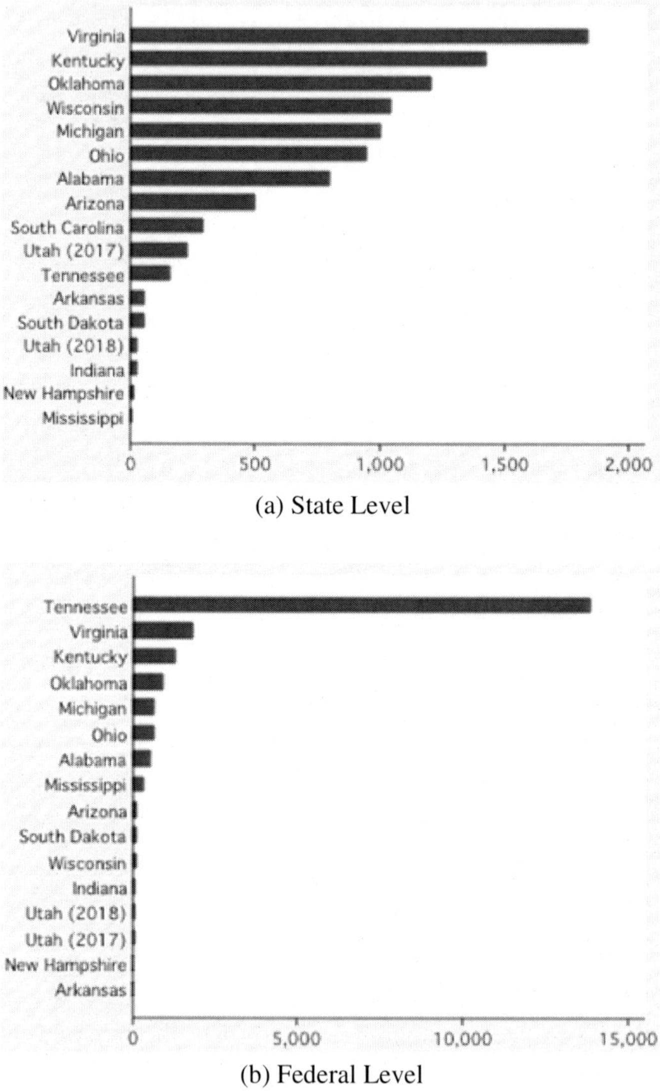

Figure 2. Comment volume on Medicaid work-requirements waivers.

Table 6. Public hearings concerning Medicaid waivers

State	N Public Hearings	Hearing in capital city?	Hearing in most populous city?
Alabama	2	Yes	No
Arizona	4	Yes	Yes (same as capital city)
Arkansas	2	Yes	Yes (same as capital city)
Indiana	2	Yes	Yes (same as capital city)
Kentucky	3	Yes	No
Michigan	3	Yes	Yes
Mississippi	2	Yes	Yes (same as capital city)
New Hampshire	3	Yes	Yes
Ohio	2	Yes	Yes (same as capital city)
Oklahoma	2	Yes	Yes (same as capital city)
South Carolina	6	Yes	Yes (same as capital city)
South Dakota	2	Yes	Yes (same as capital city)
Tennessee	3	Yes	Yes (same as capital city)
Utah (2017)	2	Yes	Yes (same as capital city)
Utah (2018)	2	Yes	Yes (same as capital city)
Virginia	4	Yes	No*
Wisconsin	2	No	Yes

*Hearing in Virginia Beach cancelled due to weather.

Source: Author's analysis of Medicaid Section 1115 waiver applications (See Appendix A for list).

Table 7. Negative binomial regression analysis of state-level comments in work requirements

Variable	Process	Population	Full Model
Executive-Branch Initiated	0.06 (.98)	--	0.12 (.69)
Enrollment Effects Mentioned? (0,1)	0.23 (1.06)	--	–0.65 (.84)
Newspaper Notice (0,1)	–0.21 (.94)	--	–0.54 (.70)
>2 Hearings (0,1)	–0.01 (.65)	--	0.28 (.54)
Traditional Medicaid Population (0,1)	--	1.33 (.58)*	1.68 (.69)*
Enrollment (Ln.)	1.10 (.75)	1.41 (.29)***	1.62 (.46)***
Log likelihood	–119.55	–117.70	–117.18
Alpha	1.13	0.95	0.91
N	17	17	17

+p < .10; *p < .05; **p < .01; ***p < .001.

Discussion

This study aimed to examine, first, the extent to which states engage in the "mobilization of bias" with respect to the development of Medicaid work-requirements waivers, and, second, the effect of this activity on public participation in the public-notice process for Section 1115 waivers created by the ACA. The results suggest a mixed picture. States have taken steps to limit public awareness of work requirements and their effects. Yet the effects of efforts to undermine participation in the public-notice process are unclear. The evidence presented here suggests that the design of the waivers themselves may have had a more substantial impact on the level of public participation during federal and state notice-and-comment periods.

Consistent with Herd and Moynihan (2019), states appear to develop policy on Medicaid work requirements through a series of low-salience political processes. Less than half the work-requirement applications surveyed were the product of standalone legislation. The development of these waivers tended to emerge from executive-branch action or omnibus state budget legislation. Thus opportunities for public participation prior to the development of state applications tend to be limited.

Once states have prepared their applications, their interpretation of federal requirements for public notice vary substantially. Consistent with the GAO's (2019) findings, the data here suggest that states' public notices on work-requirement waivers do not provide all of the information required by federal regulations. Furthermore, public notices on work-requirement waivers are more likely to lack key information about the waivers' enrollment effects when compared to a random sample of waiver applications without work requirements. Most states published notices about their waivers in newspapers, yet several states failed to publish notices in state newspapers with large circulations. Similarly, while over half the states surveyed held more than the required number of public hearings, a small number of states failed to hold hearings in large cities or the capital city.

If states' implementations of public-notice requirements had an effect on public participation, the analysis presented here does not pick it up. Negative binomial regression analyses reveal that state processes of waiver initiation, reporting of enrollment effects, and circulation of notices via newspaper had no statistically significant effects on the number of comments at the state and federal level. Holding additional public hearings had a positive and statistically significant effect on comments at the federal level only. By contrast, the design of state waivers—specifically with respect to the population covered by work requirements—had a more consistent effect on participation. All else equal, waivers that applied to traditional Medicaid populations (i.e., individuals with income below 100 percent FPL) invited a significantly larger share of public comments. This was true both at the federal and state level across several model specifications.

These findings may suggest national interest-group mobilization on work requirements blunted state efforts to conceal information about the effects of these policies and to limit participation in the public-notice process (Jarlenski et al. 2017; Keller and Packel 2014). While states effectively limited participation at the policy development stage (prior to the release of applications), interest groups routinely produced data—both in comment letters and in public reports—suggesting that work requirements would have substantial effects on Medicaid enrollment (Oklahoma Health Care Authority 2018, 144–146). Anecdotal evidence from multiple states' public notice processes reveals the mobilization of national provider and patient organizations against work requirements, including the American Academy of Family Physicians, the American Academy of Pediatrics, the American Heart Association, the Arthritis Foundation, the Cystic Fibrosis Foundation, and the American Cancer Society's Cancer Action Network. Not only did these organizations submit their own official comment letters, they coordinated the submission of form letters from numerous patient or provider-members (see, e.g., Michigan Department of Health and Human Services 2018, 2070–2333). To be sure, some of these organizations focused their energy on requesting exemptions for certain patient populations rather than opposing work requirements as such (TennCare 2018, 84–86). Nevertheless, the mobilization of these groups in the comment process contributed to successful legal challenges to work requirements in Arkansas, Kentucky, and New Hampshire (Rosenbaum and Somodevilla 2019).

If interest-group mobilization mattered, it would also help to explain why states experienced a higher comment volume when their waivers imposed work-requirements on the traditional Medicaid population. Public comments on these waivers came from organizations with a history of advocacy for low-income populations, such as the Center for Law and Social Policy, and tended to emphasize the fact that work requirements proposed in these states would take extant benefits away from vulnerable individuals (South Dakota Division of Social Services 2018, 114–118). By contrast, comments on waivers affecting only Medicaid expansion populations often emphasized that the administrative costs and burdens of imposing new work requirements outweighed any potential benefits (New Hampshire Department of Health and Human Services 2017, 27–29). Because the evidence is only anecdotal, future research should examine differences in interest-group mobilization in support of traditional Medicaid populations versus those who benefited from Medicaid expansion. It is also possible that, when compared to the traditional Medicaid population, the impositon of work requirements on so-called "able-bodied" individuals with higher incomes invites less concentrated political backlash. Further, as Lanford (Chapter 6 this volume) suggests, state-level racial resentment may inhibit the adoption of more generous Medicaid-expansion policies.

There are several limitations to this analysis. First, the data here only assess the relationship between state waiver processes and participation in the public-notice process. Thus we are observing participation at a fairly late stage of policymaking, once state waiver applications have been prepared. Yet public participation may be far less substantial at earlier stages of the process, such as the formulation of legislation or executive decisions requiring state Medicaid agencies to pursue work requirements. Future research should investigate variation in the extent of public participation "upstream" of public notice processes. Similarly, taking a cue from GAO's findings, future research may examine how state and federal officials affect the salience of Medicaid waivers through post-award monitoring and evaluation requirements (GAO 2019).

Second, the regression analyses here only tap into the relationship between elements of state waiver processes and public participation. Yet the effect of state decisions on public participation may be mediated or moderated by unobserved variables, such as interest-group mobilization or the level or quality of state media coverage (Snyder and Strömberg 2010). Given the decline in statehouse press in recent years, future research might examine the relationship between state media environments and participation in Section 1115 public-notice processes (Matsa and Boyles 2014).

Finally, caution is warranted when interpreting the regression results. Not only is the number of observations limited, variation on several key variables is constrained. Future research should leverage data about a larger set of Medicaid waivers to investigate the relationship between variation in state public-notice processes and participation.

Conclusion

Republicans at both the state and federal levels have long sought the introduction of work requirements into the Medicaid program. Yet federal officials have historically refused to invite or approve such requirements in Section 1115 waivers. The Trump administration's 2018 announcement that it would approve such waivers unleashed the largest number of applications to make work a condition of Medicaid eligibility in the program's history. Consistent with Herd and Moynihan (2019), this paper suggests that states have developed work-requirements policy through low salience processes and have taken steps to limit the scope of participation in public-notice processes. The descriptive data reflects troubling trends in the implementation of federal transparency requirements (GAO 2019). Nevertheless, the analysis here suggests that states' implementations of public-notice requirements had limited effects on participation during federal and state comment periods. States which applied work requirements to the traditional Medicaid population also invited a larger number of comments than those which did not. While no conclusive data are presented here, there is suggestive evidence that the mobilization of interest groups has served to counteract state efforts to limit the scope of conflict over Medicaid waivers. This should not minimize concerns about the quality of state public-notice processes. While interest-group mobilization has been a critical ingredient in legal challenges to Medicaid work-requirements, it has also helped to shed light on the importance of state and federal implementation of administrative procedures and the departures of public officials from public-notice requirements (Rosenbaum and Semodevilla 2019). If anything, how states implement these requirements will remain at the heart of the legal and political conflict over Section 1115.

References

Advisory Commission on Intergovernmental Relations (ACIR). 1979. *Citizen Participation in the American Federal System*. Washington, DC: ACIR.

Ali, Mir M., Judith Teich, Albert Woodward, and Beth Han. 2016. "The implications of the Affordable Care Act for behavioral health services utilization." *Administration Policy in Mental Health and Mental Health Services Research* 43(1): 11–22.

Ajkay, Nicolas, Neal Bhutiani, Bin Huang, Quan Chen, Jeffrey D. Howard, Thomas C. Tucker, Charles R. Scoggins, Kelly M. McMasters, and Hiram C. Polk Jr. 2018. "Early Impact of Medicaid Expansion and Quality of Breast Cancer Care in Kentucky." *Journal of the American College of Surgeons* 226(4): 498–504.

Antonisse, Larisa and Rachel Garfield. 2018. "*The Relationship Between Work and Health: Findings From a Literature Review*." Kaiser Family Foundation Issue Brief. https://www.kff.org/medicaid/issue-brief/the-relationship-between-work-and-health-findings-from-a-literature-review/.

Antonisse, Larisa and Robin Rudowitz. 2019. *An Overview of State Approaches to Adopting the Medicaid Expansion*. Kaiser Family Foundation Issue Brief. February 27. https://www.kff.org/

medicaid/issue-brief/an-overview-of-state-approaches-to-adopting-the-medicaid-expansion/.

Bachrach, Peter and Baratz, Morton S, 1962. "Two faces of power." *American Political Science Review* 56(4): 947–952.

Béland, Daniel, Philip Rocco, and Alex Waddan. 2016. *Obamacare Wars: Federalism, State Politics, and the Affordable Care Act.* Lawrence, KS: University Press of Kansas.

Centers for Medicare and Medicaid Services (CMS). 2018. *State Medicaid Director Letter SMD 18-002*, RE: Opportunities to Promote Work and Community Engagement Among Medicaid Beneficiaries, January 11.

Crenson, Matthew. 1971. *The Unpolitics of Air Pollution.* Baltimore, MD: The Johns Hopkins University Press.

Golden, Marissa. M. 1998. "Interest Groups in the Rule-Making Process: Who Participates? Whose Voices Get Heard?" *Journal of Public Administration Research and Theory* 8(2): 245–70.

Government Accountability Office (GAO). *2019. Medicaid Demonstrations: Approvals of Major Changes Need Increased Transparency.* GAO-19-315. https://www.gao.gov/assets/700/698608.pdf.

Grogan, Colleen M and Michael K. Gusmano. 2007. *Healthy Voices, Unhealthy Silence: Advocacy and Health Policy for the Poor.* Washington, DC: Georgetown University Press.

Hahn, Heather, Eleanor Pratt, Eva H. Allen, Genevieve M. Kenney, Diane K. Levy, Elaine Waxman. *2017. Work Requirements in Social Safety Net Programs: A Status Report of Work Requirements in TANF*, SNAP, Housing Assistance, and Medicaid. Washington, DC: Urban Institute.

Herd, Pamela, and Donald P. Moynihan. 2019. *Administrative Burden: Policymaking by Other Means.* New York: Russell Sage Foundation.

Jarlenski, Marian, Philip Rocco, Renuka Tipirneni, Amy Jo Kennedy, Nivedita Gunturi, and Julie Donohue. 2017. "Shaping Health Policy for Low-Income Populations: An Assessment of Public Comments in a New Medicaid Waiver Process." *Journal of Health Politics, Policy, and Law* 42(6): 1039–1064.

Kaiser Family Foundation (KFF). 2019. *Medicaid Waiver Tracker: Approved and Pending Section 1115 Waivers by State*. Posted June 13, 2019, https://www.kff.org/medicaid/issue-brief/medicaid-waiver-tracker-approved-and-pending-section-1115-waivers-by-state/.

Keller, Ann C., and Laura Packel. 2014. "Going for the cure: patient interest groups and health advocacy in the United States." *Journal of Health Politics, Policy, and Law* 39(2):331–367.

Kirzinger, Ashley, Bianca DiJulio, Liz Hamel, Bryan Wu, and Mollyann Brodie. 2017. "*Kaiser Health Tracking Poll - June 2017: ACA, Replacement Plan, and Medicaid*." June 23. https://www.kff.org/health-reform/poll-finding/kaiser-health-tracking-poll-june-2017-aca-replacement-plan-and-medicaid/.

Kirzinger, Ashley, Bryan Wu, and Mollyann Brodie. *2018. Kaiser Health Tracking Poll – February 2018: Health Care and the 2018 Midterms, Attitudes Towards Proposed Changes to Medicaid.* March 1. https://www.kff.org/health-reform/poll-finding/kaiser-health-tracking-poll-february-2018-health-care-2018-midterms-proposed-changes-to-medicaid/?utm_campaign=KFF-2018-February-Tracking-Poll&utm_source=hs_email&utm_medium=email&utm_content=2&_hsenc=p2ANqtz--rGDvidfxe_LmfsXS2ECGWM8lypNIT-yGfrOXwFyZpdnJ9KYFpYIVGE76yoYkcMh53-gwz2Q8mHY4WyhOfvFgunDAlNA.

Mahoney, James and Kathleen Thelen, eds. 2010. *Explaining Institutional Change: Ambiguity, Agency, Power.* New York: Cambridge University Press.

Matsa, Katerina Eva and Jan Lauren Boyles. 2014. "*America's Shifting Statehouse Press*." Pew Research Center. July 10. https://www.journalism.org/2014/07/10/americas-shifting-statehouse-press/.

Medicaid and CHIP Payment and Access Commission. 2017. Work as a Condition of Medicaid Eligibility: Key Take-Aways from TANF. *MACPAC Issue Brief.* https://www.macpac.gov/publication/work-as-a-condition-of-medicaid-eligibility-key-take-aways-from-tanf/.

Michener, Jamila. 2018. *Fragmented Democracy: Medicaid, Federalism, and Unequal Politics.* New York: Cambridge University Press.

Michigan Department of Health and Human Services. 2018. *Healthy Michigan Plan Application.*

Mississippi Division of Medicaid. 2018. *Mississippi Medicaid Workforce Training Initiative*, 1115 Revised Waiver Application.

Musumeci Marybeth, and Julia Zur. 2017. *Medicaid Enrollees and Work Requirements: Lessons from the TANF Experience.* Kaiser Family Foundation Issue Brief. 2017. https://www.kff.org/medicaid/issue-brief/medicaid-enrollees-and-work-requirements-lessons-from-the-tanf-experience/.

National Academy of State Health Policy (NASHP). 2019. *A Snapshot of State Proposals to Implement Medicaid Work Requirements Nationwide.* July 29. https://nashp.org/state-proposals-for-medicaid-work-and-community-engagement-requirements/.

New Hampshire Department of Health and Human Services. *2017. Section 1115 Demonstration Amendment.*

Oklahoma Health Care Authority. *2018. SoonerCare 1115(a) Research and Demonstration Waiver Amendment Request.*

Rosenbaum, Sara and Alexander Somodevilla. 2019. "Inside the Latest Medicaid Work Experiment Decisions: Stewart v Azar And Gresham v Azar." *Health Affairs* blog, April 2. https://www.healthaffairs.org/do/10.1377/hblog20190402.282257/full/.

Rocco, Philip, Andrew S. Kelly, and Ann C. Keller. 2018. "Politics at the Cutting Edge: Intergovernmental Policy Innovation in the Affordable Care Act." *Publius: The Journal of Federalism* 48(3): 425-453.

Schattschneider, E. E. 1956. *The Semi-Sovereign People: A Realist's View of Democracy in America.* New York: Holt, Rinehart, and Winston.

Schneider, Anne, and Helen Ingram. 1993. "Social construction of target populations: Implications for politics and policy." *American Political Science Review* 87(2): 334–347.

Snyder Jr, James M., and David Strömberg. 2010. "Press coverage and political accountability." *Journal of Political Economy* 118(2): 355–408.

Sommers, Benjamin D., Anna L. Goldman, Robert J. Blendon, E. John Orav, and Arnold M. Epstein. 2019. "Medicaid Work Requirements-Results from the First Year in Arkansas." *New England Journal of Medicine*. DOI: 1901772.

Somodevilla, Alexander, Maria Velasquez, and Sara Rosenbaum. 2019. "How Far Do Section 1115 Medicaid Experiments Designed to Restrict Eligibility and Enrollment Veer From the Norm? A 25-Year Perspective." *GW Health Policy & Management Matters*, June 13, http://gwhpmmatters.com/blog-how-far-do-section-1115-medicaid-experiments-designed-restrict-eligibility-and-enrollment-veer.

South Dakota Division of Social Services. *2018. South Dakota Career Connector 1115 Waiver Application.*

TennCare. 2018. *TennCare II Demonstration* (No. 11-W-00151/4), Amendment 38.

Thompson, Frank. 2012. *Medicaid Politics: Federalism, Durability, and Health Reform.* Washington, DC: Georgetown Universit Press.

Wen, Hefei, Jason M. Hockenberry, Tyrone F. Borders, and Benjamin G. Druss. 2017. "Impact of Medicaid expansion on Medicaid-covered utilization of buprenorphine for opioid use disorder treatment." *Medical Care* 55(4): 336–341.

Willard, Patrick and Raven Gomez. 2018. "*Medicaid Work Requirements: Lessons from the 2018 State Legislative Sessions*." FamiliesUSA.org. https://familiesusa.org/sites/default/files/product_documents/MCD_Work-Requirement_Report_0.pdf.

Yackee, Jason Webb, and Susan Webb Yackee. 2006. "A bias towards business? Assessing interest group influence on the US bureaucracy." *The Journal of Politics* 68(1): 128–139.

Zhu, Jane M., Manik Chhabra, and David Grande. 2018. "Concise research report: the future of Medicaid: state legislator views on policy waivers." *Journal of General Internal Medicine* 33(7): 999–1001.

APPENDIX A. LIST OF WAIVER DOCUMENTS SURVEYED IN MAIN ANALYSIS

State	Document Link
Alabama	https://www.medicaid.gov/Medicaid-CHIP-Program-Information/By-Topics/Waivers/1115/downloads/al/al-workforce-initiative-pa.pdf
Arizona	https://www.medicaid.gov/Medicaid-CHIP-Program-Information/By-Topics/Waivers/1115/downloads/az/az-hccc-pa6.pdf
Arkansas	https://www.medicaid.gov/Medicaid-CHIP-Program-Information/By-Topics/Waivers/1115/downloads/ar/ar-works-pa2.pdf
Indiana	https://www.medicaid.gov/Medicaid-CHIP-Program-Information/By-Topics/Waivers/1115/downloads/in/Healthy-Indiana-Plan-2/in-healthy-indiana-plan-support-20-demo-app-07202017.pdf
Kentucky	https://www.medicaid.gov/Medicaid-CHIP-Program-Information/By-Topics/Waivers/1115/downloads/ky/ky-health-pa.pdf; https://www.medicaid.gov/Medicaid-CHIP-Program-Information/By-Topics/Waivers/1115/downloads/ky/ky-health-pa2.pdf; https://www.medicaid.gov/Medicaid-CHIP-Program-Information/By-Topics/Waivers/1115/downloads/ky/ky-health-pa3.pdf
Michigan	https://www.medicaid.gov/Medicaid-CHIP-Program-Information/By-Topics/Waivers/1115/downloads/mi/mi-healthy-michigan-pa3.pdf
Mississippi	https://www.medicaid.gov/Medicaid-CHIP-Program-Information/By-Topics/Waivers/1115/downloads/ms/ms-workforce-training-initiative-pa3.pdf
New Hampshire	https://www.medicaid.gov/Medicaid-CHIP-Program-Information/By-Topics/Waivers/1115/downloads/nh/nh-health-protection-program-premium-assistance-pa3.pdf
Ohio	https://www.medicaid.gov/Medicaid-CHIP-Program-Information/By-Topics/Waivers/1115/downloads/oh/oh-work-requirement-community-engagement-pa.pdf
Oklahoma	https://www.medicaid.gov/Medicaid-CHIP-Program-Information/By-Topics/Waivers/1115/downloads/ok/ok-soonercare-pa6.pdf
South Carolina	https://www.medicaid.gov/Medicaid-CHIP-Program-Information/By-Topics/Waivers/1115/downloads/sc/sc-community-engagement-pa.pdf
South Dakota	https://www.medicaid.gov/Medicaid-CHIP-Program-Information/By-Topics/Waivers/1115/downloads/sd/sd-career-connector-pa.pdf
Tennessee	https://www.medicaid.gov/Medicaid-CHIP-Program-Information/By-Topics/Waivers/1115/downloads/tn/tn-tenncare-ii-pa6.pdf
Utah (2017)	https://www.medicaid.gov/Medicaid-CHIP-Program-Information/By-Topics/Waivers/1115/downloads/ut/ut-primary-care-network-pa3.pdf
Utah (2018)	https://www.medicaid.gov/Medicaid-CHIP-Program-Information/By-Topics/Waivers/1115/downloads/ut/ut-primary-care-network-pa4.pdf
Virginia	https://www.medicaid.gov/Medicaid-CHIP-Program-Information/By-Topics/Waivers/1115/downloads/va/va-gov-access-plan-gap-pa4.pdf
Wisconsin	https://www.medicaid.gov/Medicaid-CHIP-Program-Information/By-Topics/Waivers/1115/downloads/wi/wi-badgercare-reform-pa.pdf

Appendix B. List of Comparison Waivers for Table 3 Analysis

1. Alaska Medicaid Section 1115 Behavioral Health Demonstration Application (2018), https://www.medicaid.gov/Medicaid-CHIP-Program-Information/By-Topics/Waivers/1115/downloads/ak/behavioral-health/ak-behavioral-health-demo-pa.pdf
2. Healthy Louisiana OUD/SUD Demonstration (2017), https://www.medicaid.gov/Medicaid-CHIP-Program-Information/By-Topics/Waivers/1115/downloads/la/oud-sud-demo/la-healthy-oud-sud-demo-application-20171107.pdf
3. Iowa Wellness Plan (2013), https://www.medicaid.gov/Medicaid-CHIP-Program-Information/By-Topics/Waivers/1115/downloads/ia/Wellness-Plan/ia-wellness-plan-waiver-app-082013.pdf
4. Rhode Island Comprehensive Demonstration (2015), https://www.medicaid.gov/Medicaid-CHIP-Program-Information/By-Topics/Waivers/1115/downloads/ri/ri-global-consumer-choice-compact-pa2.pdf
5. Mass Health Extension Request (2016), https://www.mass.gov/files/documents/2016/07/uf/07-022-16-appendix-a-public-notices.pdf
6. North Carolina's Medicaid Reform Demonstration, https://www.medicaid.gov/Medicaid-CHIP-Program-Information/By-Topics/Waivers/1115/downloads/nc/nc-medicaid-reform-pa2.pdf.
7. Mississippi Family Planning Waiver Extension Application (2017), https://www.medicaid.gov/Medicaid-CHIP-Program-Information/By-Topics/Waivers/1115/downloads/ms/ms-family-planning-medicaid-expansion-project-pa2.pdf.
8. New Mexico Centennial Care 2.0, https://www.medicaid.gov/Medicaid-CHIP-Program-Information/By-Topics/Waivers/1115/downloads/nm/nm-centennial-care-pa.pdf.
9. Washington Medicaid Transformation Project (2015), https://www.medicaid.gov/Medicaid-CHIP-Program-

Information/By-Topics/Waivers/1115/downloads/wa/medicaid-transformation/wa-medicaid-transformation-state-demo-app-82415.pdf.

10. Georgia Section 1115 Family Planning Demonstration Extension (2014), https://www.medicaid.gov/Medicaid-CHIP-Program-Information/By-Topics/Waivers/1115/downloads/ga/ga-planning-for-healthy-babies-pa.pdf.

In: Medicaid: Politics, Policy, and Key Issues ISBN: 978-1-53618-133-3
Editor: Daniel Lanford

Chapter 6

MEDICAID AND RACIAL RESTRICTION: MOVING BEYOND THE WELFARE-ENTITLEMENT DICHOTOMY IN THE ANALYSIS OF INCOME-TARGETED PROGRAMS

Daniel Lanford[*]
Georgia Health Policy Center, Georgia State Univesity,
Atlanta, GA, US

ABSTRACT

Is Medicaid a residual welfare program or a popular and broad-reaching entitlement? These competing visions have long shaped our understanding of Medicaid despite the fact that scholars regularly agree neither perspective is sufficient for explaining the socio-political dynamics that go into or flow out of Medicaid politics. Key problems are twofold. First, there is the lack of systematic analyses testing hypotheses based on

[*] Corresponding Author's Email: dlanford1@gsu.edu.

these competing perspectives. Second, there is the lack of an explanatory framework that coherently ties together results that fit neither the welfare nor entitlement perspective. In this study, hypotheses are derived from the welfare and entitlement perspective and tested in two analyses. The first analysis draws on ICPSR public opinion polls to assess the influence of program design on attitudes toward Medicaid over time. The second analysis examines the influence of public opinion and non-opinion factors on actual state Medicaid expenditures over time. Results suggest that program design does influence public preferences, but not in ways that can be fully explained by the welfare or entitlement perspectives. Program size and policy legacies do not have the expected effect on public opinion, and in terms of policy outcomes, what matters is the cultural association between income-targeted programs and widespread perceptions among whites that low-income minorities will be the primary beneficiaries. Medicaid's design attracts racial and ethnic antipathy, and this has a uniquely powerful influence on policy outcomes across the study period. The analyses confirm that Medicaid is best understood neither as purely welfare nor as a popular entitlement. Instead, this paper offers a new explanation called *racial restriction*. The five qualities of a racially restricted program are discussed, and four general theoretical propositions flowing from the perspective are provided.

Keywords: racial politics, ethnic politics, stakeholder politics, welfare, policy legacy

INTRODUCTION

Medicaid is conventionally viewed either from an *entitlement perspective* or a *welfare perspective*. The first perspective is that Medicaid is not a welfare program but instead is a popular entitlement that reaches well into the middle classes, garners broad public acceptance, and continues to grow due to widespread support from beneficiaries and those who feel sympathetic toward the less fortunate (Gilens 1999; Greenstein 1991; Grogan 2014; Grogan and Patashnik 2003). From this perspective, Medicaid tends to be popular, is durable, and has considerable potential for expansion over time.

The second perspective emphasizes Medicaid's similarity to cash assistance programs commonly known as 'welfare' (Alesina, Glaeser, and

Sacerdote 2001; Disch 2012; Quadagno 1994, 2015; Skocpol 1991; Tesler 2012). Because Medicaid is limited primarily (though not exclusively) to poor and impoverished people, it is expected that the public largely views beneficiaries as undeserving loafers and minorities. Receipt of benefits is understood as heavily stigmatized, even among beneficiaries themselves. Medicaid is generally expected to receive limited public support since "everyone hates welfare" (Ellwood 1988:4). From the welfare perspective, Medicaid growth over the years has been marginal, serving largely to blunt more ambitious proposals for government health care provision.

Although few would argue that Medicaid fits neatly within either the entitlement perspective or the welfare perspective (Grogan and Patashnik 2003; Quadagno 2015), analysts, policymakers, and practitioners continue to return to these two visions in part because they offer a series of expectations about how the design of Medicaid affects public preferences toward the program and how those preferences, in turn, affect Medicaid policy outcomes.

In this study, I suggest that many of the central claims of the two perspectives are founded on expectations about public opinion and policy that have yet to be directly tested. Building on this insight, this study tests a series of hypotheses derived from both the entitlement and welfare perspectives. These tests are conducted in two separate analyses. The first analysis tests hypotheses about the factors that are expected to predict Medicaid preferences. The second analysis tests hypotheses about the factors that are expected to predict variation in actual Medicaid expenditures across the states and over time. As expected, the results do not neatly reconcile with either the entitlement perspective or the welfare perspective. In the discussion, I systematically draw upon the findings to offer a coherent explanatory framework that I call the *racial restriction perspective*. The hope is that viewing Medicaid as *racially restricted* will help us better understand the program's development and its future prospects. The racial restriction perspective also yields theoretical propositions that may be useful for understanding the relationship between program design, public opinion, and policy outcomes for social policy more generally.

LITERATURE REVIEW

Medicaid as a Popular Entitlement Program

The current discussion of Medicaid as 'welfare' has roots in debates during the early 1990s about the political viability of programs targeted to the poor versus programs that directly benefit either everyone or at least large portions of the population. One of the first to outline arguments that Medicaid was *not* a welfare program was Greenstein (1991), who suggested that most analysts' fears over the vulnerability of targeted programs were overgeneralized from cash assistance 'welfare' programs to other income-targeted programs, despite important differences in program design. A key example was Medicaid, which was targeted to the poor but also provided some benefits to other groups with more income. Greenstein argued that cash assistance 'welfare' itself was unpopular, not fundamentally because Americans are unwilling to help the poor, but because it was widely perceived as benefitting able-bodied people who should be working for an income. Greenstein pointed to surveys specifically showing greater support for Medicaid compared with cash assistance 'welfare.' Medicaid, he argued, was popular precisely *because* it benefitted low-income people with medical needs (see also Oorschot 2006; but see Barrilleaux and Rainey 2014). Gilens (1999) also found that support for Medicaid was much higher than for 'welfare' and more closely resembled support for Medicare. He suggested that the stigmatization of 'welfare' had more to do with negative racialized media coverage of 'welfare' beneficiaries than with the type of benefits provided, and he concluded that public concerns about welfare or stigmatized recipients had little to do with Medicaid. A series of policy changes in the 1990s provided support for these findings. In the 1990s, while Aid to Families with Dependent Children was dramatically restricted to its current form (Temporary Assistance for Needy Families), Medicaid expanded.

Later, under the SCHIP program (now CHIP), the federal government offered generous matching funds to states to cover health care costs for a larger pool of low-income children. This is consistent with a second version of the entitlement perspective. In this second version, Medicaid was once considered 'welfare' but is no longer widely seen as such. As Grogan (2014) observed, Medicaid had been strictly viewed as welfare in its early years but was increasingly viewed as a program for some people in the middle class. To illustrate, when New York experimented with expanded benefits soon after Medicaid was introduced in 1965 (SSA 1965), a 1968 amendment promptly restricted income eligibility to 133% of the AFDC 'welfare' eligibility limit. Yet such restrictions eventually loosened, and federal authorities gradually allowed for (and sometimes incentivized) expansions in coverage over the following decades. To various degrees, states have accepted the incentives (Grogan 2014). By 2012, New York granted Medicaid coverage to children from families at up to 400% of the federal poverty line (Snyder, Rudowitz, Garfield, and Gordon 2012). The most recent manifestation of the slow growth process came with the Affordable Care Act (ACA), which provided new incentives for extending benefits to non-guardian adults. "[O]ver time," Grogan (2014:142) argues, "Medicaid has steadily expanded and evolved from a poor people's program to more of a middle-class program."

Importantly, the design of Medicaid is understood to be linked to public opinion toward Medicaid, the political prospects of the program, and, ultimately, program growth. In the case of Medicaid, generous federal matching and substantial state discretion have potentially helped push the program in a middle-class direction (Grogan 2014). This idea is consistent with a broader argument in the social policy literature, which suggests that program growth and public opinion can be mutually reinforcing. Once a policy is in place, it is likely to create coalitions in support of that policy. Noting the resilience of many social programs despite decades of conservative attempts at welfare state retrenchment, Pierson (1996:44) emphasizes the protective power of "critical constraints on reform resulting from the role of supportive interest groups and, ultimately, voters." Broad public support is expected to produce a "ratchet" effect, whereby popular programs in particular attain a high resilience to retrenchment (Huber and Stephens 2001:29). The pattern of program longevity, or even growth, plus high public support is the foundation of the perspective that Medicaid is a popular entitlement program.

Medicaid as a Stigmatized Welfare Program

According to the welfare perspective, Medicaid began as a residual program primarily for the poor, and it largely remains exactly that (Quadagno 2015). From a welfare perspective, we would not expect public support to be consistent or lead to significant growth because key elements of the program continue to stigmatize participants. One issue is that minorities are overrepresented among the poor, and thus are overly represented in Medicaid (CMS 2014), which leaves support vulnerable to both class *and* racial fracture (Quadagno 1994). Another is that bureaucratic requirements associated with the Medicaid means tests are themselves stigmatizing and distasteful to current and potential beneficiaries (see also Herd and Moynihan, Chapter 4). Further, unlike universal programs like Social Security and Medicare, program requirements shift regularly across time and across states as state budget priorities shift. Beneficiaries must re-enroll repeatedly to retain benefits and have to report private details about life changes. Beneficiaries also encounter stigma when dealing with providers, who are increasingly rejecting Medicaid patients due to stagnant reimbursement rates and time-consuming paperwork that makes Medicaid patients less profitable compared those who are privately-insured (Quadagno 2015).

State governments also commonly treat Medicaid with disdain. While the ACA provided states with significantly expanded options for granting benefits to non-parent and non-disabled individuals of working age, half of the states initially rejected the offer, despite the fact that the federal government offered to pay the vast majority of the costs (Jacobs and Callaghan 2013; Barrilleaux and Rainey 2014; Lanford and Quadagno 2016). Several abstaining states eventually adopted some form of the expansion (often negotiating to include added restrictions), yet many states continue to reject expansion outright or experiment with smaller-scale expansions using restrictive waivers that bypass federal requirements and guard rails (KFF 2017).

There are two versions of the welfare perspective that emphasize different factors. According to the first version, attitudes toward stigmatized beneficiaries are expected to influence attitudes toward health policy, but Medicaid growth itself is not generally expected to reflect public preferences (Quadagno and Street 2005). Instead, Medicaid development is understood to be driven fundamentally by the interplay of powerful interest groups with especially high investment in the health industry (Quadagno 2004; 2015). In the 1990s, the Clinton proposal failed spectacularly due to dazzling political and public relations campaigns conducted by insurance companies who painted the reforms as government overreach, socialized medicine, and welfare medicine (Quadagno 2004). In place of the relatively ambitious Clinton reforms, Medicaid was expanded through waivers and the CHIP program.

In the period leading up to the passage of the ACA, insurers again played an important role. They agreed not to oppose the policy in return for an individual mandate that required more of the profitable working-age population to purchase private health insurance or pay a fine (Quadagno 2010). Pharmaceutical companies were also appeased by improved drug subsidies. Hospitals—many who faced new costs for uncompensated care to the poor after the Medicaid expansion was rendered optional in *NFIB v. Sebelius* (567 U.S. 2012)—also had much to gain in the form of new Medicaid patients (Ario and Jacobs 2012; Price and Eibner 2013). From this perspective then, Medicaid exists precisely because it is a welfare program that is not threatening, and perhaps even helpful to health industry stakeholders.

In the second version of the welfare perspective, Medicaid is less stigmatized than other welfare benefits because it is less racialized. Winter (2008) suggests that health policy, unlike cash assistance welfare, has rarely incited racially-tinged feelings because it has rarely been framed in racial terms. Tesler (2012), however, argues that this racialization of policy did eventually occur during the Obama administration because Obama's own racial identity made racialized understandings of welfare "chronically accessible" (Tesler and Sears 2010:6). In fact Tesler (2012:701) found racial differences in support for the Clinton health care proposals of the 1990s, but these differences were considered minor compared to differences observed later during the Obama administration.

Scholars outlining the second version of the welfare perspective have presented only preliminary analyses of the relationship between racial sentiments and health policy preferences before the Obama administration. They have also not adopted the priming perspective to directly investigate whether there is a relationship between racial and ethnic sentiments and actual policy outcomes, including Medicaid outcomes. Other scholars have, however, identified an effect of racial sentiments on actual Medicaid policy outcomes, though only in regard to the relatively recent Medicaid expansions under the ACA (Lanford and Quadagno 2016; Grogan and Park 2017).

From Typologies to Hypotheses

It should be emphasized that the entitlement and welfare perspectives do not represent an exhaustive set of any single theorists' ideas but instead represent ideal-typical explanations for the relationship between Medicaid program structure, attitudes toward Medicaid, and Medicaid policy outcomes. The entitlement perspective views Medicaid as a popular entitlement program, emphasizing high support for aid to the poor, low stigmatization of Medicaid beneficiaries, and Medicaid growth driven by program design and popular support. The welfare perspective views Medicaid as a stigmatized welfare program, emphasizing restrictive access, stigmatization of beneficiaries, and stakeholder politics.

These perspectives overlap at times, for example by acknowledging continuing growth of the Medicaid program and by acknowledging that any program understood by the public or by lawmakers as welfare faces unique political risks. However, the two perspective and their subtypes produce different predictions regarding public support for Medicaid and actual Medicaid policy outcomes. This leaves us with a limited understanding of how a policy comes to be 'welfare,' how policies respond to the phenomenon of 'welfare' as a socio-political force, and how program design ultimately shapes the prospects of a policy.

Attitudes toward Medicaid		
The Entitlement Perspective		
Version 1	H1	Income shapes attitudes toward Medicaid, with higher income associated with higher opposition to Medicaid spending.
	H2	Racial and ethnic attitudes are unrelated to Medicaid preferences (null).
Version 2	H3	The effect of income on Medicaid preferences decreases over time.
	H4	The effect of race and ethnicity on Medicaid preferences decreases over time.
The Welfare Perspective		
Version 1	H5	Income shapes attitudes toward Medicaid, with higher income associated with higher opposition to Medicaid spending.
	H6	Racial and ethnic attitudes shape Medicaid preferences with Blacks and Hispanics less likely to oppose Medicaid spending.
Version 2	H7	Racial and ethnic attitudes shape Medicaid preferences beginning with the Obama administration.
Medicaid Policy Outcomes		
The Entitlement Perspective		
Version 1	H8	Whites' feelings toward minorities are unrelated to Medicaid spending (null).
	H9	Whites' feelings toward welfare recipients are unrelated to Medicaid spending (null).
Version 2	H10	The effect of Whites' attitudes toward the poor on Medicaid spending decreases over time.
	H11	The effect of Whites' attitudes toward minorities on Medicaid spending decreases over time.
	H12	The effect of Whites' attitudes toward welfare recipients on Medicaid spending decreases over time.
	H13	State-years with more generous Medicaid policy legacies have higher Medicaid spending.
	H14	Policy legacies account for changes in the relationships between the public opinion variables and Medicaid spending over time.
The Welfare Perspective		
Version 1	H15	Public opinion is unrelated to Medicaid spending (null).
Version 2	H16	Whites' feelings toward minorities only influence Medicaid spending beginning with the Obama administration.

Figure 1. Expectations of the Entitlement and Welfare Perspectives, Formulated as Hypotheses.

At this stage of theoretical development, it is useful to move from ideal types toward more nuanced perspectives which reconcile divergent findings across and within studies. The following sections test the expectations of both perspectives reformulated as hypotheses (Figure 1). Then, in the discussion that follows the analyses, I present a synthetic theoretical explanation for the results which helps to reconcile the findings with the differing perspectives on Medicaid and which may be useful for hypothesizing about social policy more broadly.

METHODS AND ANALYSIS

This study takes two approaches to testing hypotheses derived from the perspectives described above. The first approach is to assess public support for Medicaid by examining public opinion polls of attitudes toward Medicaid. The second approach is to asses actual Medicaid policy outcomes using a unique dataset including state-level public opinion estimates derived from the ANES, state-level Medicaid expenditure data, and other state-level variables that might predict Medicaid policy outcomes. Studies in both analyses include all years for which data is available from 1986 to 2012, when Barack Obama was re-elected to the presidency and the ACA was firmly established.

Public Support for Medicaid

Data for Predictions of Medicaid Preferences

Few surveys include questions specifically about preferences toward Medicaid. However, the ICPSR public opinion poll archive contains five questions capturing attitudes toward Medicaid spending, one each in ABC News/Washington Post polls conducted in 1986, 1987, 1989, 1995, and 2011. To prevent confusion between Medicaid and Medicare among respondents, the questions are explicit, asking respondents how they feel about "Medicaid, which provides free health care for the poor." For comparative purposes, Table 1 reports public opinion toward both Medicaid and "Medicare, which helps reduce health care costs for the elderly."[1]

The ICPSR public opinion polls do not contain questions about attitudes toward the poor or toward minorities, but they do include demographic information on household income and racial/ethnic identification, which can be used to make inferences about the ways in which attitudes toward income, race, and ethnicity groups influence Medicaid preferences. Big differences in support or opposition across income and race-ethnicity groups would suggest that respondents view Medicaid as a program for low-income minority individuals rather than the general population (Bobo 2000).

Analysis of Medicaid Preferences

Do Medicaid preferences reflect generosity to the poor but not feelings toward minorities and welfare recipients? The first version of the entitlement perspective receives qualified support (see Figure 2 below for a summary of the results). Table 1 shows a positive multivariate correlation between income and preferences for cutting Medicaid in every year except 1995. However, Table 1 also demonstrates that the income-Medicaid coefficients are only marginally larger, if at all, compared with the correlation coefficients for income and preferences toward Medicare, the universal entitlement for the aged. This suggests that while attitudinal differences across income categories are important, they are not uniquely important for shaping support for Medicaid.

The first version of the entitlement perspective is further contradicted by the finding that there are wide differences in support for Medicaid across racial identity groups (Table 1). Unlike income differences, these differences are larger for Medicaid than they are for Medicare, suggesting Medicaid's income-targeted structure plays a role in creating racialized differences in support.

[1] Detailed information about question wording and coding for these items can be found in the methodological appendix, available from the author on request.

Table 1. Multivariate OLS Regression: Attitudes toward Cutting Medicaid and Medicare

	1986		1987		1989		1995		2011	
	Medicaid	Medicare	Medicaid	Medicare	Medicaid	Medicare	Medicaid	Medicare	Medicaid	Medicare
Household Income	0.08***	0.07***	0.03*	0.01	0.04*	0.03	0.00	0.03	0.12***	0.12***
Black, Non-Hispanic	-0.59***	-0.44***	-0.35***	-0.19***	-0.69***	-0.47***	-0.37*	-0.23*	-0.39*	0.18
Hispanic	-0.21	-0.25^	-0.11	-0.06	-0.24^	-0.07	0.07	0.12	0.04	0.04
Male	-0.02	0.14*	-0.01	0.05	-0.07	0.04	-0.05	0.11	0.09	-0.05
Lib.-Cons. Scale	0.52***	0.40**	0.45***	0.20**	0.69***	0.45***	0.50*	0.06	1.40***	0.97***
Constant	1.97***	1.68***	1.17***	1.16***	1.77***	1.60***	1.53***	1.17***	0.97***	0.91***
N	1380	1380	1386	1386	1397	1397	455	455	831	829

^ $p < .10$, * $p < .05$, ** $p < .01$, *** $p < .001$.

Note: The referent groups for the categorical variables are White non-Hispanic and female.

The second version of the entitlement perspective receives only mixed support in this first analysis. While this perspective allows for the stigmatization of Medicaid beneficiaries in the early years of Medicaid, the effect of attitudes toward stigmatized recipients is expected to diminish over time. This expectation is difficult to address directly since the Medicaid questions were asked differently after the 1980s (see appendix for question wording). Yet we can ask whether relative attitudes between blacks and whites toward Medicaid changed any over the study period. In fact the differences in black and white attitudes toward Medicaid spending are no smaller in 2011 than they were in 1995 or even 1987.

The data lends somewhat stronger support to the first version of the welfare perspective, since Table 1 demonstrates that income and race are both important for predicting preferences toward Medicaid. However, the second version of the welfare perspective receives only mixed support. While there is indeed evidence that racialized attitudes affected opinions of Medicaid during the Obama administration, race differences influenced preferences toward Medicaid well before 2008.

Predicting Medicaid Policy Outcomes

Dependent Variable

The federated structure of Medicaid permits wide variation in program scope across states, with some states aggressively taking advantage of federal waiver opportunities and matching funds, some states avoiding program expansion opportunities, and other states falling somewhere between (Grogan 2014; Quadagno 2015). Over time, the federal government has generally increased opportunities and incentives for expansion, and states have taken advantage of these opportunities differently in different time periods (Grogan 2014; Quadagno 2015). It is the resulting state-year variation in Medicaid expenditures that is analyzed in this section.

Medicaid policy outcomes are measured with data on state Medicaid spending from the Center for Medicare and Medicaid Services (CMS). This data is available for every year reaching back to 1980. This data includes spending directly from state budgets as well as federal matches (CMS 2011; Pew and MacArthur Foundation 2014). The federal government offers adjusted matching rates (FMAP) which incentivize states to provide services and also compensates for states' differing abilities to finance programs. The FMAP matches allow states to choose their level of generosity starting from a relatively equal starting point. Still, the matching rate is constrained to between 50 and 83 percent (KFF 2012), so the multivariate models below also control for each state's fiscal capacity using median household income data from the U.S. Census.

Two additional factors must be given special consideration when analyzing Medicaid expenditures. First, to compare expenditures over time, we must account for inflation, and since medical prices rise faster than other prices, I account for inflation using the medical price index provided by the Bureau of Labor Statistics (BLS). Second, since Medical costs are expected to vary across states as a function of cost of living, I also combine the medical price index with a state-year cost of living index (Berry, Fording, and Hanson [2000] 2009) so that each year retains the average Medical price but state differences in expenditures due to cost of living are eliminated.[2] The result is a state year index which allows for comparison of Medicaid expenditures across space and time (see the appendix for detailed information on the construction this variable).

Key Predictors

This analysis uses data from the ANES, the U.S. Census Bureau, and the American Presidency Project to produce estimates of average state-year attitudes toward the poor, attitudes toward minorities, attitudes toward welfare recipients, attitudes toward a government insurance plan, and liberal-conservative ideology. The method employed to obtain these state-year opinion estimates is a variation on the multilevel regression and poststratification (MRP) method developed, validated, and used in

[2] This study employs the revised 2009 version of the Berry-Fording-Hanson state cost of living index. It is available through the IQSS data archive, http://dvn.iq.harvard.edu/dvn/, or from one of the authors. Data for the final year, 2007, are imputed to 2008 and 2012. This is of minor concern here, since this index is only used to weight the medical price index according to the relative costs in the states.

prominent studies of political opinion (e.g., Buttice and Highton 2013; Park, Gelman, and Bafumi 2006; Lax and Phillips 2009) and Medicaid specifically (Grogan and Park 2017). The process for calculating the MRP estimates is described in detail in the methodological appendix (see also Knowles, Lowery, and Schaumberg 2010). This second analysis includes each year for which the ANES items are available: 1988, 1992, 2000, 2004, 2008, and 2012.

The MRP estimates for attitudes toward the poor and toward welfare recipients are derived from the two ANES questions employed in the first analysis which ask respondents to state how "cold" or "warm" they feel toward the poor/welfare recipients on a "feeling thermometer." Attitudes toward minorities are measured using two approaches. The first approach is to account for racial resentment with MRP estimates derived from the ANES scale for racial resentment, again using the more conservative measure of racial resentment among Whites only. The second approach is to assess racial attitudes indirectly by again assessing racial differences in opinion by including measures of the percentage of the population identifying as White (base category), Black, or Hispanic (Bobo 2000; Jacobs and Tope 2007).

We might expect that different proportions of minority and majority groups in states would produce different political pressures and, subsequently, different policy outcomes. For example, if citizens believe a program benefits Blacks, then states with more Blacks and fewer Whites might be expected to have more expansive policy compared to a state with fewer Blacks and more Whites. However, the relationship between racial composition and actual policy outcomes may be more complex. The theory of 'minority threat' suggests that, as minority populations grow, Whites, composing the electoral majority, perceive a greater degree of threat to their racial privilege and therefore evince a greater degree of racial antipathy (Blalock 1967; Bobo and Hutchings 1996). Thus, as minority proportions increase, policy viewed through a racial-ethnic lens might become less generous (rather than more generous) until the proportion of minorities becomes large enough to counterbalance the increasing opposition of Whites. The resulting U-shaped effect of minority presence on policy outcomes has been observed in ideological voting in Congress (Jacobs and

Tope 2007), and such a U-shaped effect might also be expected to influence state-year Medicaid spending if Medicaid is viewed through a racial-ethnic lens. The U-shaped effect is modelled by adding squared versions of the Black and Hispanic population proportions in the models below.

Political Ideology and Partisanship

As noted above, public liberal-conservative ideology is estimated for each state-year. This measure is included in the models below as a control along with two other controls for ideology and partisanship. The first is a measure capturing the liberal-conservative ideology of government leaders in the states. This measure is compiled by Berry, Fording, Ringquist, Hanson, and Klarner (2010). It is derived from ideological orientation ratings of state governors and state representatives to both houses of the U.S. Congress. The second measure accounts for party power in the state-years with the percentage of states' legislatures composed of Republicans. Data for this measure is obtained from the U.S. Census Bureau and the National Conference of State Legislatures.

Need

Central to the debate about Medicaid being an open-ended entitlement or a restrictive welfare program is the question of whether Medicaid responds to need. Three types of need should be particularly important. Poverty and unemployment are important since Medicaid began specifically as an anti-poverty program during Lyndon Johnson's war on poverty and still primarily targets those with low incomes. Accounting for unemployment also controls for economic booms and busts across time and geographies. The age of people in a given state should also be important, since Medicaid covers many medical expenses for the elderly when other methods of payment such as Medicare are no longer sufficient. The use of Medicaid for long term care among the elderly should be especially important. The models below therefore include a measure for the percentage of the population over age 65. Poverty and age data comes from the U.S. Census, and unemployment data comes from the BLS.

Stakeholder Groups and Time

The influence of industry stakeholder groups on health policy outcomes is a central concern for analysts interested in health politics. This is especially true for the first version of the welfare perspective. However, lobbying disclosure requirements vary considerably between states, and many states do not require lobbying disclosures at all (King 2011). Accordingly, we are left without high-quality over-time measures of state-level lobbying by the AMA, the AHA, health insurance companies, or pharmaceutical companies. Nevertheless, some idea of the size of different health industries and, accordingly, the power they would be expected to wield in state legislatures, can be estimated by determining the proportion of a state's population working within a given health industry. Data from the annual (very large) IPUMS-CPS ASEC survey (Flood, King, Ruggles, and Warren 2015), conducted by the U.S. Census and the BLS, can be used to determine the percentage of the population working in (1) the medical industry outside of hospitals, (2) hospitals, (3) the pharmaceutical industry, and (4) the insurance industry (health insurance-specific industry data cannot be isolated for this study period). These proportions are included in the multivariate models below (results do not differ substantively if the absolute presence of industry stakeholders is considered rather than the proportional presence). A variable indicating the unionized percentage of the population from unionstats.com is also included.

Controlling for State Capacity and Policy Legacies

State capacity should be controlled in the statistical model since a state's willingness to provide services must be distinguished from its ability to do so. As noted above, the federal FMAP matches largely account for the differing abilities of the states. However, three additional controls for state capacity are including in the multivariate models. First, as indicated earlier, there is a measure of median household income. Second, state capacity is also measured in terms of legislative professionalism using the Squire index. This index includes the length of a state's legislative session, legislator pay, and legislative staff resources (Squire 2012). Squire index data for 2012 are imputed as the latest values from 2009.

The third measure of state capacity is Medicaid policy legacy. Policy legacies are measured by lagging the dependent variable from the prior quadrennial. States with larger programs in the first place would naturally be expected to have larger programs down the road. Policy legacies are also expected to have a considerable influence on the prospects of a policy in the future, particularly in the first version of the entitlement perspective. Inclusion of this variable also removes any influence on Medicaid expenditures that the predictors have "built up" over time. Accordingly, the models below are especially rigorous, and the resulting predictor estimates should be considered conservative. The policy legacy variable can also be removed to test whether policy legacies help explain public opinion effects.

Also included is a measure of 'year,' which helps to account for any influence of unobserved factors that influence Medicaid spending linearly with the passage of time.

Interpreting Coefficients

Because the public opinion variables are scored on abstract scales, and because we wish to compare the effects of regular variation in the predictors, all variables without natural units are standardized in the regression models below. Standardization is indicated with a (*b*) by the variable name. Coefficients for these variables can be interpreted as the effect of a one standard deviation increase of the predictor on Medicaid expenditures in a state per person in that state, in constant Maryland 2007 medical dollars. Coefficients for the other predictors can be interpreted in their natural units (e.g., a one point increase in the percentage of a state's population composed of union members is associated with greater/fewer dollars in Medicaid expenditures). Note that in every model, significance tests are based on robust standard errors as a safeguard against underestimation of standard errors resulting from heteroscedasticity (Greene 2000). All significance tests are two-tailed.

Results from Models Predicting Medicaid Policy Outcomes

As in the analyses of Medicaid preferences, the analyses of actual Medicaid expenditures provides limited support for the first version of the entitlement perspective, which suggest Medicaid outcomes are driven by sympathy toward the poor. While attitudes toward the poor are seemingly associated with Medicaid outcomes in simpler models (Table 2, model RE2), these effects are explained-away in a more rigorous fixed effects model with the inclusion of attitudes toward minorities (Table 3, model FE2). In direct contradiction with the first version of the entitlement perspective, racial resentment and attitudinal differences between Whites and Hispanics both show strong associations with Medicaid outcomes in every model.

Looking at Table 3, we see that the public liberal-conservative ideology variable and the state partisanship variable produce effects that are opposite those which would be expected. We might think that these political ideology variables are collinear with racial stigma, resulting in odd effects for racial resentment and political ideology. Yet when the liberal-conservative ideology variable and the partisanship variable are dropped from the analysis (model FE3), the racial-ethnic stigma effects remain nearly unchanged. Likewise, when the non-significant opinion variables are dropped (model FE6), the coefficients for the racial-ethnic stigma variables remain large and statistically significant. Finally, when the public liberal-conservative ideology variable is replaced with the related Berry et al. citizen ideology measure (model FE4), the racial-ethnic stigma coefficients remain large and statistically significant.

The second version of the entitlement perspective also continues to receive limited support. None of the interactions between the public opinion variables and the year term in Tables 2 or 3 are statistically significant. Nor are interactions between the public opinion variables and the policy legacy variable statistically significant (not shown). The influence of attitudes toward minorities on Medicaid policy does not lessen significantly over time or in state-years where policy is already more generous.

Table 2. Medicaid expenditure outcomes, random effects

Predictors	RE1	RE2	RE3	RE4	RE5	RE6	RE7	RE8
Fav.-opp. gvt. health plan (*b*)	-74.84***							
x Year	3.41***							
Stigma								
Cold toward poor (*b*)		-40.04**						
x Year		2.56**						
Racial resentment, Whites (*b*)			-31.50**					
x Year			0.68					
% Black				1.17				
Squared				-0.01				
% Hispanic					-6.27*			
Squared					0.14*			
Cold toward welf. recip. (*b*)						-10.82		
x Year						0.84		
Ideology and partisanship								
Lib.-con. ideology (*b*)							-9.74	
Gvt. elites lib.-con. id. (*b*)							-18.64	
% Republican legislature							0.52	
Need								
% in poverty	5.20	3.95	9.31*	6.73	7.66	6.71	6.78	7.51
% unemployed	5.26	9.61	8.70	10.57	13.03*	10.86	9.82	11.28*
% over 65	2.91	3.30	8.65	5.54	5.26	3.96	4.23	5.20
State capacity								
Median h. income / 1000	-1.54	-1.44	-0.43	-0.44	0.64	-0.53	-1.25	-0.16
Legis. professionalism (*b*)	-7.53	-2.01	-3.66	-4.89	2.67	-3.25	-2.83	-3.62
Policy legacy (lagged DV)	0.88***	0.89***	0.88***	0.87***	0.87***	0.88***	0.87***	0.88***

Predictors	RE1	RE2	RE3	RE4	RE5	RE6	RE7	RE8
Stakeholder groups								
% in medicine (not hospitals)	45.88*	49.42**	42.35*	56.87**	49.83**	51.13**	51.56**	51.87**
% in hospitals	1.28	4.85	14.95	8.94	-0.86	10.88	5.57	10.82
% in pharmaceuticals	35.63	18.73	49.06	15.93	34.40	30.85	27.75	30.13
% in insurance	12.85	12.68	3.95	5.32	7.35	7.59	11.97	6.28
% unionized	-1.82	-0.89	-1.84	-0.46	-1.53	-1.11	-2.19	-1.14
Year	0.18	-2.51	-1.43	-1.37	-0.59	-1.95	-0.96	-1.60
N	285	285	285	285	285	285	285	285
R^2	0.89	0.88	0.88	0.88	0.88	0.88	0.88	0.88

Note: Constant not shown. (*b*) = standardized.

$*p < .05$, $**p < .01$, $***p < .001$.

Table 3. Medicaid expenditure outcomes, fixed effects

Predictors	FE1	FE2	FE3	FE4	FE5a	FE6	FE7
Fav.-opp. gvt. health plan (*b*)	-40.60*	-5.64	-15.09	-9.47	-39.45*	5.35	-3.98
x Year	0.94	0.96	2.27	2.24			0.91
Stigma							
Cold toward poor (*b*)		-30.13	-22.05	-3.53	12.84	-14.78	-38.68
x Year		2.33	2.26	1.13			3.07
Racial resentment, Whites (*b*)		-73.71***	-75.23***	-59.06**	-48.11***	-57.73***	-82.80***
x Year		1.14	1.38	0.33			1.74
% Black		22.54	11.88	40.43	13.43	32.56	12.22
Squared		-0.22	0.10	-0.37	-0.33	-0.54	0.08
% Hispanic		-29.11*	-31.27*	-29.35**	-32.06*	-32.24**	-27.61*
Squared		0.60***	0.60***	0.61***	0.53*	0.58***	0.60***
Cold toward welf. recip. (*b*)		2.14	7.31	10.31	-6.63	19.32	-5.41
x Year		-0.51	-1.49	-2.72			-0.31
Ideology and partisanship							
Lib.-con. ideology (*b*)	11.72	12.43		76.89***	28.18*	10.83	11.83
Gvt. elites lib.-con. id. (*b*)	-21.02	-28.20*	-16.91	-31.63**	-27.61*	-26.86*	-25.91*
% Republican legislature	2.32	2.67*		0.84	2.12	3.07**	2.50*
Need							
% in poverty	3.89	4.52	2.98	6.85	7.72	6.16	3.93
% unemployed	4.24	0.85	1.90	2.88	11.72	2.54	1.56
% over 65	26.43	3.88	-5.77	11.62	-6.40	7.23	5.91
State capacity							
Median h. income / 1000	-0.44	-1.24	-0.95	-1.60	1.56	-0.62	-1.12
Legis. professionalism (*b*)	-56.06	-28.43	-27.55	-9.88	-35.30	-23.63	-29.06
Policy legacy (lagged DV)	0.54***	0.49***	0.52***	0.53***	0.62***	0.43***	0.52***

Predictors	FE1	FE2	FE3	FE4	FE5a	FE6	FE7
Stakeholder groups							
% in medicine (not hospitals)	59.95*	43.60	39.29	45.40	37.61	49.56*	
% in hospitals	-31.29	-30.05	-35.10	-21.85	-11.09	-31.68	
% in pharmaceuticals	-12.17	-76.34	-62.08	-71.10	-31.33	-79.54	
% in insurance	13.44	-12.27	-6.31	4.02	1.55	-13.06	
% unionized	-8.54	-7.16	-8.63	-1.67	3.48	-6.64	-8.06
Year	4.89	9.66	11.01*	10.33*	16.92***	12.90*	9.42
N	285	285	285	285	191	285	285
R^2	0.84	0.86	0.86	0.87	0.90	0.86	0.86

Note: Constant not shown. aPre-2008. (*b*) = standardized.

$*p < .05$, $**p < .01$, $***p < .001$.

The first version of the welfare perspective receives qualified support. While attitudes toward government health care provision, the poor, and toward welfare recipients show no statistically significant independent effect on actual Medicaid outcomes in the full models, Whites' attitudes toward Blacks clearly do. Similarly, the proportion of Hispanic identifiers in the population shows the quadratic effect suggested by minority threat theory. By several measures then, racial sentiments have an influence on Medicaid outcomes, while other forms of public sentiments do not.

The second version of the welfare perspective, which predicts that racial sentiments did not affect Medicaid outcomes before the Obama administration, receives only limited support. Model FE5 in Table 3 restricts the analysis to the years before Obama's rise to national political prominence. Contrary to the expectations, model FE5 shows that Whites' attitudes toward Blacks and the proportion of Hispanics in the population both effectively predicted Medicaid outcomes before Obama rose to national prominence. Wald tests for differences in the coefficients for racial and ethnic sentiments across model FE5 and model FE6 (which is a non-interacted model for all years) indicate that coefficients in the two models are not significantly different. In other words, there is no statistical difference in the influence of attitudes toward minorities, whether the Obama years are excluded or included.

Interestingly, model FE5 shows that attitudes toward a government insurance plan had an independent influence on Medicaid expenditures prior to the Obama presidency. Put differently, sentiments toward stigmatized Medicaid beneficiaries did not drive all the observable effect of attitudes toward government health care provision on Medicaid outcomes before the Obama era (model FE5), as they did in the wider analysis (model FE2). This lends support to the second version of the welfare perspective in the sense that attitudes toward government health care provision, in general terms, themselves seem to be driven more by racial and ethnic sentiments during the Obama era. This is confirmed in Table 4 using the average state-level measure of attitudes toward a government insurance plan as the dependent variable. Wald tests show that the racial resentment coefficient is significantly larger in the analysis that includes the Obama presidency years, and this remains the case whether all predictors from Table 2 are included in the model or not. Nevertheless, Table 3 clearly demonstrates that racial and ethnic sentiments had a strong influence on Medicaid outcomes even before Obama's presidency.

Table 4. Predicting state-level attitudes toward a government health insurance plan, fixed effects

Predictors	FE8[a]	FE9	FE10[a]	FE11
Stigma				
Cold toward poor (*b*)			0.30**	0.33***
Racial resentment, Whites (*b*)	0.43***	0.62***	0.21**	0.46***
% Black			-0.11	-0.14
Squared			-0.00	-0.00
% Hispanic	0.06*	0.18***	-0.01	0.01
Squared	-0.00	-0.00**	-0.00	-0.00
Cold toward welf. recip. (*b*)			-0.21*	0.11
Ideology and partisanship				
Lib.-con. ideology (*b*)			0.10	0.15**
Gvt. elites lib.-con. id. (*b*)			0.03	0.07
% Republican legislature			0.00	-0.01
Need				
% in poverty			0.03	0.03
% Unemployed			-0.13*	-0.01
% Over 65			-0.18	0.04
State capacity				
Median h. income/1000			0.02	0.02
Legis. professionalism (*b*)			-0.35*	-0.17
Policy legacy (lagged DV)			0.00	0.00*
Stakeholder groups				
% in medicine (not hospitals)			-0.05	0.03
% in hospitals			-0.06	-0.12
% in pharmaceuticals			0.35	-0.15
% in insurance			0.02	0.03
% unionized			-0.05	-0.07**
Year			-0.03	0.02
N	191	285	191	285
R^2	0.21	0.39	0.57	0.75

Note: Constant not shown. [a]Pre-2008. (*b*) = standardized.
$*p < .05$, $**p < .01$, $***p < .001$.

Summary of Results

Most versions of the entitlement and welfare perspectives receive some support. However, none are fully supported. The first version of the entitlement perspective receives support since attitudes toward the poor apparently do influence attitudes toward Medicaid. However, these attitudes do not have an independent influence on actual Medicaid outcomes, whereas Whites' attitudes toward minorities do.

The second version of the entitlement perspective receives some support since policy legacies do seem to have a strong influence on Medicaid outcomes. However, the effect of public support does not appear to operate through policy legacies, and the link between stigmatization of beneficiaries, Medicaid preferences, and Medicaid outcomes does not appear to lessen over time.

The first version of the welfare perspective receives support since attitudes toward stigmatized minorities do appear to influence Medicaid preferences. However, public sentiments are also directly correlated with policy outcomes. Attitudes toward government health care provision appear to have a significant independent effect on Medicaid outcomes before the Obama period, and public racial-ethnic sentiments have a statistically significant association with Medicaid expenditures across the study period. The public plays an important role in shaping policy outcomes net of variations in stakeholder presence.

The second version of the welfare perspective receives support since racial and ethnic sentiments play a strong role in determining Medicaid preferences and outcomes during the Obama era. However, in contradiction to this version of the welfare perspective, Medicaid preferences and outcomes were both shaped heavily by racial sentiments before the Obama era.

	Attitudes toward Medicaid		
Result	The Entitlement Perspective		
Supported	Version 1	H1	Income shapes attitudes toward Medicaid, with higher income associated with higher opposition to Medicaid spending.
Unsupported		H2	Racial and ethnic attitudes are unrelated to Medicaid preferences (null).
Unsupported	Version 2	H3	The effect of income on Medicaid preferences decreases over time.
Unsupported		H4	The effect of race and ethnicity on Medicaid preferences decreases over time.
	The Welfare Perspective		
Supported	Version 1	H5	Income shapes attitudes toward Medicaid, with higher income associated with higher opposition to Medicaid spending.
Supported		H6	Racial and ethnic attitudes shape Medicaid preferences with Blacks and Hispanics less likely to oppose Medicaid spending.
Unsupported	Version 2	H7	Racial and ethnic attitudes shape Medicaid preferences beginning with the Obama administration.
	Medicaid Policy Outcomes		
Result	The Entitlement Perspective		
Unsupported	Version 1	H8	Whites' feelings toward minorities are unrelated to Medicaid spending (null).
Supported		H9	Whites' feelings toward welfare recipients are unrelated to Medicaid spending (null).
Unsupported	Version 2	H10	The effect of Whites' attitudes toward the poor on Medicaid spending decreases over time.
Unsupported		H11	The effect of Whites' attitudes toward minorities on Medicaid spending decreases over time.
Unsupported		H12	The effect of Whites' attitudes toward welfare recipients on Medicaid spending decreases over time.
Supported		H13	State-years with more generous Medicaid policy legacies have higher Medicaid spending.
Unsupported		H14	Policy legacies account for changes in the relationships between the public opinion variables and Medicaid spending over time.
	The Welfare Perspective		
Unsupported	Version 1	H15	Public opinion is unrelated to Medicaid spending (null).
Unsupported	Version 2	H16	Whites' feelings toward minorities only influence Medicaid spending beginning with the Obama administration.

Figure 2. Summary of results.

Discussion

As with previous studies, the present study finds that Medicaid does not fit easily within the entitlement perspective or the welfare perspective. Yet unlike earlier studies, this study distills ideal typical perspectives on Medicaid into discrete hypotheses amenable to systematic quantitative analysis. Results suggest partial but incomplete validation of both perspectives. Accordingly, the results call for a synthesis of the findings which helps to explain the relationship between Medicaid's design, Medicaid preferences, and Medicaid outcomes. Such an explanation should also be useful in understanding the politics of social policy more generally.

In light of the results, I suggest that the defining property of Medicaid is not that it is an entitlement program or a welfare program but instead that it is a *racially restricted* program. A racially restricted program has five qualities. First, it is targeted primarily to low-income individuals. This is of course different from targeting to racial minorities, where the racial content of a policy is explicit. With a racially restricted program, the public must 'fill-in-the-blanks' and draw on cultural understandings of income-targeted programs which assume the beneficiaries are primarily low-income minorities. There is no need for a policy to be explicitly racial in order for it to be racially restricted (Gilens 1999; Tesler 2012; Tesler and Sears 2010; Winter 2008). Accordingly, the second quality of a racially restricted program is that the program is widely viewed as being restricted to poor minorities regardless of participation realities. Third, while generosity toward the poor may influence policy preferences, racialized cultural understandings of means-tested policy render such programs distinctly vulnerable in the policy process. Political opponents have more room to maneuver when and where the public opposes such programs on the basis of racial sentiments than on the basis of attitudes toward the poor alone. Fourth, because generosity is subverted by public racial sentiments, need matters little for actual policy outcomes, especially in terms of need among the poor. Fifth, due to political vulnerability, the targeted program remains restricted to a form that is comparatively sensitive to industry stakeholders and comparatively insensitive to public need.

Medicaid meets the first qualification of a racially restricted program because it retains means-tests as the primary mode of determining eligibility. It is true that some children from the middle classes may obtain benefits, and some states extend benefits above the poverty line for some groups (Snyder et al. 2012). Yet the marginal growth pointed out from the entitlement perspective may paint an overly expansive picture of the program. The program generally remains restricted to the poor and near-poor, and it still always requires means-tests.

Medicaid meets the second qualification because the public still generally views Medicaid as a program primarily for poor minorities who are, in turn, cognitively associated with welfare among many Whites. People may, as the entitlement perspective suggests, view participants with a level of sympathy based on their impoverishment. Yet as the first welfare perspective suggests, racialized welfare sentiments play a key role in fracturing public support for the program.

The third qualification is also met. Despite the association anticipated by the entitlement perspective between attitudes to the poor and Medicaid preferences, income-based sympathies to the poor do not translate into policy. Instead, racial-ethnic antagonisms play a central role in shaping Medicaid policy outcomes. It would seem that racial and ethnic politics have both the cultural and political resonance necessary to influence Medicaid policy where other forms of public preferences are cast by the wayside.

Medicaid meets the fourth qualification because 'need' matters little for outcomes (see also Barrilleaux and Rainey 2014). Need among the poor in particular has little-to-no impact on Medicaid policy outcomes (Tables 2 and 3). The 'who' of 'who is impoverished to the point of need' is arbitrary and has a minor influence on policy outcomes at best. This might be surprising considering that many people view Medicaid as a program 'for the poor.' Yet it underscores the fact that racial and ethnic fracture can define a program beyond its purely bureaucratic components.

Medicaid meets the fifth qualification because it remains restrictive and stigmatizing. Medicaid is now more than 50 years old. If it is going to expand into a middle-class program, this development has been a very long time coming, and it still seems rather far off. Certainly, it has grown somewhat.

Yet it remains paltry, difficult to access, and demeaning in comparison with the universal health care systems in place in other wealthy nations. Even if Medicaid provision is considered in combination with Medicare and the private insurance system, the U.S. health care system remains over-priced, under-performing, and inaccessible to many. This is consistent with comparative research which views racial and ethnic fractures in the U.S. as a fundamental cause of relatively miserly and inefficient health care provision (Alesina, Glaeser, and Sacerdote 2001).

Importantly, the main purpose of this study is not to produce a new ideal type. Rather, the underlying goal is to produce theory about the implications of program design and public opinion for policy preferences and outcomes. I therefore present four general propositions about the relationship between program design, attitudes toward policy, and policy development. First, targeting matters for policy preferences, but it is not the size or scope of the targeted group that matters. Rather, *what matters for the relationship between income-targeted program design and policy preferences is the cultural association between income-targeted programs and the perception that poor minorities will be the primary beneficiaries of the program.* Even if a means-tested program such as Medicaid grows, the increased scope of the program is unlikely to shrink the racialized cultural connection between income targeted programs and perceptions of low-income program beneficiaries. The effect of attitudes toward the poor on policy preferences did not change significantly as Medicaid expanded margially. Instead, the effects of racial-ethnic sentiments on policy preferences grew, if they changed at all. Further, the relationship between racial-ethnic sentiments and policy outcomes was not moderated by the size of the program in the prior period (see a different but related proposition in Soss and Schram 2007).[3]

Certainly, larger programs did, later, produce larger programs again. However, this was not a result of concomitant changes in public preferences. Accordingly, my second and third propositions are that *marginal growth in income targeted programs will not boost public support* and *marginal*

[3] Whereas Soss and Schram (2007:122-123) suggest feelings about 'us' are more influential than minor differences in program scope, the present study suggests that feelings toward 'them' are most important.

growth in income targeted programs will not reduce racialized public opposition.

Fourth, public racial sentiments matter for means-tested policy outcomes. The unique power of racial and ethnic sentiments to drive Medicaid policy leads to the proposition that *racial-ethnic sentiments have the cultural and political coherency and resonance to influence targeted policy outcomes where other sorts of public sentiments remain uninfluential.* Accordingly, need will remain marginally influential as racial politics take center stage.

The cultural component of racial sentiments must be emphasized here. Racial sentiments will tend to have an influence on targeted policy outcomes over and above the influence of antagonism spurred by stakeholder mobilization. While influential parties may be able to nudge public racial sentiments one way or the other and help bind those sentiments to policy debates and outcomes, racial sentiments continue to have an influence on policy outcomes even where stakeholder mobilization appears to be neutralized.

Can these theoretical propositions be generalized to other policy areas? The answer must await future research. Nevertheless, we can briefly consider whether racial restriction is a property shared by other targeted programs and whether the theoretical propositions presented here seem to be reflected in those policies. Other well-known means-tested programs include TANF cash assistance 'welfare,' EBT 'food stamps,' the Earned Income Tax Credit (EITC), the CCDF child care block grant, and Section 8 housing. The first proposition stated above is that racialized cultural stories about means-tested program beneficiaries influence public support. A full analysis of this proposition is beyond the scope of this study and will likely be difficult in any case with existing public opinion data. Yet prior analyses show that racial sentiments do influence, or at least have at points influenced, attitudes toward 'welfare' (Gilens 1999; Winter 2008) and tax breaks (Sears and Citrin 1982; Tesler and Sears 2010). The second and third propositions are that marginal changes in the size of a targeted program are unlikely to influence public preferences, including racialized attitudes toward the program. Consistent with these propositions, Tesler and Sears

(2010) noted that racial sentiments had a considerable influence on attitudes toward tax policy well after the EITC was instituted in 1975 and expanded in the 1980s, 1990s, and early 2000s. Finally, in relation to the fourth proposition that racial sentiments have a systematically restrictive effect on actual policy outcomes, note that most income-targeted programs that have been in place since before the 1980s remain heavily constrained. There is not one example of an income-targeted social program shedding its stigma and becoming universally available.

What do the findings mean for the future of Medicaid? Central is the idea that program design interacts with cultural understandings of social policy. Design does matter but not only in the strictly bureaucratic sense of size and institutional links to industry stakeholders. From the entitlement perspective, public opinion should shift with changes in the size of a program. From the welfare perspective, opinion should change as a function of elite stakeholder interests in the program or as a function of elite discourse. There is limited support for the former expectation here and indirect support at best for the latter expectation. By contrast, understanding Medicaid as racially restricted allows us to see that there is a widespread and influential anti-minority cultural logic applied to programs that are targeted to the poor, and politicians draw on this when implementing policy.

Another implication of racial restriction is that, as policy debates take place, innovators cannot afford to ignore the cultural logics at play. Those logics ultimately do gain efficacy. To focus only on bureaucratic program design – its size or media and elite responses to program characteristics – ignores the need for policy innovators to produce a compelling cultural logic to accompany their programs. Influential conservatives have been very successful in developing a cultural logic which links program development to racial and ethnic antagonisms. Progressives hoping to expand policy without also developing a widely resonant cultural logic can look forward to continued political defeat. The importance of cultural stories in turn highlights the importance of understanding policy from a post-essentialist perspective. It is not only the program *itself* which has an influence on opinion or even on later program development. Rather, the way that people routinely *view* the policy matters.

While the findings about program design, cultural stories, and the relative political efficacy of different types of public opinion are important, this study is not without shortcomings. Data is, of course, limited. Most limiting is the lack of extensive data on state-level lobbying. One interesting application of extensive lobbying data would be new analyses building on the historical and comparative research theorizing a significant role for stakeholders in inhibiting radical but popular reforms in health policy and social policy at the state level more generally (e.g., Patashnik and Zelizer 2013; Quadagno 2004).

Future research should also investigate the link between racial attitudes and policy in more detail. It may be that important factors intervene between white racial resentment and anti-Latinx attitudes. In other words, one reason racial and ethnic attitudes matter for policy outcomes when other attitudes do not may be that some mechanism is especially likely to bind, or is effective at binding, racial and ethnic attitudes to policy outcomes. It could very well be that such attitudes are particularly important for policy outcomes because they happen to be a particularly effective tool, instrumentally leveraged for the political advantage of specific people or systems.

Conclusion

This paper analyzes the two perspectives of Medicaid as either (1) a popular entitlement program or (2) a stigmatized welfare program. The expected links between program design, policy preferences, and policy outcomes are analyzed, and results are consistent with prior studies suggesting that Medicaid fits both perspectives to some degree but neither perspective perfectly. Drawing on time-series and longitudinal quantitative analyses of policy preferences and outcomes, this study contributes to the literature not only by suggesting that Medicaid should instead be viewed as a *racially restricted* program, but also by presenting falsifiable theoretical propositions which may help to more generally explain relationships between common program design elements, public policy preferences, and policy outcomes.

Viewing Medicaid as a racially restricted program allows for improved understandings of Medicaid's development and political prospects. Its targeted nature draws support from those who feel generous toward the poor. Yet support is also limited by popular understandings of means-tested policy beneficiaries as undeserving low-income minorities. Even sustained marginal policy growth does not reliably change these understandings of Medicaid beneficiaries. In the political process, racial-ethnic fragmentation leaves Medicaid outcomes vulnerable to restrictions flowing from broader racial-ethnic conflict. Racial and ethnic sentiments ultimately play a central role in policy development, while public need, sympathy toward the poor, and other forms of public opinion matter little. We are left with a program which pales in comparison with its counterparts in Europe and is likely to remain racially restricted so long as more effective cultural logics for comprehensive reform remain elusive.

REFERENCES

Alesina, Alberto, Edward L. Glaeser, and Bruce Sacerdote. 2001. "Why Doesn't the United States Have a European-Style Welfare State?" *Brookings Papers on Economic Activity* 2:287-277.

Ario, Joel and Lawrence R. Jacobs. 2012. "In the Wake of the Supreme Court Decision, Many Stakeholders Still Support the Affordable Care Act." *Health Affairs* 31(8):1-11.

Barrilleaux, Charles and Carlisle Rainey. 2014. "The Politics of Need: Examining Governors' Decisions to Oppose the "Obamacare" *Medicaid Expansion. State Politics and Policy Quarterly* 14(4):437-460.

Berry, William D., Richard C. Fording, and Russell L. Hanson. 2000. "An Annual Cost of Living Index for the American States, 1960-1995." *The Journal of Politics* 62(2):550-567.

Berry, William D., Richard C. Fording, Russell L. Hanson, and Carl E. Klarner. 2000. "Measuring Citizen and Government Ideology in the

U.S. States: A Re-Appraisal." *State Politics & Policy Quarterly* 10(2):117-135.

Berry, William D., Even J. Ringquist, Richard C. Fording, and Russel L. Hanson. [1998] 2015. "Measuring Citizen and Government Ideology in the American States, 1960-1993." *American Journal of Political Science 42*(1):327-348.

Blalock, Hubert. 1967. *Toward a Theory of Minority-Group Relations*. New York: Wiley.

Bobo, Lawrence. 2000. "Race and Beliefs about Affirmative Action: Assessing the Effects of Interests, Group Threat, Ideology, and Racism." In *Racialized Politics: The Debate About Racism in America*, ed. D. O. Sears, J. Sidanius and L. Bobo. University of Chicago Press.

Bobo, Lawrence and Vincent L. Hutchings. 1996. "Perceptions of Racial Group Competition: Extending Blumer's Theory of Group Position to a Multiracial Social Context." *American Sociological Review* 61(6):951-972.

Buttice, Matthew K. and Benjamin Highton. 2013. "How Does Multilevel Regression and Poststratification Perform with Conventional National Surveys?" *Political Analysis* 21:449-467.

CMS. 2011. *Health Expenditures by State of Provider*. Centers for Medicare and Medicaid Services.

CMS. 2014. *2014 CMS Statistics*. Centers for Medicare and Medicaid Services.

Disch, Lisa. 2012. "A White Citizenship Movement?" In *Steep: The Precipitous Rise of the Tea Party*, ed. Christine Trost and Lawrence Rosenthal. University of California Press.

Ellwood, David. 1988. *Poor Support: Poverty in the American Family*. Basic Books.

Flood, S., King, M., Ruggles, S. and Warren, J. R. 2015. *Integrated public use microdata series, current population survey: Version 4.0*.

Gilens, Martin. 1999. *Why Americans Hate Welfare: Race, Media, and the Politics of Antipoverty Policy*. University of Chicago Press.

Greene, W. H. 2000. *Econometric Analysis, 4e*. Upper Saddle river, NJ: Prentice Hall.

Greenstein, Robert. 1991. "Universal and Targeted Approaches to Relieving Poverty: An Alternative View." In *The Urban Underclass*, edited by Christopher Jencks and Paul E. Peterson. Washington, D.C.: Brookings Institution.

Grogan, Colleen. 2014. "Medicaid: Designed to Grow." In James Morone, Theodor Litman, and Leonard Robins, Ed. *Health Politics and Policy*. Independence, KY: Engage Learning.

Grogan, Colleen and Eric Patashnik. 2003. "Between Welfare Medicine and Mainstream Entitlement: Medicaid at the Political Crossroads." *Journal of Health Politics, Policy and Law* 28(5):821-858.

Grogan, Colleen and Ethan Park. 2017. "The Racial Divide in State Medicaid Expansions." *Journal of Health Politics, Policy and Law* 42(3).

Huber, Evelyne and John Stephens. 2001. *Development and Crisis of the Welfare State: Parties and Policies in Global Markets.* Chicago, IL: University of Chicago Press.

Jacobs, David, and Daniel Tope. 2007. "The Politics of Resentment in the Post-Civil Rights Era: Minority Threat, Homicide, and Ideological Voting in Congress." *American Journal of Sociology* 112(5)1458-94).

Jacobs, Lawrence R. and Timothy Callaghan. 2013. "Why States Expand Medicaid: Party, Resources, and History." *Journal of Health Politics, Policy and Law* 38(5):1023-1050.

KFF. 2012. *Medicaid Financing: An Overview of the Federal Medicaid Matching Rate (FMAP).* Kaiser Family Foundation.

KFF. 2017. *Current Status of the Medicaid Expansion Decisions*. Kaiser Family Foundation.

King, Linda. 2011. *50-State Assessment of Lobbying Expenditure Data*. National Institute on Money in State Politics.

Knowles, Eric D., Brian Lowery, and Rebecca L. Schaumberg. 2010. "Racial Prejudice Predicts Opposition to Obama and His Health Care Reform Plan." *Journal of Experimental Social Psychology* 46:420-23.

Lanford, Daniel and Jill Quadagno. 2016. "Implementing ObamaCare: The Politics of Medicaid Expansion under the Affordable Care Act of 2010." *Sociological Perspectives* 59(3):619-639.

Lax, Jeffrey R. and Justin H. Phillips. 2009. "How Should We Estimate Public Opinion in the States?" *American Journal of Political Science* 53(1):107-21.

NFIB v. Sebelius. 2012. 567 U.S. Supreme Court.

Oorschot, Wim van. 2006. "Making the Difference in Social Europe: Deservingness Perceptions among Citizens of European Welfare States." *Journal of European Social Policy* 16(1):23-41.

Park, David K., Andrew Gelman, and Joseph Bafumi. 2006. "State-Level Opinions from National Survey: Poststratification Using Multilevel Logistic Regression." In *Public Opinion in State Politics*, ed. Cohen, Jeffrey E. Stanford University Press.

Patashnik, Eric M. and Julian E. Zelizer. 2013. "The Struggle to Remake Politics: Liberal Reform and the Limits of Policy Feedback in the Contemporary American State." *Perspectives on Politics* 11(4):1071-1087.

Pew and MacArther Foundation. 2014. *State Health Care Spending on Medicaid: A 50-state study of trends and drivers of cost.* Accessed 2015-10-22. www.pewtrusts.org/~/media/data-visualizations/interactives/2014/medicaid/downloadables/state_health_care_spending_on_medicaid.pdf.

Pierson, Paul. 1996. "The New Politics of the Welfare State." *World Politics* 48(2):143-179.

Price, Carter C. and Christine Eibner. 2013. "For States That Opt Out Of Medicaid Expansion: 3.6 Million Fewer Insured and $8.4 Billion Less In Federal Payments." *Health Affairs* 32 (6): 1030–36.

Quadagno, Jill. 1994. *The Color of Welfare*. Oxford University Press.

Quadagno, Jill. 2004. "Why the United States Has No National Health Insurance: Stakeholder Mobilization against the Welfare State, 1945-1996." *Journal of Health and Social Behavior*. 45(Extra Issue):25-44.

Quadagno, Jill. 2010. "Interest-Group Influence on the Patient Protection and Affordability Act of 2010: Winners and Losers in the Health Care Reform Debate." *Journal of Health Politics, Policy, and Law* 36(3):449-453.

Quadagno, Jill. 2015. "The transformation of Medicaid from poor law legacy to middle class entitlement." In *Medicare and Medicaid at 50*, ed. Wailoo, Keith, Julian Zelizer, and Alan Cohen. Oxford University Press.

Quadagno, Jill and Debra Street. 2005. "Ideology and Public Policy: Antistatism in American Welfare State Transformation." *The Journal of Political History* 17(1):52-71.

Skocpol, Theda. 1991. "Targeting Within Universalism." In *The Urban Underclass*, edited by Christopher Jencks and Paul E. Peterson. Washington, D.C.: Brookings Institution.

Sears, D. O. and Citrin, J. 1982. *Tax revolt: Something for nothing in California*. Harvard University Press.

Snyder, Laura, Robin Rudowitz, Rachel Garfield, and Tracy Gordon. 2012. *Why Does Medicaid Spending Vary Across States: A Chart Book of Factors Driving State Spending*. Kaiser Commission on Medicaid and the Uninsured.

Soss, Joe and Sanford F. Schram. 2007. "A Public Transformed? Welfare Reform as Policy Feedback." *American Political Science Review* 101(1):111-127.

Squire, Peverill. 2012. *The Evolution of American Legislatures: Colonies, Territories and States, 1619-2009.* Ann Arbor, MI: University of Michigan Press.

Tesler, Michael. 2012. "The Spillover of Racialization into Health Care: How President Obama Polarized Public Opinion by Racial Attitudes and Race." *American Journal of Political Science* 56(3):690-704.

Tesler, Michael. 2016. *Post-Racial or Most-Racial?* Race and Politics in the Obama Era. University of Chicago Press.

Tesler, Michal and David O. Sears. 2010. *Obama's Race: The 2008 Election and the Dream of a Post-Racial America.* Chicago University Press.

Winter, Nicholas J. G. 2008. *Dangerous Frames: How Ideas about Race and Gender Shape Public Opinion.* Chicago University Press.

SECTION III: CHALLENGES IMPLEMENTING MEDICAID

In: Medicaid: Politics, Policy, and Key Issues ISBN: 978-1-53618-133-3
Editor: Daniel Lanford

Chapter 7

MEDICAID FAMILY PLANNING EXPANSIONS: A CASE STUDY OF THE IMPLEMENTATION OF GEORGIA'S PLANNING FOR HEALTHY BABIES PROGRAM

Sarah C. Blake*
Department of Health Policy and Management
Rollins School of Public Health
Emory University, Atlanta, GA, US

ABSTRACT

For almost 50 years, Medicaid has played an important role in the provision of family planning services for low-income women and men. Beginning in the late 1990s, states began receiving federal approval to implement Medicaid demonstration programs through Section 1115 waivers to expand eligibility criteria and the scope of family planning services. In 2011, Georgia implemented an ambitious Medicaid family planning expansion, known as Planning for Healthy Babies (P4HB). This

* Corresponding Author's Email: scblake@emory.edu.

program was aimed at improving maternal and infant health outcomes through access to family planning services and interconception care. This chapter presents a case study of P4HB, investigating the causes of low enrollment and participation in its first years of implementation. Findings reveal that key health outcomes were delayed due mainly to problems in development and implementation that led to a lack of awareness and understanding about the program on the part of providers, enrollees, and other key stakeholders. This chapter concludes with a discussion of underlying challenges states would do well to address when implementing Medicaid family planning waivers.

Keywords: Medicaid, family planning, policy implementation, access to care

INTRODUCTION

Medicaid has long played an important role in providing family planning services for low-income women and men. In 1972, Congress enacted several changes to the Medicaid program to require coverage of family planning (AGI 2000). One such change was the requirement that all state Medicaid programs include “family planning services and supplies” as a mandated benefit for all enrollees. States receive an enhanced matching rate from the federal government of 90% for these services and supplies, and no cost-sharing is allowed for those seeking family planning services in the Medicaid program (IOM 2009). Consequentially, family planning services have become essential benefits in the Medicaid program, which is also now the primary funding source of family planning in the United States, accounting for approximately 75% of all publicly funded family planning expenditures (Hasstedt, Sonfeld, and Gold 2017).

Beginning in the mid-1990s, another important development occurred in federal Medicaid policy related to family planning. States began to implement Section 1115 demonstration waiver programs to expand family planning services to populations ineligible for full-scope Medicaid. These programs, which ‘waived’ certain standards of Medicaid law, increased access to Medicaid family planning services primarily for women losing

Medicaid coverage post-partum, women losing Medicaid for other reasons, and uninsured women and men with higher family incomes (Sonfield and Gold 2011). The Centers for Medicare and Medicaid Services (CMS), the federal agency that administers Medicaid, requires that Medicaid family planning waiver programs must be cost-neutral, meaning they cannot cost more to the federal government than without such a program. They are approved initially only for five years.

After the implementation of the Patient Protection and Affordable Care Act of 2010 (ACA), states were able to extend coverage for family planning and services through a state plan amendment (SPA) rather than a waiver. With this option, states can make their Medicaid family planning expansions a permanent part of their programs, but they have to meet certain requirements, including extending coverage to men, women, and adolescents at the same income eligibility as set by the state's Medicaid or CHIP coverage levels (CMS 2010).

As of May 1, 2020, 26 states have federal approval to implement Medicaid family planning expansions (Guttmacher 2020). Seventeen states operate their expansion programs through a SPA, while nine states operate their programs under a Section 1115 waiver. Of all approved Medicaid family planning expansions, 23 states provide family planning benefits to individuals based on income (most set the income threshold at 200% of the federal poverty level). Three states provide family planning benefits for women losing full-benefit Medicaid coverage either after the post-partum period (2 states) or for any reason (1 state). Twenty-one states provide family planning services to men and women, 21 states include individuals who are younger than 19 years of age, and one state (Georgia) includes 18 year olds but not younger individuals.

There is evidence to suggest positive effects of Medicaid family planning expansions. These include increased access to contraception and resulting cost savings to Medicaid from averted births (Edward, Bronstein, and Adams 2003). In some cases, women already seeking family planning services through a provider are able to switch to a more effective method or have assistance in using their current method more effectively (Gold et al. 2009). In Oregon, 29% of new clients received a more effective birth control method in 2010 (Oregon State 2010). Studies have also indicated that Medicaid family planning expansions enable women to receive more effective, long-acting reversible contraception (LARCs) and preventive screenings (Dunlop et al. 2016; Redd and Hall 2019). Furthermore, these expansions have been associated with reductions in unwanted and mistimed births (Adams, Galactionova, and Kenney 2015) and even lowered average annual birth rates across the United States (Lindrooth and McCullough 2007).

On October 27, 2010, Georgia's Medicaid program, administered through the Department of Community Health (DCH), received federal approval to implement a Section 1115 Medicaid Demonstration family planning waiver program. This program, known as Planning for Healthy Babies (P4HB), provides family planning services to uninsured and low-income women (211% or below the federal poverty level). Women meeting these income and insurance eligibility requirements and who delivered a very low birth weight (VLBW) baby are also eligible for inter-pregnancy care services (IPC) that offer primary care, chronic disease prevention, and treatment services (GDCH 2019).

Most importantly, P4HB is the first and only statewide program to use the Medicaid demonstration authority to provide IPC services to mothers of low birth-weight infants (<1500 grams). P4HB was implemented on January 1, 2011 and represents one of the most unique state health care programs aimed at both increasing women's access to family planning services and also improving maternal and child health outcomes.

When implemented, P4HB received a great deal of attention from policymakers, family planning advocates, and healthcare providers. Georgia's Medicaid family planning waiver program was under a national spotlight, and many hoped it would be a model for expanded health care for low-income women of reproductive age across the country. Early reports of P4HB's progress, however, suggested that the program was experiencing trouble. DCH estimated that 40% of eligible women in Georgia (110,620) would enroll in P4HB within the first year of the program (GDCH 2009). However, within the first six months, only 1,375 women enrolled in the family planning component and only three women enrolled in the IPC component (GDCH 2011). P4HB enrollment during this time represented less than 2% of the state's goal.

This chapter describes a case study designed to investigate the development and implementation of P4HB and identify the key factors that led to low enrollment and participation in P4HB in its first years of implementation. This study addresses three main research questions: 1) How did the development of P4HB shape its prospects for later success? 2) What resources were dedicated to achieving program goals and reaching the intended audience? and 3) What factors influenced utilization of P4HB? The findings are discussed with reference to the significance of this unique Medicaid expansion program for state efforts to improve maternal and child health.

ANALYTICAL FRAMEWORKS

Drawing on work by Mazmanian and Sabatier (1989), this study investigates the traditional "top down" approach of policy implementation to identify factors that describe how an authoritative agency and its policy planning and capabilities influence the policy implementation process. This study also draws on Aday and Andersen (1974), examining the enabling role that health services systems can play in the implementation process in terms of resources and organization. Using these two perspectives, this study is able to examine how and to what extent the barriers experienced in the early phase of P4HB's implementation might have been formally or informally influenced through the process in which the program was envisioned and articulated. The general hypothesis is that policy implementation and the factors that guide the implementation process help predict the effectiveness of program implementation. Specifically, this study hypothesizes that P4HB failed to meet its short-term programmatic objectives (enrollment and participation) and health-related outcomes (increased access to family planning and interconception care for low-income, uninsured women) due to unclear policy objectives and resulting challenges in the development and implementation phases.

Methods

An evaluative case study approach was employed to capture the development and implementation of the P4HB program. A case study is an empirical inquiry that explores a current phenomenon in depth and within its real-life context. The major purpose of conducting a case study is to uncover the "how" or "why" of a research problem (Creswell 2012; Yin 2009). Evaluative case studies usually examine what occurs within a single program and whether the program has achieved its intended results (Guba and Lincoln 1981). Evaluative case studies include examinations of processes and attempt to understand how a program has been implemented and whether it has the potential to achieve its intended goals or outcomes.

Data

A mix of qualitative and quantitative methods was used to conduct the P4HB case study. These methods included individual interviews, document reviews, focus groups (qualitative methods) and provider surveys (quantitative method). The use of both qualitative and quantitative approaches tends to allow a richer understanding of the research problem (Creswell and Clark 2007). The goal of using mixed methods was to be able to address each of the three research questions from the perspective of multiple actors involved in the implementation of P4HB.

To plan for the evaluation, a logic model was developed prior to data collection. The logic model was designed to reflect the key resources, activities, and short- and long-term objectives of P4HB. This tool was updated throughout the evaluation to reflect input from stakeholders and after acquiring new information about the program.

Interviews

Interviews were conducted in-person and by telephone with 24 study participants from the Department of Community Health, the Department of Public Health, women's health and family planning advocacy organizations, family planning providers, and representatives from care management organizations (CMOs). Interview recruitment occurred through direct email or telephone contact and through a snowballing recruitment strategy. Interviews lasted an average of one hour and addressed interviewee knowledge and experience with P4HB during the first 18 months of implementation. Interviewees volunteered their time and did not receive compensation for the interviews.

Focus Groups

Six focus groups were held with current and prospective P4HB clients. Three focus groups were held in public health departments in Atlanta, one focus group was held in a public health department in southwest Georgia, and two focus groups were held in public health departments in northwest Georgia. Two strategies were employed to recruit participants: (1) a letter mailed by CMOs to enrolled P4HB beneficiaries, and (2) flyers posted at health department family planning clinics. Information was provided for interested persons to contact the study team for more information about the focus groups. Focus groups lasted on average about 90 minutes and addressed P4HB knowledge and outreach as well as experiences with the program and publicly funded family planning services in Georgia. Participants were provided refreshments and $25 each for their time. A total of 49 women participated in the six focus groups.

Document Review

The primary goal of the document review was to have supplementary materials that provided insight into the conceptualization, policy guidance, and overall goals of the program. Secondary goals of the document review were to understand (a) what the roles and responsibilities were for implementing agencies and providers and (b) how these responsibilities were integrated with Medicaid, which holds jurisdiction over these agencies for P4HB. Lastly, the document review also provided evidence of funding and other resources allocated to the first year of the program's implementation. Documents collected fit into five categories: (1) policy development, (2) program guidelines, (3) marketing/outreach, (4) P4HB quarterly reports, and (5) provider materials.

Provider Survey

A short, 13-question survey was developed and administered via fax, via email, and in-person to both prospective and participating P4HB providers. The Georgia Department of Public Health and two provider organizations (Georgia Obstetrics and Gynecology Society and the Georgia Academy of Family Physicians) assisted with recruitment for the surveys. The goal of this survey was to assess the knowledge and experiences of providers in Georgia serving women eligible and/or enrolled in P4HB. A total of 684 surveys were distributed, with 104 completed surveys returned, yielding 15.2% response rate overall and 32.5% response rate from family physicians. Providers volunteered their time and did not receive compensation to complete the surveys.

Analysis

Data analysis included thematic coding of the qualitative data (interview and focus group transcripts, document review summaries) and descriptive analysis of the survey data. A method of "mixing" the data was then employed through the use of triangulation, which included concurrent analyses of the two types of data. This study was approved by institutional review boards at Georgia State University (GSU), Georgia Institute of Technology (Georgia Tech), Emory University, and the Georgia Department of Public Health.

Development of the P4HB Program

Defining the Policy Problem

Historically, women in Georgia have experienced poor maternal and child health outcomes compared to women in other states. Between 2007 and 2011 (prior to the implementation of P4HB), Georgia's infant mortality rate was 7.3 deaths per 1,000 live births, totalling 5,175 infant deaths. The largest proximal contributor to Georgia's infant mortality rate is low-birth weight (LBW) and very low birthweight (VLBW) births. Births of VLBW infants were approximately 2% of all births in 2009 but accounted for 50% of all infant deaths (GDCH 2009).

An important predictor of a preterm or VLBW infant is the history of a previous preterm or VLBW delivery. Prior research suggests that early access to preconception care and family planning services may reduce the incidence of low birth weight (Jourabchi et al. 2018; Dean et al. 2014).

To address the infant death problem in Georgia, DCH created the Improving Birth Outcomes Workgroup in 2008. Composed of key community and public health partners and agencies, the Workgroup embarked on an initiative to reduce Georgia's low birth weight rate from 9.5% to 8.6% over a five year time span. One interviewee indicated that the members of the Workgroup were charged with the task of "coming up with a plan that could be implemented statewide to reduce Georgia's LBW rates."

The Workgroup agreed that to reduce LBW rates, women needed to be healthy before they became pregnant, and this should be worked on from the time "a woman was born until she became of childbearing age." A second priority was to make sure women had children that were wanted and planned and appropriately timed. A third priority for the workgroup was to ensure early access to prenatal care.

For several Workgroup members interviewed for this study, improving access to family planning services for low-income women was the main focus of their plan to address Georgia's poor maternal and child health outcomes. One interviewee who represented a provider organization explained that her members experienced problems for years trying to provide family planning to women who delivered through the state's existing Medicaid pregnancy program, known as Right from the Start Medicaid (RSM). When DCH began mandatory managed care enrollment of its beneficiaries in 2006, this interviewee explained that this problem became worse. Many women were seeking services from providers who did not participate in managed care or were not part of the CMO women were assigned to, and so they experienced delays in accessing a participating managed care provider. Managed care "slowed the ability of the pregnant women to get to the obstetrician." This delay, often as long as 90 days, was not as prominent under fee-for-service Medicaid. According to the interviewee, these delays often resulted in pregnancies because women delayed the onset of family planning. "Our objective was to be able to provide them (low-income women enrolled in the RSM program) with family planning, with birth control in order to space pregnancies, in order to keep some contact with them between pregnancies."

From Concept to Design

P4HB was modeled after the Grady Memorial Hospital Interconception Care program in Atlanta, Georgia. This pilot program provided 24 months of integrated primary health care, family planning, and dental services through enhanced nurse case management and community outreach via a Resource Mother. Resource Mothers are laypersons who are trained to facilitate life skills and health education to support high-risk women (Bierman et al. 2006; Dunlop et al. 2008). Several Workgroup members had familiarity or direct experience working with the Grady program, and they wished to see it expanded on a bigger scale. A P4HB Concept Paper later developed for the Section 1115 waiver application cited the Grady program as having early success with lowering adverse pregnancy outcomes.

As initially proposed, the P4HB program would extend Medicaid eligibility for family planning services to women aged 18 to 44 years with incomes at or below 211% of the federal poverty level (FPL). Family planning (FP) services would include medically necessary services and supplies related to birth control and pregnancy prevention. Services included contraceptive management with a variety of methods, patient education, counseling, and referral to other social services and health care providers.

P4HB would also provide inter-pregnancy care (IPC) to women, at the same income level, who had previously delivered a very low birth weight baby (less than 1500 grams). IPC included primary care services, case management, Resource Mother services, and referrals to social support services. The IPC component of P4HB would also be available to women who qualify for the Low Income Medicaid (LIM) group (mothers with incomes at or below 48% FPL and who have at least one child) as well as those women enrolled in the Medicaid Aged, Blind, and Disabled (ABD) program who delivered a very low birth weight baby on or after January 1, 2011.

Resistance to P4HB as a Policy Solution

Despite consensus among the Workgroup to focus on a strategy for reducing LBW rates in the state, there was not an agreement on how the expansion program should be configured. Disagreement over its configuration was rooted in the different concerns brought to the table by key stakeholders.

Several study participants suggested that the idea of a Section 1115 Medicaid family planning waiver was conceptualized by advocates who presented the proposal to DCH officials, who initially rejected it out of concern that the Georgia legislature would not support it financially. As one interviewee explained, "[T]his was not a DCH idea...it was not a priority for DCH...it was a grass roots push…it was not on the front burner for DCH…DCH said we will not fund this program unless you get the dollars in the budget."

Nevertheless, several study participants stated that DCH eventually took the lead. Indeed, despite DCH statements that the plan was based on the Workgroup's recommendations, some advocates and providers felt excluded from the development of the Section 1115 waiver application. For example, three interviewees had proposed that Title X family planning clinics and county health departments should be explicitly included as providers of care in this new program, but this did not happen.

There was a perception among some study participants that DCH favored the private providers over the public health providers (Title X in particular) and also that the CMOs, which had already been managing DCH clients, were able to provide more input into the waiver application. One interviewee noted feeling very disappointed to read in the final waiver application sent to CMS that public health providers were "taken out" of the listed providers of care for the program.

In other examples, interviewees noted concerns about the lack of presumptive eligibility, exclusion of teens, and limited family planning services in P4HB.[1] Two interviewees expected presumptive eligibility to be included in the waiver program, just as it was a part of the RSM program. Another interviewee wished teens had been included in order to cover adolescents younger than 18 who have pre-term and LBW births. Finally, two interviewees were hopeful that P4HB would include more gynecologic care for women who have polycystic ovarian syndrome (POS) and other fertility difficulties. These services were ultimately excluded.

Funding and the Legislature

All study participants who were knowledgeable about the early phases of the development of P4HB acknowledged the importance of gaining legislative support and funding for P4HB. This process was described as occurring over one year, with advocates largely taking responsibility for lobbying the legislature, explaining the benefits of a waiver program for reducing LBW rates in Georgia, and gaining legislative support. The legislature eventually agreed to provide initial support of $25,000 in state administrative funds for the writing of the CMS Medicaid family planning waiver application. This funding was matched with state expenditures in 2009, while additional funding was allocated in 2010 for the state's share of the waiver's first-year expenses ($225,000). One interviewee explained the importance of securing this funding from the legislature, "[W]e needed to get it in the budget, you know we need to get money, because what's the

[1] Presumptive eligibility allows patients to be "presumptively eligible" for Medicaid and services to be provided at the time of application while a final determination is made of their eligibility.

point of going through this exercise of the waiver application if we're not going to be able to get it funded by the legislature."

Many advocates worked together to lobby Georgia's legislators. These advocates provided the legislators with information, explaining the potential benefits of the waiver program, the costs of LBW deliveries, the number of unintended pregnancies in the state, and the potential cost-savings of the proposed waiver programs. One interviewee said "the legislature understood that if the waiver could prevent 50% of unintended pregnancies that would eventually be paid for by DCH, this would save money."

There were different opinions about whether legislators had negative concerns for a program designed to address family planning. One interviewee was concerned that the legislature would not support the program due to the family planning waiver program failure in the 1990s and the connection of P4HB to family planning. They noted, "A family planning waiver may not have been supported as much as a program to reduce Georgia's low birth weight rates."

Another interviewee agreed that caution was necessary when discussing family planning with the legislature. "Family planning in the state had a bad connotation…it's associated with abortion, and so you had to educate folks about the word 'family planning' and that it did not mean, absolutely had nothing to do with the word abortion." This interviewee's tactic, when lobbying for P4HB, was to take "a business perspective of how this will save money...you have to come at it from a different perspective, and you have to have the Republicans buy in."

Another interviewee gave a different explanation for how legislative support for the waiver was obtained. "It really flew under the radar, and the reason it flew under the radar was because it was called Planning for Healthy Babies and it didn't say anything about family planning."

Yet other study participants do not remember such struggles with the legislature. They referred to several members of Georgia's legislature in favor of P4HB. One advocate said that even the Chairman of the Health Subcommittee of Appropriations was an early ally and supporter of the waiver, building support for the program behind the scenes with other legislators.

PROGRAM IMPLEMENTATION

The Department of Community Health estimated that 40% of eligible women in Georgia would enroll in within the first year of the P4HB program (110,620). However, within the first year, only 7,543 women had enrolled in the family planning component of the program and only 23 enrolled in the IPC component. P4HB enrollment during this time represented less than 7% of the state's goal.

Reports from key public health providers brought additional troublesome news during this time, which was that they were experiencing problems enrolling women in P4HB, and there was an overall lack of outreach about the program. Overall, signs pointed to serious problems with the early stages of the program.

Fast Tracked Implementation

The P4HB waiver application received official approval from CMS on October 29, 2010, approximately nine months after DCH submitted the initial application. From a Medicaid waiver perspective, this approval process was quick. States have been known to wait years to receive approval for such demonstration programs. Indeed, Georgia's own attempt to receive a Section 1115 waiver for Medicaid HIV services failed in the early 2000s after CMS took two years to review the application. So from an administrative perspective, the federal approval for P4HB occurred rather quickly.

Several interviewees considered this quick timeframe as a hindrance to effective implementation of the program. One CMO representative discussed the difficulty the plan encountered during the time spent preparing for the implementation of P4HB. This study participant described this time as "very intense." With just a few months to prepare, the health plan had to develop a lot of new materials, including member cards, brochures, provider guidelines, etc. The CMO representative described P4HB as a "new product…a lot of new things had to be created that impacted all areas."

The plans worked initially to "cobrand" the P4HB program materials. DCH also provided templates for many of their materials. Later, in the summer of 2012, the CMOs were given permission to develop separate materials that allowed them to tailor these materials to their plan's design scheme and layout.

An interviewee from DCH discussed all the moving parts that were in place before and after CMS approval of the waiver. Early on, in summer of 2010, DCH assembled a communications team and a data systems team to prepare for P4HB. The communications team developed the application forms, letters, flyers, posters, and report templates. However, DCH was also occupied with the Medicaid Management Information System (MMIS), then undergoing a transformation in the state. It would not be live until November 1, 2010, only two months before P4HB was to be implemented. As a precaution, DCH had a separate enrollment and billing system created just for P4HB to avoid interference with the new MMIS system's implementation. DCH also had to revise their existing contract with each of the CMOs to reflect the plans' responsibilities for this new program.

When asked why the implementation of P4HB was not postponed or delayed since so little time existed between the waiver's approval and the implementation (October 29, 2010—January 1, 2011), an interviewee from DCH explained that there was too much money at stake. The total budget for P4HB, with state and federal funds, was $2 million just for the first 6 months of the program (until the end of the 2010-2011 fiscal year, which is June 30th). This funding, or at least part of it, would have been forfeited if the program's implementation was delayed. DCH could not afford to wait.

Outreach and Education

To inform potential enrollees about P4HB, DCH developed a communications plan in 2010 which described two marketing phases. The first phase included the production of postcards and posters, as well as paid radio ads. A second marketing phase provided funds for billboards and advertisements on buses and trains over the course of six months. The marketing plan was funded by DPH for only the first year.

DCH staff also met regularly with CMOs and providers in the first year to inform them about the program. CMOs were required to create provider and client handbooks, and most also added eligibility information on their websites. In addition, RSM outreach workers attended numerous health fairs and public health events to advertise P4HB.

As noted above, utilization of services was low in the first year of P4HB implementation, and interviewees complained that a lack of appropriate and continual outreach about P4HB was a major contributor to low enrollment. One study participant explained, "I don't think it was ever effectively marketed. Now everyone's pointing fingers, like well, you're not doing your job, we don't get the information you're supposed to be providing." This interviewee thought DCH should have done more marketing, and that other agencies, such as Women Infants Children (WIC), and the Department of Family and Children Services (DFACS) should have been responsible for more outreach.

Several study participants explained that their concern about outreach was voiced early to DCH before the waiver application was completed. Multiple study participants had recommended to DCH that outreach be a billable service. As one interviewee noted:

> …then you're going to have more likelihood of outreach activities occurring to ensure enrollment utilization keep a focus on including outreach as a component of the waiver. One of the things I have learned from DCH consultants that I had spoken with is that it is actually one of the most important things to include in any waiver…I asked about that…and I was told that yes, you know…and the truth is it (the waiver application) didn't include outreach, which I think is a big problem.

Findings from the focus groups suggest that outreach about P4HB occurred mainly through word of mouth. A majority of the focus group participants were told about P4HB either by a health clinic worker or by someone they knew, such as a family member or friend. Many women found out about P4HB at the clinic when they came in for their children's WIC or health services, or to get on birth control. About two-thirds of the participants regularly accessed family planning services at public health clinics, and this presented the first opportunity to learn about P4HB. About a quarter of the participants, however, had not enrolled in P4HB and had not heard about the program. Outreach and education even at public health clinics was limited.

Other sources of data also reflect problems associated with limited outreach about P4HB. CMO P4HB enrollee survey results from 2011 revealed that women learned about the program through word of mouth from health department staff or at WIC offices (28%), and from various mailings (22%). Findings from our evaluation's survey reflect that over one-third (38%) of all providers received no information about P4HB, while about a quarter (26.1%) indicated they received information and/or materials about P4HB from DCH. One fifth of these providers (18.5%) reported receiving information from DPH, and another fifth received information from a CMO.

Enrollment

All interviewees reported that there were barriers to enrolling women in P4HB in the early phases of implementation. A key problem was awareness and understanding. One interviewee who was a provider said there was little outreach to providers or women about P4HB. The interviewee also thought Title X family planning providers weren't doing enough to enroll clients. "I think that it (P4HB) has been perceived as a threat to them and that they were perceiving it as 'oh this mean women [has] come to us and we'll lose head count.'"

One interviewee who was a public health provider stated "anyone we think might be eligible, we try and get them on the program." Nevertheless, public health departments were initially instructed only to hand out brochures and flyers to eligible clients.

About nine months into the first year of P4HB, when DCH realized few women were enrolled in the program, public health departments were asked to take a more active role in assisting women to enroll in the program. All public health departments now provide women P4HB applications and instruct them about how to complete the application process. However, only half of the public health providers interviewed for this study faxed completed applications to DCH for eligible clients. The others tell women they must either fax their applications, seek assistance through local welfare offices, or complete the P4HB application process online.

Study participants from all three CMOs suggested that the lack of awareness and understanding about P4HB was a problem and critical barrier to enrolling more women into the program. One CMO representative indicated that enrollment of IPC women is the plan's main challenge. Even though the plan has instituted more on-site outreach and education at area hospitals, women are still not electing to enroll. These women "are not concerned about applying for a program that could possibly stop them, prevent them from having another pregnancy. They're more concerned about the health of their baby at that time." Another CMO representative echoed the same concern. This interviewee suggested that women who are eligible for the IPC component have "competing priorities…they have a preemie that they're dealing with. They have all sorts of family and social issues that they are dealing with." This interviewee confessed that their health plan was still trying to find a way to make more eligible women aware of P4HB, the IPC component, and the value this new program offers.

The low IPC enrollment was also a concern for another study participant who felt that IPC enrollment should be coordinated through newborn intensive care units (NICUs) and perinatal health centers, while women are in the hospital and before they are discharged.

Focus group participants reported various enrollment experiences. Most women started their application online or at a health clinic with the assistance of a staff person. Several participants described applying at a local welfare office. It appears also that some women may have been automatically enrolled after their eligibility ended for RSM or PeachCare, the state's State Children's Health Insurance Program. Many women described finding out that they were enrolled in P4HB after seeking services at their providers' offices or receiving a card in the mail. These women were surprised and often confused about being on P4HB. They were not sure whether or not the program was the same as full-scope Medicaid. One focus group participant described her surprise finding out she was auto enrolled after losing Peach Care.

> They just sent mine in the mail and I didn't really know what it was…I called them [Medicaid] on the phone and you just want to know what's going on- why are they sending me a card that I don't know about? I thought it was a scam at first.

Another young woman indicated she did receive information prior to the auto enrollment. "I just kept getting [e]mails from the Planning for Healthy Babies Program telling me that I'm eligible and that I'm in the program and things like that, but then I wasn't really sure. And then I think they sent me a card." So whether or not these women received information prior to the auto enrollment process, it is clear that they did not understand the program or exactly what the enrollment process meant.

Utilization

Many interviewees believed that P4HB was underperforming in the first year of implementation because women were not being enrolled and thus not accessing the covered services. As one interviewee stated, "Medicaid simply thought, 'if you build it, they will come.' Well, they haven't come." Some interviewees indicated that even participants who were enrolled in P4HB were not using the services, which several feared is because these participants did not know they were enrolled in the program or did not understand what services are covered in the program.

As noted earlier, many study participants felt that there was a lot of confusion about the nature and scope of P4HB. One reason they gave was that they felt it marketed a false identity as a maternal and child health ("healthy babies") program. Based on its title, women have little reason to expect that it provides family planning and inter-pregnancy care services.

One interviewee stated that the name "Planning for Healthy Babies" is "awful." Originally, the name discussed for the program was "Family Planning for Healthy Babies," but for political reasons, the term "family planning" was omitted. The interviewee further stated "we believe [the name] is deceptive in terms of people who don't want to be pregnant...why would they ever think 'I need to enroll in a program called Planning for Healthy Babies'?"

Two study participants working in public health explained how the confusion over the name of the program led to delays in utilization of services. One provider mentioned that women come to her clinic already enrolled in P4HB. "There's a good many women that are coming in who think it is not just for planning and spacing their babies, but to help them have a healthy baby." These women think P4HB is for women who are pregnant. These women come in for pregnancy testing, most already knowing they are pregnant, and then have to be disenrolled from P4HB after their pregnancy test is positive.

In addition to confusion over the name and scope of the P4HB program, several providers reported that very few P4HB women sought health care during the first year of implementation. One public health provider indicated she only began to see P4HB clients at her clinic in June 2012, 18 months after the implementation of the program. Another public health provider felt that perhaps P4HB clients switched initially to seeing private health care providers the first year, and then after being unhappy with their care, or simply not having the same kind of relationship with their private physician as they did with their public health nurse, these clients came back to public health after the first year of P4HB.

Satisfaction

Another important finding from the focus groups was that most of the P4HB participants seek family planning services from public health providers. A majority of the P4HB enrollees sought family planning services from local public health clinics prior to their enrollment in the program, and once enrolled, preferred to continue using their usual health care providers. These participants expressed preferences for their providers because they were conveniently located, familiar to them, and because the participants had been seeking services from them for a long time.

Despite the confusion over the name and scope of the program, focus groups with current P4HB enrollees revealed overall satisfaction with the program. When they were asked what health care services they accessed since enrollment in the program, most reported seeking traditional family planning services. Women received contraception, annual exams (Pap smears), STD testing, and pregnant testing through P4HB. In a few cases, women accessed other related services, including the HPV vaccine, ultrasound, and diagnostic MRI. One participant was diagnosed and treated for cervical cancer while on the P4HB program. She has also received follow-up care since being treated.

Utilization Data Insight into the P4HB Implementation

An anticipated mechanism for improving maternal and child health outcomes through P4HB was that the program would increase the overall use of family planning services/supplies among low-income women and promote more consistent use of effective contraceptive methods among program users. With such improved family planning utilization, Georgia could lower the number of overall Medicaid paid pregnancies and deliveries/births and hence, costs, such that the state and federal government will ultimately realize a net cost savings despite increased spending on family planning and inter-pregnancy care services. As indicated in Table 1 below, which shows data from the P4HB Year 1 Annual Report (GDCH 2011), the enrollment in the first year of P4HB was significantly lower than anticipated.[2]

[2] In Table 1, those eligible only for family planning benefits are uninsured female citizens ages 18-44 with income < 200% FPL residing in Georgia. The estimated number of uninsured women in this age and income range is 257,895 for 2009. Since this number has likely grown since 2009, our estimate of this eligible population is likely understated. Those eligible for IPC

Table 1. Eligibility and enrollment

Demonstration Group	Enrolled in 4th Quarter 2011	Population Eligible in Community[1,2]	Percent Eligible Enrolled
FP Only	7,543	257,895	2.9%
FP Only (adjusted)	7,543	140,522[4]	5.3%
IPC/Resource Mother Only	23	1,420	1.6%

These very low participation rates among the eligible population of women suggest the need for far more intensive education and outreach as well as significant efforts to make the application process more user-friendly and accessible in the community.

DISCUSSION

This study suggests that development and implementation are critical in the policy process because they shape how a program's goals or objectives are transferred into practice. This study reflects upon whether this process occurred as planned, and if not, what barriers existed to implementation. This study also described the top-down approach, where an authorizing agency maintains control, affecting the development and implementation

include uninsured women 18-44 with income < 200% FPL residing in Georgia with a live birth infant under 1500 grams at delivery. Women enrolled in RSM with a VLBW infant should be the denominator for this calculation. Those eligible for Resource Mother only include LIM and ABD Classes of Eligibility women with a VLBW infant. We combine the enrollment counts for IPC and Resource Mother for the numerator and use all Medicaid paid VLBW births (N = 1,420) as the denominator. The count of women ever enrolled in the FP only component of the Demonstration includes the number reported earlier even though some of these women would have been disenrolled during the first three months of the Demonstration. We use the 7,543 number for consistency with the early parts of the report. The second row, FP Only (adjusted), is adjusted for women in need of family planning services based on a report from the Guttmacher Institute. Their estimate is that only 54.5% of women in the age group 13-44 were actually in need of family planning services. We therefore multiplied the Population Eligibility in the Community from the first row by .545 to get 140,522 in row 2, column 3 (Sonfield, Aldrich, and Gold 2008; http://www.guttmacher.org/pubs/win/contraceptive-needs-2008.pdf.).

process. There are three major findings. They concern collaboration at all stages, statutory coherence, and the 'field of dreams' approach.

Collaboration at All Stages

First, collaboration is important during all stages of implementation. The findings reflect the need for ongoing collaboration among practice partners during all stages of the development and implementation process. Interviewees, especially the advocates, felt there was a lack of engagement in the development and implementation of P4HB after a decision was made to apply for a Medicaid family planning waiver. These interviewees, many of whom helped obtain legislative support and funding for P4HB, felt shut out when the concept paper for the program was issued by DCH without their review.

These and other study participants, including those at other state agencies, wished they were also able to collaborate while the program was being implemented. Such collaboration may have enabled them to provide outreach and education to their own constituents and to be able to educate others about the purpose and scope of the program. These interviewees also believed that they should have been included as advisory council members so that they could provide feedback and ongoing counseling about the program.

More extensive provider collaboration may also have promoted successful development, enabling providers to influence the outreach and enrollment process that was identified as problematic in this study. Some providers were informed of the initial concept of P4HB, but few were consulted during the planning process, and none appeared to be actively engaged in the design of P4HB. In fact, one provider whose IPC program became the model for P4HB's inter-pregnancy care component was never consulted about P4HB.

We observed through our interviews and provider surveys that many providers have the potential to serve P4HB consumers as well as to enroll them. However, there seemed to be a lack of education and outreach to these providers about the program and about how to assist clients with enrollment. Provider participation and engagement should be an ongoing process during the development and implementation of a program where providers are critical for its success.

Statutory Coherence

The second major finding is that statutory coherence does not necessarily result in successful policy implementation. The articulation of a program's goals and objectives through the provision of legal resources or a regulation does not necessarily guarantee implementation as intended. While the goals and objectives created for the P4HB program were rather precise and clear, these objectives were not necessarily well translated into program guidelines and materials. Not all implementing agencies understood the full scope of these goals and objectives or their role in implementing the program. P4HB struggled to achieve its initial program goals in part because providers and patients were confused about the nature and scope of the program. Only the CMOs seemed to have effectively obtained the program's goals and objectives, though many are still trying to find ways to enroll eligible clients and encourage current P4HB clients to utilize services.

One component of implementation that did largely reflect statutory intentions was finance. Financial resources from the legislature funded the waiver application and first-year operational expenses. Marketing funds were also allocated through an interagency agreement between DPH and DCH for the first year of P4HB, though the latter funds were expended by the end of the first year of the program, and additional funding has not been secured.

The "Field of Dreams" Approach

The quote from the popular film *Field of Dreams* states, "if you build it, they will come." Yet the idea that you can create a health care program, give it a name, and expect patients to enroll was not realized with the P4HB program. This study shows how, even with certain enabling factors such as insurance (via P4HB), access to care is not guaranteed and neither is successful program implementation.

One of the goals of the P4HB program was to expand access to Medicaid via the waiver program for low-income and uninsured women. Due to the factors identified in this study, it appears such access was far less than it could have been under different conditions. Key factors were the lack of understanding and awareness (by consumers and providers) of the nature and scope of the program. Also, the decision by DCH to auto enroll certain women into P4HB did not appear to increase utilization, as many women in the focus groups expressed surprise that they were enrolled and had not sought services through the program. Notably, other states such as Alabama and Mississippi have attempted this enrollment tactic and found that most auto enrolled women do not make use of their new coverage (Sonfield, 2011).

Findings from this study suggest that more expansive outreach and education is needed, and such efforts should continue throughout the life of the program. Due to poor outreach efforts, utilization was affected, and enrollment into P4HB was very low in both the FP and IPC components. These findings reflect a well-known problem common among social service programs such as Medicaid: agencies face serious compliance and administrative burdens that ultimately affect and limit participation among clients and providers. (Herd and Moynihan 2018; Herd et al. 2013; Fairbrother et al. 2004).

Recent studies of state Medicaid family planning waiver programs have highlighted the importance of outreach and branding for increasing enrollment and utilization. As noted by Sonfield, Aldrich, and Gold (2008), effective family planning waiver programs tend to conduct outreach to clients. Strategies include mass media campaigns (radio, TV ads) and the use of internet and web-based education, though Sonfield and colleagues explain that such expensive outreach efforts usually wane after the start of the waiver programs, just as they did in Georgia.

Successful states also tend to focus much of their outreach activities on community-level efforts, reaching consumers through local health programs and providers. Successful states also brand their family planning programs using creative names to reflect the purpose or goal of the program. States have used names like "Women's Health Waiver," and "Contraceptive Care" or Ccare, to denote the purpose and goal of their programs. As mentioned previously, the Georgia waiver program did not include family planning in its title due to concerns on the part of DCH and other proponents of the program over the conservative Georgia legislature, where some legislators are suspect of family planning policy. The lack of clear branding may have back-fired to cause poor utilization of Georgia's Medicaid family planning waiver program.

Implications for Policy and Practice

While these study findings cannot be generalized beyond Georgia's Planning for Healthy Babies (P4HB) program without considerations for context, results still offer insight for public policy and public health research. For states considering a Medicaid family planning waiver program specifically or even more broadly, for example a broader Section 1115 Medicaid expansion such as currently being considered in Georgia, the findings provide evidence about the facilitators and barriers to effective policy development and implementation. In particular, challenges can occur when development and implementation occurs through a top-down approach. In addition, having a coherent statute or regulation or even formal guidance about how a program will be structured does not guarantee successful implementation. Finally, when a state builds a program but does not collaborate effectively with available and willing stakeholders, the program may not be implemented as intended.

There are six major lessons that other states can learn from this study (1) formal program guidelines and legal tools (regulations in particular) should reflect input and consensus among all collaborating individuals and entities; (2) formal program guidelines should be explicit in the purpose and goals of the program or policy, as well as the allocation and availability of resources. Guidelines should also reflect eligibility, recruitment, enrollment, disenrollment, and service coverage and utilization; (3) resources should be available prior to and after implementation. These resources should include financial, human, and material resources to effectively reach the intended audience (or consumers); (5) consumer materials should be developed with input from the consumers and incorporated at an appropriate health literacy level; and (6) programs should be branded to inform consumers about the nature of the program and the intended audience.

CONCLUSION

As the health care community grows increasingly aware of the risk factors for maternal morbidity and mortality, more attention has been placed on improving women's health through early access to family planning and interpregnancy care. The CDC's Healthy People 2020 goals address family planning as a means to improve preconception health, reduce adolescent teen pregnancy and unintended pregnancy, and lower adverse infant health outcomes (CDC 2019). As the largest source of public funding for family planning, Medicaid plays an important role in providing access to family planning services for vulnerable population. Medicaid programs can be more effectively implemented not only through favorable legislation but also through collaborative development and implementation of policy.

REFERENCES

Adams, EK, Galactionova, Kenney, GM. Mediaid family planning waivers in 3 states: Did they reduce unwanted births? *Inquiry 2015: 52*; pii: 004695801558915.

Aday, LA and Andersen RA. A Framework for the Study of Access to Medical Care. *Health Services Res* 9:208-9, 1974.

Bierman, J, Dunlop, AL, Brady, C, Dubin, C, and Brann, AW. Promising Practices in Preconception Care for Women at Risk for Poor Health and

Pregnancy Outcomes. Matern Child Health J (2006): 10:S21-S28. doi: 10.1007/s10995-006-0097-8.

Centers for Disease Control and Prevention. *Healthy People 2020 Goals: Family Planning*. 2019 https://www.healthypeople.gov/2020/topics-objectives/topic/family-planning.

Centers for Medicare and Medicaid Services (CMS). *Family Planning Services Option and New Benefit Rules for Benchmark Plans*. July 2, 2010.

Creswell, J. and V. Plano Clark. *Designing and Conducting Mixed Methods Research*. Thousand Oaks, CA, Sage Publications. 2007.

Creswell, JW. *Qualitative Inquiry & Research Design: Choosing among Five Approaches*. Thousand Oaks, Sage. 2012.

Dean SV, Lassi ZS, Iman AM, Bhutta ZA. Preconception care: closing the gap in the continuum of care to accelerate improvements in maternal, newborn and child health. *Reprod Health.* 2014;*11* (Suppl 3):S1. Available at: http://www.ncbi.nlm.nih.gov/pmc/articles/ PMC4196556/ pdf/1742-4755-11-S3-S1.pdf. Accessed March 3, 2016.

Dunlop, AL, Adams, EK, Blake, SC, Hawley, J, Joski, P, Adams, EK. Georgia's Medicaid Family Planning Waiver: Working together with Title X to Enhance Contraception Access. *Women's Health Issues,* 2016.://dx.doi.org/10.1016/j.whi.2016.07.006

Dunlop, AL, Dubin, C, Raynor, BD, Bugg, GW, Schmotzer, B, Brann, SW. Interpregnancy Primary Care and Social Support for African American Women at Risk for Recurrent Very-low-birthweight Delivery: A Pilot Intervention. Matern Child Health J. (2008); 12:461-468. doi 10.1007/s10995-007-0279-z.

Edwards, J, Bronstein, J and Adams, K. *Evolution of Medicaid Family Planning Expansion*. Virginia: The CAN Corporation, 2003.

Fairbrother, G, Dutton, MJ, Bachrach, D, Newell, K, Boozang, P, and Cooper, R. Costs of Enrolling Children in Medicaid and SCHIP. *Health Affairs*, 2004: 23(1): 237-243.

Georgia Department of Community Health (GDCH). *Planning for Healthy Babies: Eligibility, 2019*. https://medicaid.georgia.gov/eligibility.

Georgia Department of Community Health (GDCH). *Planning for Healthy Babies Concept Paper*. December 17, 2009. https://dch.georgia.gov/sites/dch.georgia.gov/files/imported/vgn/images/portal/cit_1210/33/52/156793595PlanningforHealthyBabiesProgram121709Final.pdf.

Georgia Department of Community Health (GDCH). *Planning for Healthy Babies P4HB annual report, 2011*. https://medicaid.georgia.gov/sites/medicaid.georgia.gov/files/related_files/document/Annual%20Report%20for%20Program%20Year%201%20FINAL%2012.26.12.pdf.

Gold, RB, Sonfield, A, Frost, JJ, and Richards, CL. *Next Steps for American's Family Planning Program: Leveraging the Potential for Medicaid and Title X in an Evolving Health Care System*, New York: Guttmacher Institute, 2009.

Guba, EG and Lincoln, YS. *Effective Evaluation*. San Francisco, CA: Jossey-Bass Publishers. 1981.

Guttmacher Institute. *State Laws and Policies: Medicaid Family Planning Eligibility Expansions*. May 1, 2020. https://www. guttmacher.org/state-policy/explore/medicaid-family-planning-eligibility-expansions.

Hasstedt, K, Sonfield, Gold, RB. 2017. *Public Funding for Family Planning and Abortion Services, FY 1980-2015*. https://www. guttmacher.org/report/public-funding-family-planning-abortion-services-fy-1980-2015.

Herd P, and Moynihan DP. 2018. *Administrative Burden: Policymaking by Other Means*. Russell Sage Foundation.

Herd P, DeLeire T, Harvey H, Moynihan DP. Shifting Administrative Burden to the State: The Case of Medicaid Take-Up. *Public Administration Review*. 2013;73 (s1) :S69-S81.

Institute of Medicine (US) Committee on a Comprehensive Review of the HHS Office of Family Planning Title X Program: Stith Butler A, Wright Clayton E, editors. *A Review of the HHS Family Planning Program; Mission, Management, and Measurement of Results*. Washington (DC): National Academies Press (US), 2009.

Jourabchi, Z, Sharif, S, Lye, MS, Saeed, A, Khor, G, Tajuddin, S. Association between Preconception Care and Birth Outcomes. *Am J Health Promotion*. 2018. doi: 10.1177/0890117118779808.

Lindrooth, RC, McCullough, JS. The effect of Medicaid family planning expansion on unplanned births. *Women's Health Issues*. 2007; 17:66-74.

Mazmanian, DA and Sabatier, PA. *Implementation and Public Policy*. Lanham MD: University Press of America, 1989.

Oregon Health. *State of Oregon Family Planning Facts 2010, 2010*. http://public.health.oregon.gov/HealthyPeopleFamilies/ReproductiveSexualHealth/Resources/Documents/County_Data_Sheets/Edited%20FINAL%20State%20of%20Oregon%202010_03-08-11.pdf.

Redd, SK and Hall, KS. Medicaid Family Planning Expansions: The Effect of State Plan Amendments on Postpartum Contraceptive Use. *J Women's Health*. 2019; 28(4):551-559. http://doi.org/10.1089/jwh.2018.7129.

Sonfield, A, Aldrich, C, and Gold, RB. *State Government Innovation in the Design and Implementation of Medicaid Family Planning Expansions*. Guttmacher Institute. March 2008.

Sonfield, A, and Gold, RB. *Medicaid Family Planning Expansions: Lessons Learned and Implications for the Future*. December 2011.

Sonfield, A, and Gold, RB. *Medicaid Family Planning Expansions: Lessons Learned and Implications for the Future*. Guttmacher Institute. December 2011.

The Alan Guttmacher Institute (AGI). *Fulfilling the promise: Public policy and U.S. family planning clinics*. New York: AGI. 2000.

Yin, RK. Case study research: *Design and methods*. 4th edition. Thousand Oaks: Sage Publications, 2009.

In: Medicaid: Politics, Policy, and Key Issues ISBN: 978-1-53618-133-3
Editor: Daniel Lanford

Chapter 8

MEDICAID COVERAGE ACROSS THE INCOME DISTRIBUTION UNDER THE AFFORDABLE CARE ACT

***Charles Courtemanche*[1], *James Marton*[2] *and Aaron Yelowitz*[1,*]**
[1]Department of Economics, University of Kentucky, Lexington, KY, US
[2]Department of Economics, Georgia State University, Atlanta, GA, US

ABSTRACT

This chapter examines trends in Medicaid enrollment across the income distribution after the ACA's Medicaid expansion. Using data from the American Community Survey between 2012 and 2017, we compare Medicaid coverage over time in 9 states that expanded Medicaid in 2014 with no previous expansion for able-bodied, working-age adults with 12 states that had not expanded Medicaid by 2019 and also had no previous expansion for such adults. A difference-in-differences model is used to

[*] Corresponding Author's Email: aaron@uky.edu.

formalize this comparison. Similar to many previous studies, we find that Medicaid coverage increased dramatically for income-eligible adults under 138% of the federal poverty level ("FPL"). In addition, we show that Medicaid participation increased by 3.0 percentage points for those with incomes above 138% of the FPL from a pre-ACA baseline of 2.7% among this group. While we cannot say with certainty why these individuals were able to participate in Medicaid, we offer several potential explanations that should be the subject of future work. For example, consistent with our finding that improper enrollment rose more rapidly in some expansion states than others, it is possible that the ACA Medicaid expansions were administered differently at the state or local level than federal rules would require, similar to differences between effective tax rates and statutory tax rates in many transfer programs.

Keywords: Medicaid, Affordable Care Act, Effective Tax Rates, Health Care Finance

INTRODUCTION

Large gains in health insurance coverage were documented early in the rollout from the main components of the Affordable Care Act (ACA) in 2014 (Gruber and Sommers 2019). As originally envisioned in 2010, the ACA aimed to provide Medicaid coverage across all states for the poor, and state-run exchanges with private coverage for those who were more affluent. The intent was to provide different sources of health insurance coverage and different subsidies based on a person's economic circumstances. Lower-income individuals were meant to get larger subsidies. Medicaid generally provides more heavily subsidized coverage in comparison to Marketplace coverage and was targeted to those with incomes under 138% of the federal poverty level ("FPL") – roughly $35,000 for a family of four in 2019. Higher-income individuals were meant to get smaller subsidies. Private coverage, with less generous subsidies, was targeted to those with incomes between 138% and 400% of the FPL. While subsidized Marketplace coverage was made available nationally, the Supreme Court ruled in 2012 that the Medicaid expansion was optional for states. As a result, only 27 states (including the District of Columbia) expanded Medicaid in 2014

(Courtemanche et al. 2017). These new sources of subsidized coverage, along with other reforms to the non-group insurance market (such as community rating, guaranteed issue, and minimum coverage requirements) and the individual mandate represent the major 2014 components of the ACA.

Among states opting to expand Medicaid in 2014, the coverage gains in Kentucky were particularly noteworthy. Kentucky experienced the largest percentage point gain in insurance coverage out of all the states in 2014, primarily from increases in Medicaid enrollment (Courtemanche, Marton, and Yelowitz 2016). These gains received national attention. Artiga, Tolbert, and Rudowitz (2016) argue that "Kentucky has had one of the most successful ACA implementation experiences among states." Rosenbaum, Schmucker, and Rothenberg (2016) note that "among states that have implemented the Affordable Care Act's Medicaid expansion, Kentucky has been singular in its success." Atkin and Israel (2015) call Kentucky "the nation's most unlikely Obamacare success story." A state-commissioned study showed that Kentucky's Medicaid enrollment exceeded expectations (Deloitte 2015). Remarkably, the report notes that first-year Medicaid expansion enrollment in Kentucky exceeded estimates of the entire pool of potentially eligible enrollees. Yelowitz (2016) found that coverage gains across the income distribution in Kentucky did not always conform to predictions based on self-reports of income in the American Community Survey ("ACS") and programmatic rules. Specifically, 38% of new adults enrolled in Medicaid in Kentucky in 2014 – roughly 73,000 adults – appeared to be income-ineligible, with the vast majority instead qualifying for subsidized private coverage through the Marketplace.

The purpose of this chapter is to examine the impact of the ACA across the income distribution in multiple states, as opposed to focusing on one state, over the first four years of the rollout. Thus our findings contribute to the literature on the impact of the ACA broadly and the literature on the initial implementation of the ACA more specifically. Although many studies show the ACA's success in terms of reducing the number of uninsured individuals, a more nuanced definition of success is whether the ACA was carried out in the way it was intended. The intent was to provide different sources of health insurance coverage based on a person's economic circumstances. Contrary to this intent, our findings suggest that many working-age adults who were seemingly eligible for private coverage instead enrolled in Medicaid.

Using data from the ACS Public Use Microdata Sample ("PUMS") between 2012 and 2017, we examine 21 states where alternative routes for higher-income, abled-bodied, working-age adults to qualify for Medicaid were essentially non-existent prior to the implementation of the ACA in 2014. Of these 21 states, 9 of them implemented Medicaid expansions to 138% of the FPL in 2014, while 12 of them never implemented expansions (as of 2019). Our analysis goes through 2017, allowing us examine whether or not the impact of the ACA across the income distribution varied over time. We compare insurance changes among working-age adults from these two sets of states over time using a difference-in-differences ("DD") regression framework.

We find that the Medicaid expansions implemented in 2014 led to a 3.0 percentage point increase in Medicaid enrollment among working-age adults with incomes at or above 138% of the FPL, a sizable effect from a baseline rate of 2.7%. This translates into approximately 522,000 seemingly income-ineligible enrollees across the 9 states, and 47% of the entire gain in insurance coverage for these relatively higher income adults. In addition, this enrollment effect persists for individuals relatively far from the Medicaid threshold of 138% of the FPL and for full-time, full-year ("FTFY") workers, albeit with smaller baseline participation and marginal effects. The impact of the Medicaid expansions grows over time, with impacts two to three times as large in 2017 as 2014. Some of the Medicaid expansion states – in particular New Mexico, Kentucky, and West Virginia – have much larger enrollment effects than other expansion states. To summarize, many seemingly income-ineligible working-age adults in expansion states enroll in Medicaid rather than the subsidized private, Marketplace coverage.

While we cannot say with certainty why these individuals were able to participate in Medicaid, we offer several potential explanations that should be explored further in future work. One possible reason – echoed in longstanding literature on effective tax rates in welfare programs (Ziliak 2007) – is that the way ACA rules are enforced in states or localities differs from formal federal policy. This could arise, in part, due to the elevated federal match rate on new adults from the Medicaid expansion, which was 100% from 2014-2016, and 95% in 2017 (falling to 90% in 2020 and beyond). Without states assuming significant share of the costs for improperly enrolled adults, their incentives to aggressively monitor eligibility are diminished (Blase and Yelowitz 2019). Recent federal and state audits show program integrity issues related to eligibility, especially with the expansion population (U.S. Department of Health and Human Services 2017a,b, 2018a,b,c, 2019a,b; Louisiana Department of Health 2018; State of Oregon 2017; State of Montana 2018). The federal audits highlight systemic errors including neglecting to obtain proper documentation from applicants, failing to properly verify income eligibility, misclassifying individuals, and failing to properly verify citizenship. The state audits highlight weaknesses in preventive controls, detection, and monitoring. For example, several state audits mention reliance on the Federally Facilitated Marketplace to make final eligibility determinations. In addition, the Centers for Medicare and Medicaid Services ("CMS") has reported improper Medicaid payments amounting to $57 billion in 2019, or 14.9% of total federal spending on the program (CMS 2019).[1] It is also possible that our findings are partly attributable to issues with the ACS data, such as measurement error in insurance coverage, income, or eligibility for Medicaid.

---

[1] Blase and Yelowitz (2019) and Yelowitz and Blase (2019) argue that improper payments likely exceeded $75 billion in the 2019 CMS report, rather than the widely-reported $57 billion. The improper payment rate for fiscal year 2018 was likely at least 20%, given the construction of the three-year moving average for the improper payment rate and the selection of states.

INSTITUTIONAL BACKGROUND

Although the intent of the ACA is to provide near-universal health insurance coverage, the rules affect some subgroups more than others. Neither the elderly nor children should be dramatically affected by the ACA (Courtemanche et al. 2017, Courtemanche et al. 2018a, Courtemanche et al. 2018b, Courtemanche et al. 2019a, Courtemanche et al. 2019b). Virtually all elderly had coverage through Medicare (perhaps with supplemental coverage from other sources). In 2013, 98% of elderly had insurance coverage, with 94% having government coverage (Smith and Medalia 2014). Children tend to be covered at higher rates than working-age adults are, because comprehensive safety net programs (implemented long before the ACA) lead to high insurance coverage rates. In 2013, 93% of children had insurance coverage, with 41% receiving government health insurance. Medicaid and Children's Health Insurance Program (CHIP) expansions from the 1980s and 1990s allowed children with household incomes under certain multiples of the FPL to obtain public coverage at minimal cost regardless of family structure (Yelowitz 1995). Under Medicaid, newborns were eligible up to 185% of the FPL, children aged 1 to 5 were eligible up to 133% of the FPL, and children aged 6 to 18 were eligible up to 100% of the FPL. Many states expanded beyond these minimums through CHIP, often to 200% of the FPL or higher.[2]

We expect the largest impacts of the ACA on working-age adults, where working-age is defined as ages 19 to 64. Prior to the ACA, the main avenue for working-age adults to obtain health insurance was through private, employer-sponsored health insurance. In 2013, 82% of working-age adults had insurance coverage, with 68% having private coverage (Smith and

[2] The CHIP program often had monthly premiums which could affect enrollment among uninsured children (Marton 2007; Kenney et al. 2007a, 2007b; Marton, Ketsche, and Zhou 2010; Marton, Searcy, and Ghandhi 2010; Marton and Talbert 2010). Given the relative ease of sign-up – even prior to the ACA – such uninsured children might be viewed as "conditionally covered" (meaning they can become insured relatively easily if they get sick; see Marton and Yelowitz 2015). Some of the rise in Medicaid / CHIP enrollments – in both expansion and non-expansion states – could be due to the individual mandate and other outreach efforts compelling eligible children to enroll, known as a "woodwork effect" (Frean, Gruber, and Sommers 2017).

Medalia 2014). The non-group (individual) market was very small prior to the ACA. A small percentage of individuals involved with the armed forces obtained private insurance through the military, called Tricare. In many states, able-bodied, childless, working-age adults did not qualify for Medicaid. Medicaid was generally restricted to narrow categories of adults. Pregnant women with incomes below 185% of the FPL were eligible for Medicaid. The disabled could potentially qualify for Medicaid through Supplemental Security Income ("SSI"), with a national income limit of approximately 77% of the FPL, or they may qualify for Medicare after two years on disability insurance; approximately 57% of disabled adults received government health insurance in 2013. Parents or caretakers could qualify for Medicaid, with income thresholds as high as 57% of the FPL (Kaiser Family Foundation 2013). In addition, foster care children up to age 26, individuals in the Breast and Cervical Cancer Treatment Program, the Medically Needy (Spend Down) Program, the Transitional Medical Assistance program, and the Nursing Facility Services Program also received Medicaid.[3]

The 2014 rollout of the main components of the ACA dramatically changed opportunities for working-age adults. The ACA provided a number of reforms, primarily to the non-group (individual) market and to the Medicaid program. As discussed in Courtemanche et al. (2017), 27 states (including the District of Columbia) expanded their Medicaid programs to 138% of the FPL in the beginning of 2014. For working-age adults in Medicaid expansion states, the vast majority of uninsured individuals became newly eligible for Medicaid in 2014 if their incomes were below this

---

[3] Some of these less prominent programs have income thresholds exceeding 138% of the FPL, yet apply to very narrow groups. The Breast and Cervical Cancer Early Detection Program had a threshold of 250% of the FPL (Kaiser Family Foundation 2019a). However, national enrollment in the program ranged from 56,938 women in 2013, to 46,143 in 2014, to 26,577 in 2015. For children who were in foster care on their eighteenth birthday, Medicaid eligibility would extend to age 26 starting in 2014 under the ACA (Pergamit et al. 2012). In 2010, approximately 28,000 youth aged out of foster care nationally, again suggesting little impact on the overall estimates. See Palmer et al. (2017) for additional details about eligibility for Medicaid through foster care. Other programs – such as Transitional Medicaid Assistance – are considerably larger (reaching 3.7 million working parents in 2011), but end coverage for parents and other adults at 138% of the FPL after the implementation of the ACA (Schneider 2018). Although dated, the Medically Needy program applied to approximately 929,000 adults (and 2,836,000 individuals) in 2009, yet had income thresholds far below 138% FPL in virtually all states (Kaiser Family Foundation 2012).

threshold. Relative to private coverage, Medicaid generally provides more generous subsidies with respect to copayments and deductibles and has no monthly premiums (Marton 2007). In non-expansion states, adults with incomes under 100% of the FPL can purchase private health insurance via the Marketplace, but do not receive a subsidy (i.e., they do not qualify for the premium tax credit). Insurance is still community rated and guaranteed issue, thereby providing implicit subsidies to those with high medical expenses. Adults in non-expansion states with incomes of 100% to 138% of the FPL can purchase a highly subsidized Marketplace plan.[4]

Importantly, working-age adults with incomes at or above 138% of the FPL were generally not eligible for Medicaid. In all states, adults with incomes of 138% to 400% of the FPL are eligible to purchase private, non-group health insurance via the Marketplace, with a sliding-scale subsidy from the premium tax credit. Various cost-sharing provisions from the Marketplace plans are less generous once income exceeds 250% of the FPL. Those with incomes above 400% of the FPL can purchase unsubsidized insurance from the Marketplace (or pay the penalty associated with the individual mandate).

DATA

We use individual data from the ACS PUMS one-year estimates, conducted by the U.S. Census Bureau, to examine changes in insurance coverage and insurance sources from 2012 to 2017. The ACS is a widely used data source because of its large sample size, mandatory respondent participation, breadth of questions on sources of insurance, focus on contemporaneous coverage, and uniformity of questions over time.

We focus on working-age adults aged 19 to 64 in the 2012 to 2017 ACS, giving us four years of data after the rollout of the biggest pieces of the ACA. We analyze 21 states – which we call "new expanders" and "never

[4] No individual mandate exists for this group; consumers can claim a coverage exemption even though some privately subsidized plans involve virtually no cost to the consumer (U.S. Department of Treasury, 2019).

expanders." The new expanders were 9 states that expanded Medicaid in 2014 and had not implemented earlier broad-based Medicaid expansions for adults. They include Arkansas, Kentucky, Michigan, Nevada, New Hampshire, New Mexico, North Dakota, Ohio, and West Virginia. None of these states implemented the expansions early, and none had subgroups (other than pregnant women) eligible for coverage above 138% of the FPL. Of these nine expansion states, several had approved Section 1115 waivers often related to work requirements.[5] These waivers did not affect the income threshold for eligibility; thus, we should not expect increases in Medicaid coverage above that threshold. The never expanders were 12 states that did not expand by 2019 (and had not implemented earlier expansions). They include Alabama, Florida, Georgia, Kansas, Mississippi, Missouri, North Carolina, Oklahoma, South Carolina, South Dakota, Texas, and Wyoming. In these states, the Medicaid income eligibility threshold was between 17 to 54% of the FPL for adult caretakers in families. For childless adults, none of these states extended eligibility for coverage. Consequently, all 21 states had weak health insurance safety nets for working-age adults prior to the ACA, and there is little reason to expect increased Medicaid take-up at incomes higher than 138% of the FPL in any state after the rollout.[6]

The insurance questions in the ACS form the core of the analysis and have both advantages and drawbacks. The focus on current coverage in the ACS leads to less confusion than with other public surveys such as the Current Population Survey, which asks respondents to recall coverage in the previous calendar year (Klerman et al. 2009).[7] In addition, the ACS is continuously fielded during the year. One drawback with the public version of the ACS is that the respondent's interview date within the year is

---

[5] Kaiser Family Foundation (2019b).

[6] As noted in Courtemanche et al., (2017), 18 of the 27 Medicaid expansion states in 2014 had some form of partial expansion prior to 2014. In addition, two non-adopting states (Tennessee and Wisconsin) are excluded because they had a previous, partial Medicaid expansion; see Kaestner et al., (2017). Of states that have expanded Medicaid coverage outside of the traditional "categorically eligible" group (low-income children, pregnant women, disabled, blind, and elderly SSI recipients, adult caretakers), only three jurisdictions (Indiana, Minnesota, and Washington DC) have income limits exceeding 138% of the FPL after 2013, and none are included in our analysis (Kaiser Family Foundation, 2019c).

[7] The ACS asks: "Is this person CURRENTLY covered by any of the following types of health insurance or health coverage plans?" (U.S. Department of Commerce, 2019).

unknown. However, virtually all changes from the ACA occurred at the beginning 2014, limiting the need for precise interview timing. As discussed below, this includes the rollout of the Medicaid expansions for almost all of the selected states we consider.

ACS respondents may report more than one source of coverage. In our tables below, we create categories for seven sources of coverage, where the first six sources are defined as having coverage from that source *only*. The sources are employer-sponsored health insurance ("ESHI"), non-group (individual), Tricare, Medicaid, Medicare, and VA. The final category is defined as "multiple," meaning the individual reports coverage in at least two of the coverage sources. In practice, approximately 8% of the sample reports multiple contemporaneous sources, and this percentage changes very little over the time. Adding up all seven sources of coverage gives the overall insurance coverage rate.

Several limitations to measuring health insurance coverage with the ACS should be noted. Prior work has shown that private, non-group coverage is overstated in the ACS, both as a sole type of comprehensive coverage and as reported in combination with other coverage types. Substantive differences in individual coverage exist between survey estimates and administrative counts from the National Association of Insurance Commissioners (Abraham, Karaca-Mandic, and Boudreaux 2013). Mach and O'Hara (2011) find that the population that reports non-group health insurance coverage in combination with other sources is small, but it seems to be misreported, especially in combination with employer-based insurance. Our results below reveal gains in non-group coverage were small in Medicaid-expansion states after the reform (for adults above the Medicaid eligibility threshold), and these studies suggest that even those small gains may be overstated.

In addition, the ACS survey instrument does not include any state-specific names for Medicaid, and the survey instrument was not updated to reflect newly available Marketplace coverage. Thus, there is concern that ACS respondents may be confused about their coverage type, leading to additional misreporting on household surveys post-2013, after the major ACA provisions were implemented. Existing evidence suggests that public health insurance coverage tends to be underreported in such surveys. Lurie and Pearce (2019) compared health insurance sources from the Internal Revenue Service tax form 1095 to measures from various surveys for 2016. For individuals younger than age 65, administrative tax data revealed 75.6 million covered life years from all public insurance sources, while the point of interview measure in the ACS revealed 66.6 million individuals. Boudreaux et al. (2019) found that "starting in 2014, there was a large [Medicaid] undercount in expansion states that was absent in non-expansion states," leading to "downwardly biased estimates of expansion on means-tested coverage in the ACS relative to administrative records." The undercount exceeded 10% in expansion states for every year between 2014 and 2016, with ACS data missing approximately 3.9 million Medicaid enrollees. In contrast, non-expansion states had Medicaid enrollment counts far closer to administrative sources.

We first examine changes in coverage. In the calculations below, it should be noted that population changes from year-to-year (as well as within income groupings). To allocate gains in coverage to specific sources, we use average population across all years for working-age adults. Our insurance sources (including uninsured and multiple sources) add up to 100% in each year. We approximate the change (in overall coverage or attributable to a specific source) by multiplying the percentage point change by average population, or by comparing that source-specific change to the percentage point change in the overall insured population. Table 1 shows health insurance coverage from 2012 to 2017 for the 9 states that expanded Medicaid in 2014. Across these states, total population averaged 22.8 million and insurance coverage increased by 10.4 percentage points from 2012 to 2017, leading to 2.4 million more adults having coverage. Medicaid coverage increased by approximately 1.7 million, translating into approximately 69% of the total gains. Overall, there were also modest gains from employer coverage and non-group coverage (387,000 and 319,000, respectively), responsible for 16% and 13% of the gains, respectively. Employer coverage could increase due to improving economic conditions, the individual mandate, and the ACA's employer mandate (effective 2015). Non-group (individual) insurance should increase due to the establishment of subsidized Marketplace coverage and the individual mandate. There was modest growth in Medicare coverage and a modest reduction in Tricare and VA coverage.

We break out the 22.8 million adults in these 9 states between 2012 and 2017 into 5.4 million with incomes under 138% of the FPL, 4.3 million with incomes between 138% to 249% of the FPL, and 13.1 million with incomes at or above 250% of the FPL.[8] For poor Medicaid-eligible adults (<138% of the FPL), Medicaid is responsible for 92% of the insurance gains from 2012 to 2017. Overall coverage grew in these 9 states by 21.3 percentage points overall. Approximately 1.1 million low-income adults gained Medicaid. There were small and offsetting changes in employer and non-group coverage.

For the near-poor (138% to 249% of the FPL) in these 9 states, one would expect that many of the 4.3 million would not be Medicaid eligible during the year, but would be eligible for subsidized private coverage through the Marketplace. Insurance coverage increased by 13.7 percentage points among this near-poor group. Overall, the descriptive estimates would suggest that 458,000 in this group (that are seemingly income-ineligible) gained Medicaid coverage, representing 78% of the overall gain in coverage. Gains in non-group individual coverage were one-fifth as large – around 103,000 adults – in these 9 states between 2012 and 2017.

Given that Medicaid enrollment gains might be explained to some degree by income variation around the 138% of the FPL cut-off, we also examine those with incomes at or above 250% of the FPL (roughly $65,000 for a family of four in 2019). For the 13.1 million non-poor (i.e., income ≥ 250% of the FPL) in these 9 states, overall insurance coverage grew by 4.0 percentage points, translating into around 525,000 more insured overall. Even among this higher income group, Medicaid grew by 342,000, and represented 65% of the change in coverage. Gains in non-group, individual coverage were one-half as large – around 157,000 adults. Employer coverage grew modestly, and there were small changes in other categories between 2012 and 2017.

[8] Throughout the analysis, individuals who were not assigned a poverty level in the ACS PUMS data were grouped with those under 138% of the FPL.

Table 1. New expanders, coverage for working-age adults

					Private Sources			Public Sources			
Income bin	Year	Population	Any coverage	Uninsured	ESHI	Non-group	Tricare	Medicaid	Medicare	VA	Multiple
All	2012	22,846,118	18,319,724 (26,483) 80.2%	4,526,394 (26,483) 19.8%	12,712,229 (35,496) 55.6%	1,245,129 (17,128) 5.5%	217,383 (7,249) 1.0%	1,802,104 (18,825) 7.9%	344,938 (8,044) 1.5%	148,388 (5,092) 0.6%	1,849,551 (19,840) 8.1%
	2013	22,833,979	18,420,892 (25,656) 80.7%	4,413,087 (25,656) 19.3%	12,745,386 (35,231) 55.8%	1,308,355 (16,797) 5.7%	204,640 (6,711) 0.9%	1,918,004 (17,792) 8.4%	355,518 (7,373) 1.6%	140,927 (5,065) 0.6%	1,748,062 (17,274) 7.7%
	2014	22,834,946	19,588,965 (23,764) 85.8%	3,245,981 (23,764) 14.2%	12,968,409 (33,739) 56.8%	1,540,242 (15,281) 6.7%	193,115 (6,156) 0.8%	2,603,561 (21,102) 11.4%	381,567 (7,972) 1.7%	135,201 (4,658) 0.6%	1,766,870 (15,731) 7.7%
	2015	22,811,536	20,403,388 (20,177) 89.4%	2,408,148 (20,177) 10.6%	12,905,551 (29,436) 56.6%	1,675,035 (16,924) 7.3%	194,350 (6,396) 0.9%	3,244,624 (23,852) 14.2%	388,930 (8,543) 1.7%	115,896 (4,790) 0.5%	1,879,002 (18,660) 8.2%
	2016	22,770,361	20,632,784 (20,063) 90.6%	2,137,577 (20,063) 9.4%	12,943,081 (36,223) 56.8%	1,693,985 (18,674) 7.4%	195,914 (6,676) 0.9%	3,415,042 (27,140) 15.0%	378,102 (8,664) 1.7%	106,092 (4,247) 0.5%	1,900,567 (16,688) 8.3%
	2017	22,764,726	20,613,557 (21,258) 90.6%	2,151,169 (21,258) 9.4%	13,045,964 (41,855) 57.3%	1,575,986 (20,395) 6.9%	189,218 (6,918) 0.8%	3,446,529 (25,481) 15.1%	376,991 (7,997) 1.7%	108,827 (3,879) 0.5%	1,870,040 (16,277) 8.2%
<138% FPL (or missing)	2012	5,623,770	3,486,137 (15,387) 62.0%	2,137,633 (15,387) 38.0%	1,090,955 (12,513) 19.4%	266,930 (6,339) 4.7%	37,225 (2,250) 0.7%	1,312,116 (13,394) 23.3%	158,833 (5,572) 2.8%	54,192 (2,715) 1.0%	565,886 (10,171) 10.1%

Table 1. (Continued)

					Private Sources			Public Sources			
Income bin	Year	Population	Any coverage	Uninsured	ESHI	Non-group	Tricare	Medicaid	Medicare	VA	Multiple
	2013	5,614,596	3,565,434 (14,196) 63.5%	2,049,162 (14,196) 36.5%	1,099,141 (14,619) 19.6%	295,350 (6,230) 5.3%	35,780 (2,751) 0.6%	1,403,359 (14,513) 25.0%	152,771 (4,864) 2.7%	49,542 (2,832) 0.9%	529,491 (10,279) 9.4%
	2014	5,508,264	4,063,643 (14,482) 73.8%	1,444,621 (14,482) 26.2%	1,094,395 (14,752) 19.9%	345,795 (8,844) 6.3%	36,913 (3,194) 0.7%	1,796,167 (14,367) 32.6%	170,737 (5,695) 3.1%	45,139 (2,576) 0.8%	574,497 (8,947) 10.4%
	2015	5,365,608	4,356,251 (13,443) 81.2%	1,009,357 (13,443) 18.8%	1,022,556 (12,108) 19.1%	347,018 (8,771) 6.5%	30,246 (2,412) 0.6%	2,142,545 (17,824) 39.9%	167,561 (5,805) 3.1%	36,519 (2,519) 0.7%	609,806 (10,135) 11.4%
	2016	5,201,206	4,321,325 (14,569) 83.1%	879,881 (14,569) 16.9%	993,119 (13,680) 19.1%	345,588 (7,288) 6.6%	35,697 (3,113) 0.7%	2,165,387 (16,750) 41.6%	161,572 (5,395) 3.1%	31,557 (2,505) 0.6%	588,405 (10,180) 11.3%
	2017	5,024,634	4,187,283 (11,749) 83.3%	837,351 (11,749) 16.7%	917,624 (12,272) 18.3%	303,886 (8,257) 6.0%	27,672 (1,969) 0.6%	2,159,666 (18,316) 43.0%	160,896 (5,733) 3.2%	32,994 (2,232) 0.7%	584,545 (10,140) 11.6%
138%-249% FPL	2012	4,266,176	3,067,751 (13,293) 71.9%	1,198,425 (13,293) 28.1%	1,962,182 (15,908) 46.0%	239,058 (6,345) 5.6%	43,018 (3,362) 1.0%	305,727 (8,296) 7.2%	105,314 (3,915) 2.5%	42,375 (2,675) 1.0%	370,077 (8,528) 8.7%
	2013	4,332,888	3,147,580 (13,449) 72.6%	1,185,308 (13,449) 27.4%	2,034,852 (16,179) 47.0%	238,936 (6,405) 5.5%	39,311 (2,953) 0.9%	327,046 (7,459) 7.5%	108,712 (4,637) 2.5%	39,711 (2,527) 0.9%	359,012 (7,994) 8.3%

					Private Sources			Public Sources			
Income bin	Year	Population	Any coverage	Uninsured	ESHI	Non-group	Tricare	Medicaid	Medicare	VA	Multiple
	2014	4,428,554	3,531,693 (11,840) 79.7%	896,861 (11,840) 20.3%	2,117,241 (16,865) 47.8%	341,320 (7,393) 7.7%	37,253 (2,550) 0.8%	501,347 (9,935) 11.3%	118,209 (4,467) 2.7%	36,599 (2,519) 0.8%	379,724 (8,156) 8.6%
	2015	4,287,873	3,619,892 (10,544) 84.4%	667,981 (10,544) 15.6%	1,997,111 (15,456) 46.6%	366,294 (6,840) 8.5%	39,780 (3,014) 0.9%	667,695 (11,089) 15.6%	115,016 (4,236) 2.7%	32,448 (2,139) 0.8%	401,548 (8,274) 9.4%
	2016	4,186,655	3,596,347 (9,840) 85.9%	590,308 (9,840) 14.1%	1,926,423 (14,595) 46.0%	359,789 (8,597) 8.6%	34,292 (2,744) 0.8%	731,500 (12,840) 17.5%	114,543 (5,164) 2.7%	29,247 (2,560) 0.7%	400,553 (7,873) 9.6%
	2017	4,175,478	3,573,777 (9,922) 85.6%	601,701 (9,922) 14.4%	1,930,603 (16,943) 46.2%	335,983 (7,616) 8.0%	30,252 (2,493) 0.7%	746,776 (11,941) 17.9%	118,114 (4,373) 2.8%	25,374 (2,096) 0.6%	386,675 (8,672) 9.3%
≥250% FPL	2012	12,956,172	11,765,835 (16,846) 90.8%	1,190,337 (16,846) 9.2%	9,659,092 (24,820) 74.6%	739,141 (13,486) 5.7%	137,141 (5,949) 1.1%	184,261 (6,860) 1.4%	80,790 (4,178) 0.6%	51,821 (2,834) 0.4%	913,589 (13,480) 7.1%
	2013	12,886,495	11,707,879 (13,515) 90.9%	1,178,616 (13,515) 9.1%	9,611,392 (21,966) 74.6%	774,070 (12,325) 6.0%	129,551 (5,713) 1.0%	187,599 (6,091) 1.5%	94,035 (3,572) 0.7%	51,674 (3,369) 0.4%	859,560 (11,349) 6.7%
	2014	12,898,128	11,993,630 (15,447) 93.0%	904,498 (15,447) 7.0%	9,756,773 (25,601) 75.6%	853,129 (12,387) 6.6%	118,948 (4,215) 0.9%	306,047 (7,045) 2.4%	92,621 (3,857) 0.7%	53,464 (3,130) 0.4%	812,648 (10,049) 6.3%
	2015	13,158,055	12,427,245 (12,125) 94.4%	730,810 (12,125) 5.6%	9,885,884 (21,161) 75.1%	961,724 (13,209) 7.3%	124,324 (5,397) 0.9%	434,383 (9,684) 3.3%	106,353 (3,963) 0.8%	46,930 (3,346) 0.4%	867,649 (11,844) 6.6%

Table 1. (Continued)

					Private Sources			Public Sources			
Income bin	Year	Population	Any coverage	Uninsured	ESHI	Non-group	Tricare	Medicaid	Medicare	VA	Multiple
	2016	13,382,500	12,715,113	667,387	10,023,539	988,609	125,927	518,154	101,987	45,288	911,609
			(13,215)	(13,215)	(22,764)	(14,717)	(5,519)	(12,596)	(4,375)	(2,531)	(12,055)
			95.0%	5.0%	74.9%	7.4%	0.9%	3.9%	0.8%	0.3%	6.8%
	2017	13,564,614	12,852,498	712,116	10,197,737	936,118	131,295	540,089	97,981	50,459	898,821
			(13,548)	(13,548)	(26,827)	(15,384)	(6,081)	(10,925)	(3,677)	(2,887)	(12,778)
			94.8%	5.2%	75.2%	6.9%	1.0%	4.0%	0.7%	0.4%	6.6%

Source: Authors' tabulation of the 2012-2017 American Community Survey data for working-age adults aged 19-64.

Notes: Individuals reporting more than one source of coverage are included in the final column. All numbers are weighted using ACS person weight. There are between 218,973 and 223,542 unweighted observations in the 2012-2017 ACS, respectively. Standard errors are in parentheses and computed using ACS replicate weights. Approximately 3% of adults did not have a poverty line measure; they are included in the 0-137% of FPL category. "New expanders" includes 9 states that expanded Medicaid in 2014 but not before: Arkansas, Kentucky, Michigan, Nevada, New Hampshire, New Mexico, North Dakota, Ohio, and West Virginia.

To summarize the main findings of Table 1, we are focusing on the 9 states that expanded their Medicaid program via the ACA in 2014 and previously lacked a deep safety net in terms insurance coverage for working-age adults above 138% of the FPL. Overall, more than 2.4 million adults gained coverage in these 9 states between 2012 and 2017; a 10.4 percentage point increase. Medicaid coverage alone increased 7.2 percentage points, or approximately 1.7 million working-age adults. Of these, approximately 800,000 individuals appeared to gain Medicaid coverage for which they were seemingly income-ineligible, or about 43% of the overall gain in Medicaid coverage.[9] In principle, many would be eligible for subsidized private coverage through the Marketplace.

Table 2 reports changes in health insurance coverage over time for the 12 states that did not expand Medicaid via the ACA by 2019. Total population averaged 56.8 million and insurance coverage increased by 7.1 percentage points, leading to approximately 4.0 million more working-age adults having coverage between 2012 and 2017. Medicaid coverage increased by 227,000 (0.4 percentage points), translating into approximately 6% of the total gains over these six years. Overall, there were also larger contributions from employer coverage and non-group coverage, responsible for 52% and 45% of the insurance gains, respectively. Employer coverage grew by 3.7 percentage points, and non-group coverage grew by 3.2 percentage points, translating into 2.1 million and 1.8 million newly covered, respectively.

Within these 12 non-expansion states, we break out the average population of 56.8 million into 13.7 million with incomes under 138% of the FPL, 11.5 million with incomes between 138% to 249% of the FPL, and 31.6 million with incomes at or above 250% of the FPL, as we did with the expansion states. For poor working-age adults in non-expansion states (i.e., with incomes under 138% of the FPL), Medicaid is responsible for 18% of the insurance gains from 2012 to 2017 (versus 92% in expansion states). Overall insurance coverage grew by 10.2 percentage points (far less than in expansion states), and Medicaid coverage grew by 1.8 percentage points.

---

[9] The enrollment of 800,000 ineligible working-age adults comes from the time-series descriptive analysis in Table 1; the DD estimate from Table 3 suggests 522,000 ineligible adults.

Approximately 246,000 low-income adults gained Medicaid. There were sizable gains for employer and individual coverage, 2.7 and 4.0 percentage points, translating to gains in coverage of 370,000 and 548,000, respectively.

For near-poor working-age adults in these 12 states, one would expect that many of the 11.5 million would not be Medicaid eligible, yet many would be eligible for subsidized Marketplace plans. Insurance coverage increased by 9.4 percentage points (again, smaller than for this group in expansion states), and Medicaid coverage increased by 1.2 percentage points (dramatically lower than the 10.7 percentage point gain in expansion states). Overall, the estimates would suggest nearly 1.1 million working-age adults in this near-poor group gained coverage between 2012 and 2017. Of these, 137,000 gained Medicaid coverage, representing 13% (rather than 78%) of the overall gain in coverage, though they are seemingly income-ineligible for Medicaid. Gains in non-group individual coverage were more than four times as large – around 631,000 adults.

For the 31.6 million non-poor working-age adults in these 12 non-expansion states, coverage grew by 2.9 percentage points (versus 4.0 percentage points for this group in the 9 expansion states), translating into around 917,000 more insured. Among this income group, Medicaid coverage grew by 158,000, and represented 17% (rather than 65% in the 9 expansion states) of the change in coverage. Gains in non-group individual coverage were four times as large – around 632,000 adults. None of these states expanded Medicaid by 2019, and none had significant safety net insurance coverage for non-elderly childless adults.

Overall, the descriptive coverage estimates in Table 2 for the non-expansion states find approximately 4.0 million non-elderly adults gained some form of insurance coverage between 2012 and 2017. Of these, 227,000 (6%) gained coverage via Medicaid. Although gains in Medicaid were very small in non-expansion states compared to expansion states, among those gaining coverage via Medicaid, 54% appeared to be income-ineligible.

Table 2. Never expanders, coverage for working-age adults

					Private Sources			Public Sources			
Income bin	Year	Population	Any coverage	Uninsured	ESHI	Non-group	Tricare	Medicaid	Medicare	VA	Multiple
All	2012	55,635,019	40,709,840 (50,033) 73.2%	14,925,179 (50,033) 26.8%	27,376,530 (52,753) 49.2%	3,412,407 (28,457) 6.1%	1,052,882 (15,984) 1.9%	3,349,568 (23,239) 6.0%	750,194 (9,636) 1.3%	385,706 (8,668) 0.7%	4,382,554 (24,090) 7.9%
	2013	55,998,623	41,189,966 (58,367) 73.6%	14,808,657 (58,367) 26.4%	27,816,700 (62,198) 49.7%	3,617,657 (24,869) 6.5%	1,094,482 (16,508) 2.0%	3,367,270 (27,439) 6.0%	787,122 (12,448) 1.4%	363,549 (8,596) 0.6%	4,143,181 (28,139) 7.4%
	2014	56,565,140	43,667,078 (54,778) 77.2%	12,898,062 (54,778) 22.8%	28,825,375 (58,907) 51.0%	4,856,881 (32,214) 8.6%	1,059,742 (14,645) 1.9%	3,527,730 (25,901) 6.2%	837,832 (11,217) 1.5%	362,894 (7,936) 0.6%	4,196,624 (28,039) 7.4%
	2015	57,119,240	45,705,274 (44,433) 80.0%	11,413,966 (44,433) 20.0%	29,652,814 (56,714) 51.9%	5,795,369 (31,267) 10.1%	1,073,413 (16,993) 1.9%	3,670,208 (25,961) 6.4%	843,600 (11,224) 1.5%	345,017 (9,253) 0.6%	4,324,846 (25,921) 7.6%
	2016	57,486,065	46,533,211 (40,148) 80.9%	10,952,854 (40,148) 19.1%	30,147,158 (51,462) 52.4%	5,900,180 (33,750) 10.3%	1,052,202 (14,228) 1.8%	3,746,626 (33,836) 6.5%	871,908 (12,768) 1.5%	338,294 (8,083) 0.6%	4,476,837 (28,312) 7.8%
	2017	58,034,073	46,619,659 (51,447) 80.3%	11,414,414 (51,447) 19.7%	30,718,967 (62,735) 52.9%	5,423,516 (38,958) 9.3%	1,064,780 (13,853) 1.8%	3,706,317 (27,433) 6.4%	875,647 (12,588) 1.5%	335,280 (8,456) 0.6%	4,495,151 (28,384) 7.7%
<138% FPL (or missing)	2012	14,374,649	7,427,499 (26,950) 51.7%	6,947,150 (26,950) 48.3%	2,482,120 (20,247) 17.3%	744,420 (13,689) 5.2%	230,398 (6,273) 1.6%	2,296,687 (17,214) 16.0%	319,132 (7,466) 2.2%	135,437 (5,199) 0.9%	1,219,307 (14,263) 8.5%

Table 2. (Continued)

					Private Sources			Public Sources			
Income bin	Year	Population	Any coverage	Uninsured	ESHI	Non-group	Tricare	Medicaid	Medicare	VA	Multiple
	2013	14,253,377	7,476,924 (28,671) 52.5%	6,776,453 (28,671) 47.5%	2,564,616 (21,295) 18.0%	798,858 (10,881) 5.6%	239,765 (7,028) 1.7%	2,272,089 (20,539) 15.9%	341,919 (8,407) 2.4%	126,681 (4,761) 0.9%	1,132,995 (13,203) 7.9%
	2014	14,031,179	8,052,753 (32,618) 57.4%	5,978,426 (32,618) 42.6%	2,687,855 (22,255) 19.2%	1,113,416 (15,067) 7.9%	219,867 (6,513) 1.6%	2,329,305 (20,978) 16.6%	356,156 (7,498) 2.5%	121,445 (4,750) 0.9%	1,224,709 (12,977) 8.7%
	2015	13,622,028	8,309,675 (23,498) 61.0%	5,312,353 (23,498) 39.0%	2,696,228 (20,658) 19.8%	1,342,915 (16,138) 9.9%	215,844 (5,427) 1.6%	2,363,173 (19,358) 17.3%	356,172 (8,181) 2.6%	112,507 (4,062) 0.8%	1,222,834 (12,510) 9.0%
	2016	13,171,371	8,238,949 (24,439) 62.6%	4,932,422 (24,439) 37.4%	2,700,006 (20,777) 20.5%	1,323,627 (14,070) 10.0%	215,805 (5,627) 1.6%	2,320,541 (23,577) 17.6%	355,719 (8,593) 2.7%	105,054 (4,119) 0.8%	1,218,196 (14,093) 9.2%
	2017	12,761,687	7,903,956 (23,081) 61.9%	4,857,731 (23,081) 38.1%	2,558,115 (19,889) 20.0%	1,179,932 (15,571) 9.2%	219,028 (5,818) 1.7%	2,275,268 (19,745) 17.8%	349,170 (7,175) 2.7%	97,812 (3,891) 0.8%	1,224,631 (14,140) 9.6%
138%-249% FPL	2012	11,165,078	7,116,303 (22,799) 63.7%	4,048,775 (22,799) 36.3%	4,446,949 (23,266) 39.8%	609,411 (10,769) 5.5%	192,318 (7,634) 1.7%	662,318 (10,739) 5.9%	238,980 (5,776) 2.1%	104,560 (5,044) 0.9%	861,766 (12,647) 7.7%
	2013	11,417,744	7,340,073 (25,504) 64.3%	4,077,671 (25,504) 35.7%	4,647,329 (23,514) 40.7%	659,775 (11,793) 5.8%	211,087 (6,520) 1.8%	671,135 (12,834) 5.9%	236,606 (6,835) 2.1%	92,783 (3,682) 0.8%	821,355 (12,505) 7.2%

					Private Sources			Public Sources			
Income bin	Year	Population	Any coverage	Uninsured	ESHI	Non-group	Tricare	Medicaid	Medicare	VA	Multiple
	2014	11,675,999	8,108,375 (24,876) 69.4%	3,567,624 (24,876) 30.6%	4,895,215 (22,748) 41.9%	1,046,697 (16,582) 9.0%	204,733 (5,984) 1.8%	740,483 (11,368) 6.3%	258,411 (6,855) 2.2%	95,480 (5,072) 0.8%	867,355 (12,274) 7.4%
	2015	11,595,625	8,493,879 (24,842) 73.3%	3,101,746 (24,842) 26.7%	4,931,573 (22,367) 42.5%	1,365,267 (15,589) 11.8%	204,526 (6,570) 1.8%	774,828 (12,280) 6.7%	243,285 (5,721) 2.1%	91,190 (4,671) 0.8%	883,210 (12,542) 7.6%
	2016	11,458,342	8,487,632 (22,384) 74.1%	2,970,710 (22,384) 25.9%	4,832,866 (23,838) 42.2%	1,357,962 (18,396) 11.9%	196,185 (7,021) 1.7%	834,637 (14,264) 7.3%	249,681 (6,412) 2.2%	84,040 (4,612) 0.7%	932,260 (12,493) 8.1%
	2017	11,544,025	8,436,219 (26,727) 73.1%	3,107,806 (26,727) 26.9%	4,889,265 (26,981) 42.4%	1,264,765 (18,074) 11.0%	200,738 (7,277) 1.7%	814,830 (12,857) 7.1%	266,724 (6,676) 2.3%	88,149 (4,305) 0.8%	911,751 (13,120) 7.9%
≥250% FPL	2012	30,095,292	26,166,036 (30,730) 86.9%	3,929,256 (30,730) 13.1%	20,447,461 (38,170) 67.9%	2,058,578 (20,004) 6.8%	630,162 (13,278) 2.1%	390,562 (7,894) 1.3%	192,083 (5,784) 0.6%	145,712 (5,291) 0.5%	2,301,480 (18,479) 7.6%
	2013	30,327,502	26,372,969 (27,595) 87.0%	3,954,533 (27,595) 13.0%	20,604,757 (37,837) 67.9%	2,159,024 (19,234) 7.1%	643,631 (12,219) 2.1%	424,042 (11,060) 1.4%	208,599 (6,317) 0.7%	144,086 (5,410) 0.5%	2,188,830 (20,137) 7.2%
	2014	30,857,962	27,505,951 (29,281) 89.1%	3,352,011 (29,281) 10.9%	21,242,306 (38,551) 68.8%	2,696,767 (23,594) 8.7%	635,143 (10,482) 2.1%	457,944 (8,930) 1.5%	223,264 (6,459) 0.7%	145,967 (5,033) 0.5%	2,104,559 (20,601) 6.8%
	2015	31,901,587	28,901,715 (24,529) 90.6%	2,999,872 (24,529) 9.4%	22,025,009 (35,542) 69.0%	3,087,190 (23,706) 9.7%	653,045 (13,750) 2.0%	532,208 (10,212) 1.7%	244,143 (6,626) 0.8%	141,324 (5,299) 0.4%	2,218,800 (18,624) 7.0%

Table 2. (Continued)

					Private Sources			Public Sources			
Income bin	Year	Population	Any coverage	Uninsured	ESHI	Non-group	Tricare	Medicaid	Medicare	VA	Multiple
	2016	32,856,352	29,806,625 (25,099) 90.7%	3,049,727 (25,099) 9.3%	22,614,288 (39,368) 68.8%	3,218,589 (26,387) 9.8%	640,213 (12,315) 1.9%	591,450 (11,194) 1.8%	266,504 (7,435) 0.8%	149,201 (5,030) 0.5%	2,326,381 (18,465) 7.1%
	2017	33,728,361	30,279,484 (31,974) 89.8%	3,448,877 (31,974) 10.2%	23,271,588 (45,614) 69.0%	2,978,818 (28,231) 8.8%	645,018 (11,623) 1.9%	616,217 (13,249) 1.8%	259,756 (6,881) 0.8%	149,319 (5,950) 0.4%	2,358,769 (21,444) 7.0%

Source: Authors' tabulation of the 2012-2017 American Community Survey data for adults aged 19-64.

Notes: Individuals reporting more than one source of coverage are included in the final column. All numbers are weighted using ACS person weight. There are between 530,103 and 542,848 unweighted observations in the 2012-2017 ACS, respectively. Standard errors are in parentheses and computed using ACS replicate weights. Approximately 3% of adults did not have a poverty line measure; they are included in the 0-137% of FPL category. "Never expanders" includes 12 states that had not expanded Medicaid by 2019: Alabama, Florida, Georgia, Kansas, Mississippi, Missouri, North Carolina, Oklahoma, South Carolina, South Dakota, Texas, and Wyoming.

METHODS

In this section we describe a DD model to formalize the comparison in changes in Medicaid coverage across the income distribution between the 9 expansion states from Table 1 and 12 non-expansion states from Table 2 before versus after the ACA Medicaid expansion. The DD specification takes the form:

$$M_{ist} = \beta_0 + \beta_1(POST_t * EXPAN_s) + \beta_2 POST_t + \beta_3 EXPAN_s + \beta_4 X_{ist} + \varepsilon_{ist} \quad (1)$$

where M_{ist} is an indicator for whether individual *i* living in state *s* had Medicaid coverage in year *t*, $POST_t$ indicates whether time *t* is in the post-treatment period (2014 or later), $EXPAN_s$ indicates whether state *s* participated in the ACA's Medicaid expansion in 2014, X_{ist} is a set of individual-level controls, and ε_{ist} is the error term. Standard errors are robust to heteroskedasticity and clustered by state. All models use person-weights provided in the ACS. The individual controls in X_{ist} include the respondent's age, gender, education, race/ethnicity, difficulty with English, citizenship, foreign born indicator, marital status, changes in family structure, military service, disability, annual work hours, and receipt of various income sources. In some specifications we include location and year fixed effects (denoted α_{as} and τ_t, respectively), in which case we do not separately include the $POST_t$ and $EXPAN_s$ dummies. These location fixed effects control for the individual's public-use microdata area (PUMA) of residence. There are 985 PUMAs (nested within states) represented by the individuals in our sample from our 21 states of interest in the ACS. In addition, we also explore state-specific impacts of Medicaid expansions, in which case we replace $EXPAN_s$ with state-specific indicators for Medicaid expansions.

The key coefficient of interest is β_1 which represents the average effect of the Medicaid expansion on Medicaid coverage for working-age adults in expansion states. The coefficient estimate has a causal interpretation under the assumption that, conditional on the other covariates, changes in Medicaid coverage post 2013 would have been the same in expansion and non-expansion states if the Medicaid expansion had not occurred. Figure 1 plots the trends in Medicaid coverage over time between the 9 expansion and 12 non-expansion states in our sample. For all income groups, the trends in coverage prior to expansion in 2014 look remarkably similar.

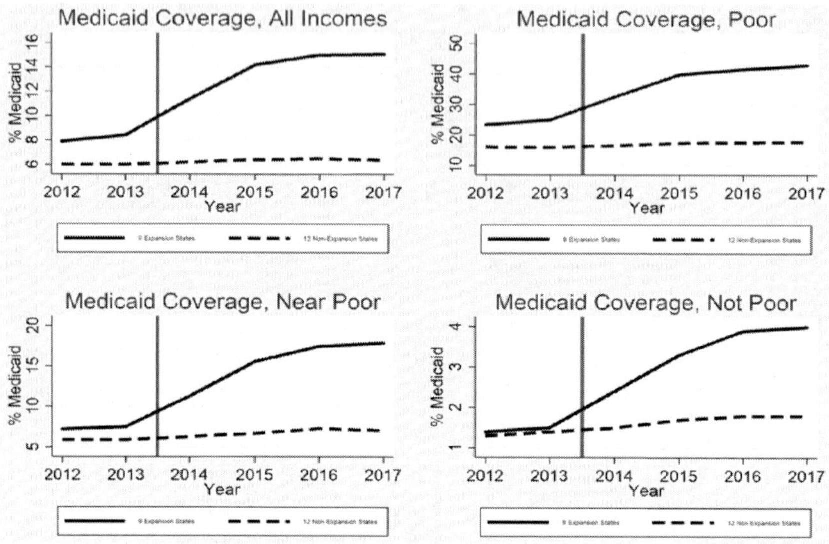

Figure 1. Trends in Medicaid coverage.

To test the identifying assumption of our DD model more formally, we estimate an event study model given by:

$$M_{ist} = \gamma_0 + \gamma_1 \sum_{t=2012}^{2017}(YEAR_t * EXPAN_s) + \gamma_2 EXPAN_s + \gamma_3 X_{ist} + \alpha_s + \tau_t + \varepsilon_{ist} \quad (2)$$

Here we replace the $POST_t$ indicator with a vector of individual year indicators, with 2013 being the reference year. If the model is valid, we would expect the interaction of the year indicator for 2012 and the Medicaid expansion indicator to be statistically insignificant, or at least for its coefficient estimate to be small relative to those from the post-treatment years. This specification also allows us to see the year over year impact of the ACA Medicaid expansion by examining the coefficient estimates for the interactions of the year indicators for 2014, 2015, 2016, and 2017 with the Medicaid expansion indicator.

RESULTS

Table 3 examines the impact of Medicaid expansions on Medicaid coverage among adults across the income distribution. As with the earlier tables, Medicaid coverage is defined as the individual having that source as a unique form of coverage (rather than having multiple sources). Overall, there were 1,094,667 working-age adults aged 19 to 64 with incomes below 138% of the FPL (or missing), and 3,440,670 adults with incomes at or above 138% of the FPL in our ACS sample. In principle, if the ACS data accurately measured income and health insurance coverage sources and the Medicaid statutory rules were fully enforced, we would not expect any Medicaid participation among higher income adults. In practice, Medicaid coverage was reported to be 2.7% for higher income adults (in 2012 and 2013, prior to the rollout; coverage was 18.2% for lower-income adults). This suggests that other avenues may exist to qualify for Medicaid for higher-income adults, such as categorical eligibility from pregnancy, disability, or public assistance programs. As a check on the results, we also restrict the sample to 2,906,015 higher-income respondents who do not report a birth in the past year, disability, or receipt of income from SSI, Social Security, or public assistance. The baseline participation rate in 2012 and 2013 is much lower at 1.4%.

Columns 1, 3, 5, 7, and 9 of Table 3 estimate DD models for five groups, without additional covariates. The groups are income-eligible adults (under 138% FPL), ineligible adults (138% FPL or higher), ineligible adults near the Medicaid income threshold (138 to 249% of the FPL), ineligible adults far from the threshold (250% of the FPL or higher), and ineligible adults far from threshold and FTFY workers. Columns 2, 4, 6, 8, and 10 include individual covariates, as well as fixed effects for local area and year.

In the top panel, focusing on the income-eligible sample, column 1 reveals baseline Medicaid participation of 18.2%. The Medicaid expansions (in the 9 states) increased participation by 13.6 percentage points, with similar results when covariates are included in column 2.

Column 3 reveals baseline Medicaid participation among the ineligible population prior to the ACA reforms was 2.7%, and the Medicaid expansions increased participation by an additional 3.0 percentage points (standard error = 0.4). Including individual covariates – some of which are highly predictive of Medicaid participation – has very little impact on the rise in participation from the pre- to post-period; column 4 reveals expansions increase participation by 3.0 percentage points among ineligibles. Some individual characteristics – especially the presence of SSI income, public assistance income, social security, or disability status – are extremely important determinants of Medicaid participation for this group of seemingly ineligible adults. These factors are suggestive of alternative pathways to qualify for Medicaid among working-age adults, namely via the pregnancy expansions, disability programs, and welfare programs. Other factors that are linked to sizable increases in Medicaid participation include lack of a high school diploma and being a recent mover. Holding other characteristics constant, working-age adults without a diploma (with a diploma or GED) are 4.4 percentage points (1.8 percentage points) more likely to participate in Medicaid than those with at least some college. The bottom panel of Table 3 focuses on the subset of respondents who are highly unlikely to qualify for Medicaid through categorical eligibility. Although the pre-ACA participation rate was just 1.4%, the coefficient estimates are nearly as large as the full sample with incomes at or above 138% of the FPL. Virtually all of the increase in participation for income-ineligible adults is coming from those with no obvious path to qualify for Medicaid.

Returning to the top panel, the next two groupings separate out individuals into those who might be considered close to the Medicaid threshold (138% to 249% of the FPL), and those who are far from it (≥250% of the FPL). To the extent that income is volatile during the year, one might expect that those whose incomes were close to the threshold may have qualified for at least part of the year, and may currently have Medicaid coverage. In contrast, it would be far less likely that those with particularly high incomes would qualify, even with volatility. Both Brooks (2019) and Solomon and Broaddus (2019) argue that income volatility could explain improper enrollment, since income is measured annually in the ACS.[10] People who had low income in the month they applied for Medicaid would

[10] Yelowitz (2019) addresses the criticisms of both Brooks (2019) and Solomon and Braddus (2019).

likely have been properly enrolled even if it turns out that their annual income exceeds 138% of the FPL. A key reason we look at higher income thresholds is that, at higher income thresholds, income volatility is less of a concern. Sommers and Rosenbaum (2011) note that income volatility could be important for adult Medicaid enrollment with incomes under 200% of the FPL. Looking at the population of adults who were initially ineligible for Medicaid based on monthly income, they estimate that nearly 30% of this population would have experienced a decline in income within six months that would make them eligible for Medicaid. Their analysis examined Medicaid eligibility, not Medicaid enrollment; respondents who experience an income decline may still have coverage from another source, such as employer-sponsored health insurance. Importantly, the authors suggest that people with income above 200% of the FPL for the year are unlikely to qualify for Medicaid during that year: "*Most people with incomes of 200–400 percent of poverty receive insurance through their employers and are unlikely to participate in Medicaid or exchange plans in large numbers; therefore, they were not included in the sample.*" Focusing on our DD results in Table 3, we observe increases of 7.2 and 1.6 percentage points in the top panel, respectively, for those near and far from the Medicaid eligibility threshold. Excluding those who may be categorically eligible in the bottom panel leads to nearly identical marginal effects (from a much lower baseline Medicaid participation rate).

The final two columns – columns 9 and 10 – further restrict the sample to a subset of individuals with income at or above 250% of the FPL and who report FTFY work (defined as working 40 or more hours per week and 50 or more weeks per year). Prior to the expansion, Medicaid coverage was 0.4% for FTFY workers (compared with 1.4% for respondents above 250% of the FPL), and the percentage with employer-sponsored health insurance was 77.6% (compared to 69.9% for respondents above 250% of the FPL). The impact of the Medicaid expansion on coverage remains highly significant. The expansion raised Medicaid coverage for FTFY workers with income above 250% of the FPL by 0.8 percentage points (200% above the base rate).

Tables 4 and 5 present two versions of our event study specification, with Table 4 reporting event study results for the full sample, while Table 5 excludes those who might be categorically eligible. Among income-eligible adults, the event study specification shows the marginal impact of the expansions was more than twice as large in 2017 as in 2014 in column 1. For the income-ineligible population, Medicaid participation grew over time as well. The marginal impacts either doubled or tripled from 2014 to 2017, depending on the sample and specification. For example, among the sample that excludes categorically eligible individuals with income at or above 250% of the FPL (Table 5, column 8), the marginal impact increased from 0.7 percentage points in 2014 to 1.8 percentage points in 2017, from a baseline participation rate of 0.7%. The "placebo" coefficients for the 2012 interaction are sometimes statistically significant, but in all cases much smaller than the magnitudes for the post-treatment interactions. Focusing on FTFY workers with incomes exceeding 250% of the FPL, the results once again show much larger increases in potentially improper Medicaid enrollment in 2017 (1.0 percentage points) relative to 2014 (0.4 percentage points).

Another concern about our approach with the ACS is the complexity of household size for calculating Medicaid eligibility. Brooks (2019) notes: "*The ACS household requests information for everyone in the household, including non-married partners, in-laws, roommates, and other individuals who should not be counted in determining the household size or income for Medicaid.*" Table 6 replicates the DD findings, restricted to nuclear families, in which all individuals in the household are a household head or couple and their children. Once again, we find significant effects of the expansion on seemingly income-ineligible enrollment. Overall, the expansions lead to a 2.2 percentage point increase in Medicaid coverage for nuclear families with incomes at or above 138% of the FPL (from a baseline rate of 1.8%), and 1.2 percentage point increase for those at or above 250% of the FPL (from a baseline rate of 0.8%).

In Table 7, we examine state-specific responses to the Medicaid expansion. Instead of one coefficient – $POST_t * EXPAN_s$ – we now include indicator variables for each expansion state interacted with $POST_t$. Although the estimated effects on potentially improper enrollment are always significant, the magnitudes vary across states. For example, New Mexico, Kentucky, and West Virginia saw increases of 4.4 percentage points or more for individuals at or above 138% of the FPL, while North Dakota and New Hampshire saw increases of 1.2 percentage points or less. The heterogeneous effects potentially suggest issues at the state-level with weaknesses in preventive controls, detection, and monitoring, issues we return to below.

Finally, Table 8 re-estimates the models, excluding respondents with imputed values on any variable used in the analysis. The results are modestly smaller. The Medicaid expansions increase potentially improper enrollment by 2.6 percentage points among the sample with income at or above 138% of the FPL (relative to 3.0 percentage points with the full sample). The baseline participation rates are somewhat smaller as well, and all of the results continue to be significant and sizable relative to the pre-ACA means.

In summary, there is strong evidence that Medicaid participation increased for groups for whom Medicaid was not intended to be the source of insurance coverage. Neither excluding those who might be categorically eligible, nor focusing on those whose income was far from the threshold alters the fundamental results. The estimated program effect grows over time. The estimated magnitudes from the DD analysis in Table 3 are non-trivial. If the coefficient estimates from the DD analysis are applied to the full sample of ineligible adults in the 9 expansion states (from Table 1), approximately 308,000 working-age adults with incomes between 138% to 249% of the FPL joined Medicaid due to the ACA expansions, while 223,000 adults with incomes at or above 250% of the FPL joined due to the expansions.[11]

[11] In Table 9, we present average population sizes for expansion and non-expansion states by income category and other data screens (e.g., excluding categorically eligible, etc.). One can use these to estimate improper enrollment levels from the marginal effects in the other tables.

Table 3. Medicaid-only take-up among working-age adults

	Income <138% FPL		Income ≥138% FPL		Income between 138%-249% FPL		Income ≥250% FPL		Income ≥250% FPL FTFY workers	
	(1)	(2)	(3)	(4)	(5)	(6)	(7)	(8)	(9)	(10)
Sample 1										
POST*EXPAN	0.136*** (0.017)	0.137*** (0.017)	0.030*** (0.004)	0.030*** (0.004)	0.072*** (0.007)	0.072*** (0.007)	0.016*** (0.002)	0.017*** (0.002)	0.008*** (0.001)	0.008*** (0.001)
EXPAN	0.082*** (0.022)	---	0.003 (0.003)	---	0.015* (0.007)	---	0.001 (0.002)	---	0.001 (0.001)	---
POST	0.014*** (0.005)	---	0.005*** (0.001)	---	0.009*** (0.003)	---	0.004*** (0.001)	---	0.002*** (0.001)	---
R^2	0.0435	0.1947	0.0054	0.1223	0.0157	0.1313	0.0029	0.1041	0.0019	0.0272
N	1,094,667		3,440,670		833,817		2,606,853		1,625,347	
$\overline{MEDICAID_{Pre}}$	0.182		0.027		0.063		0.014		0.004	
Sample 2										
POST*EXPAN	0.154*** (0.021)	0.154*** (0.021)	0.026*** (0.003)	0.027*** (0.003)	0.070*** (0.008)	0.071*** (0.008)	0.014*** (0.002)	0.014*** (0.002)	0.007*** (0.001)	0.007*** (0.001)
EXPAN	0.061** (0.024)	---	0.003 (0.003)	---	0.012 (0.007)	---	0.001 (0.001)	---	0.001 (0.001)	---
POST	0.016** (0.006)	---	0.005*** (0.001)	---	0.012*** (0.003)	---	0.003*** (0.001)	---	0.002*** (0.001)	---
R^2	0.0521	0.1286	0.0068	0.0371	0.0202	0.0548	0.0037	0.0236	0.0019	0.0138
N	729,595		2,906,015		641,749		2,264,266		1,520,695	
$\overline{MEDICAID_{Pre}}$	0.117		0.014		0.036		0.007		0.003	

Notes: Authors' analysis of 2012-2017 American Community Survey from 21 states. *Sample 1* includes all adults aged 19 to 64. *Sample 2* excludes adults who might be categorically eligible for Medicaid based on the following variables: had baby in previous year, disabled, social security receipt, public assistance receipt, SSI receipt. $\overline{MEDICAID_{Pre}}$ is the mean of the dependent variable, pre-treatment (2012-2013). Columns (2), (4), (6), (8), and (10) include controls for individual characteristics, local areas fixed effects, and year fixed effects. Specifications with individual characteristics control for respondent's age, sex, education, race/ethnicity, English difficulty, citizenship, foreign-born, marital status, military service, disability, annual hours of work, recent changes (marital status, births, and moves), and income sources (social security, wages, earnings, interest, other income, public assistance, retirement, self-employment or SSI). All specifications include person weights from ACS. Standard errors in parentheses and clustered at state level. *** = p<0.01, ** = p<0.05, * = p<0.10.

Table 4. Medicaid-only take-up among working-age adults, event study

	Income<138% FPL		Income≥138% FPL		Income between 138%-249% FPL		Income ≥250% FPL		Income ≥250% FPL FTFY workers	
	(1)	(2)	(3)	(4)	(5)	(6)	(7)	(8)	(9)	(10)
Sample 1										
2017*EXPAN	0.161*** (0.020)	0.159*** (0.020)	0.037*** (0.004)	0.038*** (0.004)	0.092*** (0.009)	0.092*** (0.009)	0.021*** (0.002)	0.022*** (0.002)	0.010*** (0.002)	0.010*** (0.002)
2016*EXPAN	0.150*** (0.021)	0.150*** (0.021)	0.035*** (0.004)	0.036*** (0.004)	0.085*** (0.009)	0.086*** (0.009)	0.020*** (0.002)	0.021*** (0.002)	0.010*** (0.001)	0.010*** (0.001)
2015*EXPAN	0.135*** (0.019)	0.135*** (0.019)	0.029*** (0.003)	0.030*** (0.003)	0.072*** (0.008)	0.071*** (0.008)	0.016*** (0.002)	0.016*** (0.002)	0.007*** (0.001)	0.007*** (0.001)
2014*EXPAN	0.070*** (0.015)	0.070*** (0.016)	0.015*** (0.003)	0.015*** (0.003)	0.033*** (0.008)	0.033*** (0.008)	0.008*** (0.002)	0.009*** (0.002)	0.004*** (0.001)	0.004*** (0.001)
2013*EXPAN	---	---	---	---	---	---	---	---	---	---
2012*EXPAN	-0.017*** (0.005)	-0.018*** (0.004)	-0.001 (0.001)	-0.001 (0.001)	-0.004* (0.002)	-0.004 (0.002)	0.001 (0.001)	0.000 (0.001)	-0.001 (0.001)	-0.001 (0.001)
R^2	0.0454	0.1957	0.0061	0.1227	0.0174	0.1322	0.0034	0.1043	0.0022	0.0274
N	1,094,667		3,440,670		833,817		2,606,853		1,625,347	
$\overline{MEDICAID_{Pre}}$	0.182		0.027		0.063		0.014		0.004	

Notes: Authors' analysis of 2012-2017 American Community Survey from 21 states. *Sample 1* includes all adults aged 19 to 64. $\overline{MEDICAID_{Pre}}$ is the mean of the dependent variable, pre-treatment (2012-2013). Columns (2), (4), (6), (8), and (10) include controls for individual characteristics, local areas fixed effects, and year fixed effects. Specifications with individual characteristics control for respondent's age, sex, education, race/ethnicity, English difficulty, citizenship, foreign-born, marital status, military service, disability, annual hours of work, recent changes (marital status, births, and moves), and income sources (social security, wages, earnings, interest, other income, public assistance, retirement, self-employment or SSI). All specifications include person weights from ACS. Standard errors in parentheses and clustered at state level. *** = p<0.01, ** = p<0.05, * = p<0.10.

Table 5. Medicaid-only take-up among working-age adults (exclude categorically needy)

	Income<138% FPL		Income≥138% FPL		Income between 138%-249% FPL		Income ≥250% FPL		Income ≥250% FPL FTFY workers	
	(1)	(2)	(3)	(4)	(5)	(6)	(7)	(8)	(9)	(10)
Sample 2										
2017*EXPAN	0.182***	0.179***	0.033***	0.034***	0.091***	0.091***	0.018***	0.018***	0.009***	0.009***
	(0.025)	(0.024)	(0.004)	(0.004)	(0.010)	(0.010)	(0.002)	(0.002)	(0.001)	(0.001)
2016*EXPAN	0.171***	0.171***	0.032***	0.033***	0.086***	0.087***	0.018***	0.018***	0.009***	0.009***
	(0.026)	(0.025)	(0.004)	(0.004)	(0.010)	(0.010)	(0.002)	(0.002)	(0.001)	(0.001)
2015*EXPAN	0.158***	0.159***	0.025***	0.026***	0.066***	0.066***	0.014***	0.015***	0.006***	0.006***
	(0.023)	(0.024)	(0.004)	(0.004)	(0.008)	(0.008)	(0.002)	(0.002)	(0.001)	(0.001)
2014*EXPAN	0.077***	0.077***	0.012***	0.012***	0.028***	0.029***	0.007***	0.007***	0.003***	0.003***
	(0.017)	(0.017)	(0.003)	(0.003)	(0.008)	(0.008)	(0.002)	(0.002)	(0.001)	(0.001)
2013*EXPAN	---	---	---	---	---	---	---	---	---	---
2012*EXPAN	-0.017***	-0.019***	-0.001	-0.001	-0.005*	-0.005*	0.000	0.000	-0.001	-0.001
	(0.004)	(0.004)	(0.001)	(0.001)	(0.003)	(0.003)	(0.001)	(0.001)	(0.001)	(0.001)
R^2	0.0552	0.1303	0.0076	0.0376	0.0229	0.0563	0.0042	0.0238	0.0022	0.0139
N	729,595		2,906,015		641,749		2,264,266		1,520,695	
$\overline{MEDICAID_{Pre}}$	0.117		0.014		0.036		0.007		0.003	

Notes: Authors' analysis of 2012-2017 American Community Survey from 21 states. *Sample 2* excludes adults who might be categorically eligible for Medicaid based on the following variables: had baby in previous year, disabled, social security receipt, public assistance receipt, SSI receipt. $\overline{MEDICAID_{Pre}}$ is the mean of the dependent variable, pre-treatment (2012-2013). Columns (2), (4), (6), (8), and (10) include controls for individual characteristics, local areas fixed effects, and year fixed effects. Specifications with individual characteristics control for respondent's age, sex, education, race/ethnicity, English difficulty, citizenship, foreign-born, marital status, military service, disability, annual hours of work, recent changes (marital status, births, and moves), and income sources (social security, wages, earnings, interest, other income, public assistance, retirement, self-employment or SSI). All specifications include person weights from ACS. Standard errors in parentheses and clustered at state level. *** = p<0.01, ** = p<0.05, * = p<0.10.

Table 6. Medicaid-only take-up among working-age adults, nuclear families only

	Income<138% FPL		Income≥138% FPL		Income between 138%-249% FPL		Income ≥250% FPL		Income ≥250% FPL FTFY workers	
	(1)	(2)	(3)	(4)	(5)	(6)	(7)	(8)	(9)	(10)
Sample 1										
POST*EXPAN	0.148*** (0.017)	0.149*** (0.018)	0.022*** (0.003)	0.023*** (0.003)	0.063*** (0.007)	0.064*** (0.007)	0.012*** (0.002)	0.012*** (0.001)	0.006*** (0.001)	0.006*** (0.001)
EXPAN	0.098*** (0.029)	---	0.002 (0.002)	---	0.014** (0.006)	---	0.000 (0.001)	---	0.000 (0.001)	---
POST	0.017*** (0.005)	---	0.004*** (0.001)	---	0.010*** (0.003)	---	0.003*** (0.000)	---	0.001*** (0.000)	---
R^2	0.0526	0.1993	0.0043	0.1021	0.015	0.115	0.0023	0.0848	0.0013	0.0229
N	494,577		2,637,704		534,685		2,103,019		1,308,305	
$\overline{MEDICAID}_{Pre}$	0.199		0.018		0.052		0.008		0.003	
Sample 2										
POST*EXPAN	0.180*** (0.023)	0.180*** (0.023)	0.020*** (0.003)	0.020*** (0.003)	0.063*** (0.007)	0.064*** (0.007)	0.010*** (0.001)	0.011*** (0.001)	0.005*** (0.001)	0.006*** (0.001)
EXPAN	0.078** (0.034)	---	0.001 (0.002)	---	0.011 (0.006)	---	0.000 (0.001)	---	0.000 (0.001)	---
POST	0.022*** (0.005)	---	0.004*** (0.001)	---	0.012*** (0.003)	---	0.002*** (0.000)	---	0.001*** (0.000)	---
R^2	0.0675	0.1447	0.0053	0.0283	0.0193	0.05	0.0028	0.0165	0.0014	0.012
N	310,677		2,244,824		409,276		1,835,548		1,225,945	
$\overline{MEDICAID}_{Pre}$	0.130		0.009		0.030		0.004		0.002	

Notes: Authors' analysis of 2012-2017 American Community Survey from 21 states. *Sample 1* includes all adults aged 19 to 64. *Sample 2* excludes adults who might be categorically eligible for Medicaid based on the following variables: had baby in previous year, disabled, social security receipt, public assistance receipt, SSI receipt. $\overline{MEDICAID}_{Pre}$ is the mean of the dependent variable, pre-treatment (2012-2013). Columns (2), (4), (6), (8), and (10) include controls for individual characteristics, local areas fixed effects, and year fixed effects. Specifications with individual characteristics control for respondent's age, sex, education, race/ethnicity, English difficulty, citizenship, foreign-born, marital status, military service, disability, annual hours of work, recent changes (marital status, births, and moves), and income sources (social security, wages, earnings, interest, other income, public assistance, retirement, self-employment or SSI). All specifications include person weights from ACS. Standard errors in parentheses and clustered at state level. *** = p<0.01, ** = p<0.05, * = p<0.10.

Table 7. Medicaid-only take-up among working-age adults, state-specific impacts

	Income<138% FPL		Income≥138% FPL		Income between 138%-249% FPL		Income ≥250% FPL		Income ≥250% FPL FTFY workers	
	(1)	(2)	(3)	(4)	(5)	(6)	(7)	(8)	(9)	(10)
Sample 1										
POST*Arkansas	0.109*** (0.005)	0.110*** (0.004)	0.033*** (0.001)	0.035*** (0.001)	0.063*** (0.003)	0.068*** (0.003)	0.020*** (0.001)	0.021*** (0.001)	0.011*** (0.000)	0.011*** (0.000)
POST*New Hampshire	0.075*** (0.005)	0.079*** (0.005)	0.011*** (0.001)	0.012*** (0.001)	0.042*** (0.003)	0.043*** (0.003)	0.006*** (0.001)	0.007*** (0.001)	0.003*** (0.000)	0.003*** (0.000)
POST*New Mexico	0.203*** (0.005)	0.194*** (0.005)	0.056*** (0.001)	0.054*** (0.001)	0.104*** (0.003)	0.103*** (0.003)	0.033*** (0.001)	0.032*** (0.001)	0.017*** (0.000)	0.017*** (0.000)
POST*Ohio	0.116*** (0.005)	0.113*** (0.005)	0.026*** (0.001)	0.027*** (0.001)	0.073*** (0.003)	0.071*** (0.003)	0.013*** (0.001)	0.014*** (0.001)	0.006*** (0.000)	0.006*** (0.000)
POST*Kentucky	0.207*** (0.005)	0.213*** (0.005)	0.046*** (0.001)	0.047*** (0.001)	0.101*** (0.003)	0.102*** (0.003)	0.025*** (0.001)	0.026*** (0.001)	0.013*** (0.000)	0.014*** (0.000)
POST*Michigan	0.103*** (0.005)	0.105*** (0.004)	0.022*** (0.001)	0.023*** (0.001)	0.055*** (0.003)	0.055*** (0.003)	0.013*** (0.001)	0.014*** (0.001)	0.007*** (0.000)	0.007*** (0.000)
POST*Nevada	0.169*** (0.005)	0.170*** (0.004)	0.032*** (0.001)	0.032*** (0.001)	0.066*** (0.003)	0.068*** (0.003)	0.019*** (0.001)	0.018*** (0.001)	0.008*** (0.000)	0.008*** (0.000)
POST*North Dakota	0.028*** (0.005)	0.017*** (0.005)	0.008*** (0.001)	0.006*** (0.001)	0.034*** (0.003)	0.023*** (0.003)	0.003*** (0.001)	0.003*** (0.001)	0.003*** (0.000)	0.003*** (0.000)
POST*West Virginia	0.212*** (0.005)	0.210*** (0.005)	0.044*** (0.001)	0.044*** (0.001)	0.101*** (0.003)	0.099*** (0.003)	0.023*** (0.001)	0.023*** (0.001)	0.010*** (0.000)	0.011*** (0.000)
R^2	0.0486	0.1955	0.0069	0.1226	0.0179	0.1316	0.0038	0.1042	0.0025	0.0273
N	1,094,667		3,440,670		833,817		2,606,853		1,625,347	
$\overline{MEDICAID_{Pre}}$	0.182		0.027		0.063		0.014		0.004	

Table 8. Medicaid-only take-up among working-age adults, exclude imputed values

	Income<138% FPL		Income≥138% FPL		Income between 138%-249% FPL		Income ≥250% FPL		Income ≥250% FPL FTFY workers	
	(1)	(2)	(3)	(4)	(5)	(6)	(7)	(8)	(9)	(10)
Sample 1										
POST*EXPAN	0.159*** (0.021)	0.157*** (0.021)	0.025*** (0.004)	0.026*** (0.004)	0.075*** (0.007)	0.074*** (0.008)	0.011*** (0.002)	0.012*** (0.002)	0.004*** (0.001)	0.004*** (0.001)
EXPAN	0.093*** (0.026)	---	0.003 (0.002)	---	0.014* (0.007)	---	0.001 (0.001)	---	0.000 (0.000)	---
POST	0.017*** (0.005)	---	0.004*** (0.001)	---	0.011*** (0.003)	---	0.003*** (0.001)	---	0.001*** (0.000)	---
R^2	0.0580	0.2322	0.0053	0.1585	0.0188	0.1614	0.0022	0.1561	0.0011	0.0156
N	678,751		2,320,863		514,941		1,805,922		1,142,741	
$\overline{MEDICAID_{Pre}}$	0.177		0.020		0.053		0.009		0.001	
Sample 2										
POST*EXPAN	0.176*** (0.023)	0.175*** (0.024)	0.022*** (0.003)	0.023*** (0.003)	0.071*** (0.008)	0.072*** (0.008)	0.010*** (0.002)	0.010*** (0.002)	0.003*** (0.001)	0.003*** (0.001)
EXPAN	0.067** (0.027)	---	0.002 (0.002)	---	0.010 (0.007)	---	0.001 (0.001)	---	0.000 (0.000)	---
POST	0.015** (0.006)	---	0.004*** (0.001)	---	0.011*** (0.003)	---	0.002*** (0.001)	---	0.001*** (0.000)	---
R^2	0.0656	0.1546	0.0065	0.0373	0.0227	0.0618	0.0031	0.0213	0.0011	0.0102
N	468,094		2,011,037		407,832		1,603,205		1,079,064	
$\overline{MEDICAID_{Pre}}$	0.112		0.010		0.029		0.004		0.001	

Notes: Authors' analysis of 2012-2017 American Community Survey from 21 states. *Sample 1* includes all adults aged 19 to 64. *Sample 2* excludes adults who might be categorically eligible for Medicaid based on the following variables: had baby in previous year, disabled, social security receipt, public assistance receipt, SSI receipt. $\overline{MEDICAID_{Pre}}$ is the mean of the dependent variable, pre-treatment (2012-2013). Columns (2), (4), (6), (8), and (10) include controls for individual characteristics, local areas fixed effects, and year fixed effects. Specifications with individual characteristics control for respondent's age, sex, education, race/ethnicity, English difficulty, citizenship, foreign-born, marital status, military service, disability, annual hours of work, recent changes (marital status, births, and moves), and income sources (social security, wages, earnings, interest, other income, public assistance, retirement, self-employment or SSI). All specifications include person weights from ACS. Standard errors in parentheses and clustered at state level. *** = p<0.01, ** = p<0.05, * = p<0.10.

Table 9. Average population (from 2012-2017) used to measure potentially improper medicaid enrollment

Income Bin	Population Included	Expan Avg Pop	Expan Avg Pop (no imputes)	Non-Expan Avg Pop	Non-Expan Avg Pop (no imputes)
All	Group 1 - All 19-64	22,810,278	15,273,671	56,806,360	36,557,923
Income<138% FPL or missing	Group 1 - All 19-64	5,389,680	3,390,260	13,702,382	8,556,835
Income between 138%-249% FPL	Group 1 - All 19-64	4,279,604	2,723,161	11,476,136	6,977,861
Income ≥250% FPL	Group 1 - All 19-64	13,140,994	9,160,250	31,627,843	21,023,228
All	Group 2 - Exclude Cat Elig.	18,168,038	12,454,439	46,745,217	30,682,169
Income<138% FPL or missing	Group 2 - Exclude Cat Elig.	3,462,713	2,197,028	9,726,668	6,178,263
Income between 138%-249% FPL	Group 2 - Exclude Cat Elig.	3,282,918	2,138,580	9,203,103	5,699,852
Income ≥250% FPL	Group 2 - Exclude Cat Elig.	11,422,406	8,118,831	27,815,446	18,804,055
All	Group 3 - and FTFY	9,810,015	6,821,109	25,880,126	16,939,828
Income<138% FPL or missing	Group 3 - and FTFY	594,332	359,035	2,055,163	1,211,092
Income between 138%-249% FPL	Group 3 - and FTFY	1,667,300	1,083,532	4,903,486	2,973,103
Income ≥250% FPL	Group 3 - and FTFY	7,548,383	5,378,542	18,921,477	12,755,634
All	Group 4 - and nuclear	7,328,824	5,318,855	18,489,131	12,799,746
Income<138% FPL or missing	Group 4 - and nuclear	329,902	207,781	1,132,719	703,498
Income between 138%-249% FPL	Group 4 - and nuclear	1,006,219	686,400	2,831,579	1,850,460
Income ≥250% FPL	Group 4 - and nuclear	5,992,703	4,424,674	14,524,833	10,245,789

Notes: Authors' tabulation of the 2012-2017 American Community Survey. The averages for Group 1 (including imputed values) can be derived from Tables 1 and 2 for expansion and non-expansion states, respectively.

DISCUSSION

As mentioned above, we find large impacts of the ACA Medicaid expansion on Medicaid coverage among the intended recipients, working-age adults with incomes below 138% of the FPL. In addition, perhaps somewhat surprisingly, we also find increases in Medicaid coverage among adults with income between 138 and 250% of the FPL, as well as those with income at or above 250% of the FPL. The impact of the Medicaid expansions on potentially improper enrollment varies across the expansion states, with larger effects in New Mexico, Kentucky, and West Virginia. The impact is also larger in later years, suggesting that potentially improper enrollment cannot be explained by short-run implementation problems. We conclude this chapter with some discussion of potential explanations for these findings, which should be the focus of future work.

One important possibility has to do with program integrity. It is possible that the ACA legislative rules are simply not being carried out as intended. For decades, prominent researchers have found that the "effective tax rate" on income to be far below the statutory level specified by program rules for welfare programs like Aid to Families with Dependent Children, primarily from income that is disregarded in eligibility calculations (Ziliak 2007). One possible reason for this divergence could be caseworker error or discretion. Moffitt (1979) notes that caseworkers might make mistakes when applying complex regulations to calculating benefits. Favorable errors that understate income are less likely to be pointed out by the welfare participant (McKinnish, Sanders, and Smith 1999). Edin and Jencks (1992) emphasize the role of caseworker discretion, noting that caseworkers often knew about clients' unreported supplemental income, but choose not to pursue the issue with them. Both issues – error and discretion – could arise in the ACA context. In 2015, there were more than 4,600 ACA assister programs helping approximately 5.9 million consumers (Pollitz, Tolbert, and Ma 2015), and these were funded through a variety of mechanisms. These programs helped an estimated 630,000 consumers apply for coverage. The assister programs employed 30,400 full time equivalent staff and volunteers. Given the magnitude and complexity of the ACA rollout, both the skills and motivations of such workers in terms of furthering their clients' interests will surely vary, and could plausibly explain some of our findings.

These concerns are supported by recent federal and state audits (although the audits primarily focus on states not in our analysis). The Office of Inspector General ("OIG") at the Department of Health and Human Services has published results from a series of audits covering part of the 2014-2015 period in four states (California, Colorado, Kentucky, and New York) for beneficiaries enrolled in the expansion. The OIG has also released reports on similar determinations for non-newly eligible adults in California, Kentucky, and New York. All the reports show that there are serious problems with eligibility-verification systems. Consistent errors include neglecting to verify income eligibility properly, misclassifying individuals into incorrect category classifications, failing to properly verify citizenship, and other issues. Some of these enrollment errors lead to incorrect and often higher federal reimbursement for individuals who would qualify for Medicaid under a category other than "new adults," while others lead to complete ineligibility for Medicaid. The OIG estimated more than 366,000 ineligible and 79,000 potentially ineligible beneficiaries in California, more than 85,000 ineligible and 13,000 potentially ineligible beneficiaries in Colorado, more than 47,000 ineligible beneficiaries in New York, and nearly 35,000 potentially ineligible beneficiaries in Kentucky (Blase and Yelowitz 2019; Yelowitz 2019).[12]

There are also explanations related to the quality of the ACS data. One potential explanation for these findings could be mismeasurement of either income or insurance coverage in the ACS. With respect to insurance coverage, the fact that healthcare.gov is designed to be a one-stop-shop for insurance coverage that routes applicants to either Marketplace or Medicaid coverage as appropriate could lead to some confusion in terms of the applicant's final source of coverage. The fact that multiple private insurance companies sell both Marketplace and Medicaid managed care plans may also contribute to this confusion. In addition, while the ACS health insurance survey question clearly asks individuals to self-report their current sources of coverage, survey respondents may answer the question in different ways, such as their longest source of coverage during the year. Of course, both of these explanations may be just as likely to lead to individuals under-reporting Medicaid coverage as over-reporting it.

---

[12] State-level audits in Louisiana, Oregon, and Montana also find serious issues with improper enrollment.

In terms of income, the ACS asks individuals to self-report income from a variety of sources over the previous 12 months. All major household surveys have been found to have some degree of measurement error in income, and the ACS is no exception (Moore, Stinson, and Welniak, Jr. 1997; Czajka 2012; Czajka and Denmead 2014). Comparisons of income measures constructed using survey responses with administrative records show that surveys tend to understate total income for most sources. It is not clear if under-reporting in a survey context such as the ACS would carry over into the application process for transfer programs such as Medicaid, but it may be possible given that in both cases individuals are reporting income data to government. It could also be the case that individuals may be basing their survey answers on forecasts of future income rather than a recounting of income over the previous 12 months or may not recall accurately all sources of income. While under-reporting seems more common, if some of these reasons lead individuals to overstate their income in the ACS, then they may appear to be income-ineligible for Medicaid.

A related possibility is that people have trouble forecasting their income when determining their eligibility for ACA coverage. For example, an individual applying during the open enrollment period in late 2013 would forecast their 2014 income, and Marketplace subsidies such as the premium tax credit would be advanced ahead of time based on their forecast (Yelowitz 2016). If an individual under-forecasts their income, then they may qualify for Medicaid coverage despite ultimately realizing a higher level of income during the year.

References

Abraham, Jean M., Pinar Karaca-Mandic, and Michel Boudreaux. 2013. "Sizing Up the Individual Market for Health Insurance: A Comparison of Survey and Administrative Data Sources." *Medical Care Research and Review* 70(4): 418–33.

Artiga, Samantha, Jennifer Tolbert, and Robin Rudowitz. 2016. "Implementation of the ACA in Kentucky: Lessons Learned to Date and the Potential Effects of Future Changes." Kaiser Family Foundation Issue Brief, Kaiser Family Foundation, April. http://files.kff.org/

attachment/issue-brief-implementation-of-the-aca-in-kentucky-lessons-learned-to-date-and-the-potential-effects-of-future-changes . Accessed December 1, 2019.

Atkin, Emily, and Josh Israel. 2015. "Kentucky Is Obamacare's Undeniable Success Story. This Man Is Trying to Burn It All Down." *ThinkProgress*, September 14. https://thinkprogress.org/kentucky-is-obamacares-undeniable-success-story-this-man-is-trying-to-burn-it-all-down-56c7d60933ac#.olltoebkd . Accessed December 1, 2019.

Blase, Brian C., and Aaron Yelowitz. 2019. "*The ACA's Medicaid Expansion: A Review of Ineligible Enrollees and Improper Payments*." Mercatus Research, Mercatus Center at George Mason University, Arlington, VA, November 2019.

Boudreaux, Michel, James M. Noon, Brett Fried, and Joanne Pascale. 2019. "Medicaid Expansion and the Medicaid Undercount in the American Community Survey." *Health Services Research* 54(6): 1263–72.

Brooks, Tricia. 2019. "What Some Researchers Get Wrong about Medicaid's Income Eligibility Requirements." *Health Affairs Blog*, September 19, 2019. https://www.healthaffairs.org/do/10.1377/hblog 20190918.358911/full/ . Accessed December 1, 2019.

Centers for Medicare and Medicaid Services, "*Fiscal Year (FY) 2019 Medicare Fee-for-Service Improper Payment Rate Is Lowest since 2010*." https://www.cms.gov/newsroom/press-releases/fiscal-year-fy-2019-medicare-fee-service-improper-payment-rate-lowest-2010-while-data-points . Accessed December 1, 2019.

Courtemanche, Charles, James Marton, and Aaron Yelowitz. 2016. "Who Gained Insurance Coverage in 2014, the First Year of Full ACA Implementation?" *Health Economics* 25(6): 778–84.

Courtemanche, Charles, James Marton, Benjamin Ukert, Aaron Yelowitz, and Daniela Zapata. 2017. "Impacts of the Affordable Care Act on Health Insurance Coverage in Medicaid Expansion and Non-Expansion States." *Journal of Policy Analysis and Management* 36(1): 178–210.

Courtemanche, Charles, James Marton, Benjamin Ukert, Aaron Yelowitz, and Daniela Zapata. 2018a. "Early Effects of the Affordable Care Act on Health Care Access, Risky Health Behaviors, and Self-Assessed Health," *Southern Economic Journal,* 84(3): 660–691.

Courtemanche, Charles, James Marton, Benjamin Ukert, Aaron Yelowitz, and Daniela Zapata. 2018b. "Effects of the Affordable Care Act on Health Care Access and Self-Assessed Health after 3 Years," *Inquiry: The Journal of Health Care Organization, Provision and Financing,* 55: 1–10.

Courtemanche, Charles, James Marton, Benjamin Ukert, Aaron Yelowitz, and Daniela Zapata. 2019a. "Effects of the Affordable Care Act on Health Behaviors after 3 Years," *Eastern Economic Journal,* 45(1): 7–33.

Courtemanche, Charles, James Marton, Benjamin Ukert, Aaron Yelowitz, Daniela Zapata, and Ishtiaque Fazlul. 2019b. "The Three-Year Impact of the Affordable Care Act on Disparities in Insurance Coverage," *Health Services Research*, 54(S1): 307–316.

Czajka, John L. 2012. "Measuring Income Simply: Observations from a Comparative Analysis of Survey Income Data." *Presentation to the Population Health Subcommittee, NCVHS, Mathematica Policy Research*, March 9. http://www.ncvhs.hhs.gov/wp-content/uploads/2014/05/120308p12.pdf. Accessed December 1, 2019.

Czajka, John L., and Gabrielle Denmead. 2014. "*Getting More from Survey Income Measures: Empirically-Based Recommendations for Improving Accuracy and Efficiency*." https://s3.amazonaws.com/sitesusa/wpcontent/uploads/sites/242/2014/05/Czajka_2012FCSM_III-D.pdf. Accessed July, 2019.

Deloitte Development LLC. 2015. "*Commonwealth of Kentucky Medicaid Expansion Report: 2014*." Deloitte Development LLC, February. http://jointhehealthjourney.com/images/uploads/channel-files/Kentucky_Medicaid_Expansion_One-Year_Study_FINAL.pdf. Accessed December 1, 2019.

Edin, Kathryn, and Christopher Jencks. 1992. "Reforming Welfare." In *Rethinking Social Policy: Race, Poverty, and the Underclass,* edited by Christopher Jencks, 204–35. Cambridge: Harvard University Press.

Frean, Molly, Jonathan Gruber, and Benjamin D. Sommers. 2017. "Premium Subsidies, the mandate, and Medicaid expansion: Coverage effects of the Affordable Care Act." *Journal of Health Economics* 53: 72–86.

Gruber, Jonathan, and Benjamin D. Sommers. 2019. "The Affordable Care Act's Effects on Patients, Providers and the Economy: What We've Learned so Far." *Journal of Policy Analysis and Management* 38(4): 1028–1052.

Kaiser Family Foundation. 2012. "*The Medicaid Medically Needy Program: Spending and Enrollment Update*." https://www.kff.org/wp-content/uploads/2013/01/4096.pdf . Accessed December 1, 2019.

Kaiser Family Foundation. 2013. "*Medicaid Eligibility for Adults as of January 1, 2014*." Kaiser Family Foundation Fact Sheet. https://kaiserfamilyfoundation.files.wordpress.com/2013/10/8497-medicaid-eligibilityfor-adults-as-of-january-1-2014.pdf. Accessed September, 2016.

Kaiser Family Foundation. 2019a. "*Medicaid and Breast Cervical Cancer Treatment Program*." https://www.kff.org/other/state-indicator/medicaid-breast-and-cervical-cancer-treatment-program-enrollment/. Accessed December 1, 2019.

Kaiser Family Foundation. 2019b. "*Waivers with Eligibility and Enrollment Restrictions: Approved and Pending as of November 11, 2019*." https://www.kff.org/medicaid/issue-brief/medicaid-waiver-tracker-approved-and-pending-section-1115-waivers-by-state/#Table3. Accessed December 1, 2019.

Kaiser Family Foundation. 2019c. "*Trends in Medicaid Income Eligibility Limits*." https://www.kff.org/data-collection/trends-in-medicaid-income-eligibility-limits/ . Accessed December 1, 2019.

Kaestner, Robert, Bowen Garrett, Jiajia Chen, Anuj Gangopadhyaya, and Caitlyn Flemming. 2017. "Effects of ACA Medicaid Expansions on Health Insurance Coverage and Labor Supply." *Journal of Policy Analysis and Management* 36(3): 608–642.

Kenney, Genevieve, R. Andrew Allison, Julia Costich, James Marton, and Joshua McFeeters. 2007a. "The Effects of Premium Increases on

Enrollment in SCHIP Programs: Findings from Three States." *Inquiry* 43(4): 378–92.

Kenney, Genevieve, James Marton, Joshua McFeeters, and Julia Costich. 2007b. "Assessing Potential Enrollment and Budgetary Effects of SCHIP Premiums: Findings from Arizona and Kentucky." *Health Services Research* 42(6 pt. 2): 2354–72.

Klerman, Jacob A., Michael Davern, Kathleen Call, Victoria Lynch, and Jeanne Ringel. 2009. "Understanding the Current Population Survey's Insurance Estimates and the Medicaid Undercount." *Health Affairs* 28(6): 991–1001.

Lurie, Ithai Z., and James Pearce. 2019. "Health Insurance Coverage from Administrative Tax Data" (*Working Paper 117*, Department of the Treasury, Office of Tax Analysis, Washington, DC, 2019). https://www.treasury.gov/resource-center/tax-policy/tax-analysis/Documents/WP-117.pdf. Accessed December 1, 2019.

Louisiana Department of Health, "Medicaid Eligibility: Wage Verification Process of the Expansion Population," *Medicaid Audit Unit Report*, November 8, 2018. http://app.lla.state.la.us/PublicReports.nsf/0/1CDD30D9C82860828625834000 65E5F6/$FILE/0001ABC3.pdf. Accessed December 1, 2019.

Mach, Annie, and Brett O'Hara. 2011. "Do People Really Have Multiple Health Insurance Plans? Estimates of Nongroup Health Insurance in the American Community Survey." *SEHSD Working Paper Number 2011-28*. Social, Economic, and Housing Statistics Division, United States Census Bureau, January. https://www.census.gov/content/dam/Census/library/working-papers/2011/demo/SEHSD-WP2011-28.pdf . Accessed December 1, 2019.

Marton, James. 2007. "The Impact of the Introduction of Premiums into a SCHIP Program." *Journal of Policy Analysis and Management* 26(2): 261–79.

Marton, James, Patricia Ketsche, and Mei Zhou. 2010. "SCHIP Premiums, Enrollment, and Expenditures: A Two State, Competing Hazard Analysis." *Health Economics* 19(7): 772–91.

Marton, James, Cynthia S. Searcy, and Jennifer Ghandhi. 2010. "Disparate Effects of CHIP Premiums on Disenrollment for Minorities," in *Current Issues in Health Economics*, edited by Daniel Slottje and Rusty Tchernis. United Kingdom: Emerald Group.

Marton, James, and Jeffrey Talbert. 2010. "SCHIP Premiums, Health Status, and the Insurance Coverage of Children." *Inquiry* 47(3): 199–214.

Marton, James, and Aaron Yelowitz. 2015. "Health Insurance Generosity and Conditional Coverage: Evidence from Medicaid Managed Care in Kentucky." *Southern Economic Journal* 82(2): 535–55.

McKinnish, Terra, Seth Sanders, and Jeffrey Smith. 1999. "Estimates of Effective Guarantees and Tax Rates in the AFDC Program for the Post-OBRA Period." *Journal of Human Resources* 34(2): 312–45.

Moffitt, Robert. 1979. "Cumulative Effective Tax Rates and Guarantees in Low-Income Transfer Programs." *Journal of Human Resources* 14(1): 122–9.

Moore, Jeffrey C., Linda L. Stinson, and Edward J. Welniak, Jr. 1997. "Income Measurement Error in Surveys: A Review." *Census Working Paper SM97-05*, United States Census Bureau. https://www.census.gov/content/dam/Census/library/working-papers/1997/adrm/sm97-05.pdf . Accessed December 1, 2019.

Palmer, Makayla, James Marton, Aaron Yelowitz, and Jeffrey Talbert. 2017. "Medicaid Managed Care and the Health Care Utilization of Adolescent Foster Children." *Inquiry: The Journal of Health Care Organization, Provision and Financing* 54:1–9.

Pergamit, Michael R., Marla McDaniel, Vicki Chen, Embry Howell, and Amelia Hawkins. 2012. "*Providing Medicaid to Youth Formerly in Foster Care Under the Chafee Provision: Informing Implementation of the Affordable Care Act*." U.S. Department of Health and Human Services, Office of the Assistant Secretary for Planning and Evaluation. https://aspe.hhs.gov/system/files/pdf/76721/rpt.pdf. Accessed December 1, 2019.

Pollitz, Karen, Jennifer Tolbert, and Rosa Ma. 2015. "*2015 Survey of Health Insurance Marketplace Assister Programs and Brokers*," Kaiser Family Foundation Issue Brief, Kaiser Family Foundation, August.

https://nationaldisabilitynavigator.org/wp-content/uploads/resources-links/KFF_2015-survey-marketplace-assister-programs.pdf. Accessed December 1, 2019.

Rosenbaum, Sara, Sara Schmucker, and Sara Rothenberg. 2016. "Will Kentucky Roll Back Its Medicaid Expansion?" *To the Point*, The Commonwealth Fund, July 8. http://www.commonwealthfund.org/publications/blog/2016/jul/will-kentucky-roll-back-its-medicaid-expansion. Accessed December 1, 2019.

Schneider, Andy. 2018. "*Gutting Medicaid Transitional Medical Assistance: Watch What We Waive, Not What We Say*." Georgetown University Health Policy Institute, Center for Children and Families. https://ccf.georgetown.edu/2018/03/15/gutting-medicaid-transitional-medical-assistance-watch-what-we-waive-not-what-we-say/. Accessed December 1, 2019.

Smith, Jessica C., and Carla Medalia. 2014. "Health Insurance Coverage in the United States: 2013." *Current Population Reports P60-250*, United States Census Bureau, September. https://www2.census.gov/library/publications/2014/demographics/p60-250.pdf. Accessed December 1, 2019.

Solomon, Judith, and Matt Broaddus. 2019. "*New Claims by Opponents of Medicaid Expansion Rest on Faulty Analysis*," Center on Budget and Policy Priorities, September 2019.

Sommers, Benjamin D. and Sara Rosenbaum. 2011. "How Changes in Eligibility may move Millions Back and Forth between Medicaid and Insurance Exchanges." *Health Affairs* 30(2): 228–236.

State of Montana, Department of Public Health and Human Services, Legislative Audit Division, "*Performance Audit: State Efforts to Mitigate Fraud, Waste, and Abuse in the Montana Medicaid Program*," https://leg.mt.gov/content/Publications/Audit/Report/17P-02.pdf, June 2018. Accessed December 1, 2019.

State of Oregon, "Oregon Health Authority Should Improve Efforts to Detect and Prevent Improper Medicaid Payments," *Report 2017-25*, November 2017, https://sos.oregon.gov/audits/Documents/2017-25.pdf. Accessed December 1, 2019.

U.S. Department of Commerce, U.S. Census Bureau. 2019. "*The American Community Survey*." https://www2.census.gov/programs-surveys/acs/methodology/questionnaires/2014/quest14.pdf. Accessed December 1, 2019.

U.S. Department of Health and Human Services, Office of Inspector General, "Kentucky Did Not Correctly Determine Medicaid Eligibility for Some Newly Enrolled Beneficiaries," *Report A-04-15-08044*, May 2017a.

U.S. Department of Health and Human Services, Office of Inspector General, "Kentucky Did Not Always Perform Medicaid Eligibility Determinations for Non-Newly Eligible Beneficiaries in Accordance with Federal and State Requirements," *Report A-04-16-08047*, August 2017b.

U.S. Department of Health and Human Services, Office of Inspector General, "New York Did Not Correctly Determine Medicaid Eligibility for Some Newly Enrolled Beneficiaries," *Report A-02-15-01015*, January 2018a.

U.S. Department of Health and Human Services, Office of Inspector General, "California Made Medicaid Payments on Behalf of Newly Eligible Beneficiaries Who Did Not Meet Federal and State Requirements," *Report A-09-16-02023*, February 2018b.

U.S. Department of Health and Human Services, Office of Inspector General, "California Made Medicaid Payments on Behalf of Non–Newly Eligible Beneficiaries Who Did Not Meet Federal and State Requirements," *Report A-09-17-02002*, December 2018c.

U.S. Department of Health and Human Services, Office of Inspector General, "New York Did Not Correctly Determine Medicaid Eligibility for Some Non-Newly Eligible Beneficiaries," *Report A-02-16-01005*, July 2019a.

U.S. Department of Health and Human Services, Office of Inspector General, "Colorado Did Not Correctly Determine Medicaid Eligibility for Some Newly Enrolled Beneficiaries," *Report A-07-16-04228*, August 2019b.

U.S. Department of Treasury, Internal Revenue Service. 2019. "*2018 Instructions for Form 8965*." https://www.irs.gov/pub/irs-pdf/i8965.pdf. Accessed December 1, 2019.

Yelowitz, Aaron. 1995. "The Medicaid Notch, Labor Supply and Welfare Participation: Evidence from Eligibility Expansions." *Quarterly Journal of Economics* 110(4): 909–39.

Yelowitz, Aaron. 2016. "How Did the ACA Affect Health Insurance Coverage in Kentucky?" *Schnatter Institute Working Paper*. John H. Schnatter Institute for the Study of Free Enterprise, University of Kentucky. http://isfe.uky.edu/sites/ISFE/files/research-pdfs/Schnatter.2017.Yelowitz.pdf . Accessed December 1, 2019.

Yelowitz, Aaron. 2019. "Improper Medicaid Enrollment Following ACA Expansion," *Health Affairs*, November 15, 2019.

Yelowitz, Aaron, and Brian Blase. 2019. "*Medicaid Improper Payments are Much Worse than Reported.*" Cato at Liberty, https://www.cato.org/blog/medicaid-improper-payments-are-much-worse-reported. Accessed December 1, 2019.

Ziliak, James. 2007. "Making Work Pay: Changes in Effective Tax Rates and Guarantees in US Transfer Programs, 1983–2002." *Journal of Human Resources* 42(3): 619–42.

SECTION IV: PROGRAM CHANGE

In: Medicaid: Politics, Policy, and Key Issues ISBN: 978-1-53618-133-3
Editor: Daniel Lanford

Chapter 9

CHANGES IN MEDICAID FOR PEOPLE WITH DISABILITY

Madonna Harrington Meyer[*] and J. Dalton Stevens
Syracuse University, Syracuse, NY, US

ABSTRACT

US disability rates have increased. Has Medicaid coverage of people with disability also increased? We take an historical approach to examine how, despite general trends toward welfare retrenchment and devolution, legislation has expanded Medicaid eligibility. In addition to benefits available to all Medicaid recipients, those with disability may be deemed eligible for special services. Eligibility for Medicaid varies by age, state, and numerous pathways to eligibility. Applicants often endure a daunting array of barriers. Effectiveness is mixed; generally those with disability who have Medicaid coverage have better access to health care and better health outcomes than the uninsured, but many barriers interfere with access to and quality of care. We conclude by evaluating policy proposals aimed at retrenching and expanding Medicaid for people with disability.

[*] Corresponding Author's Email: mhm@maxwell.syr.edu.

Keywords: disability, Medicaid, welfare policy, administrative burden, and health care

INTRODUCTION

US disability rates have increased. Has Medicaid kept pace? In this paper, we take an historic look at how Medicaid has responded to disability. We explore how, despite an overall mood of welfare retrenchment and devolution, Medicaid has expanded such that more people with disability rely on Medicaid than ever in history. Over 10 million non-elderly people with disability – 48% of children with special health care needs and 48% of nonelderly adults with disability – are covered by Medicaid (Rudowitz, Orgera, and Hinton 2019; Musumeci, and Chidambarm 2019).

We also demonstrate that for those who are able to secure coverage, mandatory and optional benefits are wide and deep. We examine how eligibility varies by age, state, and pathway to eligibility. We then turn to the administrative hurdles that people with disability face when trying to access, use, and retain Medicaid. We note that those with disability who have Medicaid coverage have better access to care and better health outcomes than the uninsured, but they face many barriers that shape access to and quality of care. We conclude by evaluating the potential impact of recent policy proposals for people with disability, some aimed at retrenchment and some aimed at expansion.

Defining and Measuring Disability

Disability is somewhat difficult to define and measure since it is neither an individual nor static phenomena – disability varies by social factors including age, time period, gender, race, income, education, and geographic location. People may have more than one, onset may occur at birth or at any later time, and the experiences of disability often change over the life course.

Conventionally, disability is understood as health conditions that impair body functions, limit activities, and restrict social participation (Schalock, Luckasson, and Shogren 2007). They fall into four broad categories: physical disabilities such as multiple sclerosis or traumatic brain injuries; mental health conditions such as schizophrenia or substance abuse disorders; intellectual or developmental disabilities such as Down syndrome or Autism; and sensory disabilities such as loss of hearing or vision (Albrecht 2012; Musumeci and Foutz 2017).

Over time the characterization of disability has shifted from an emphasis on the individual to an emphasis on society more broadly. For centuries, people and social institutions tended to view disability from an *individualistic* model that regarded disability as a trait of the individual that required correction (Priestley 2003). Throughout the early 1900s, people with disability were often kept out of sight and, therefore, out of mind. Many were placed in asylums, sterilized, or ridiculed in exhibitions; few could afford humane or effective medical interventions. After decades of activism by people with disability, their families, and those involved in the Civil Rights Movement, a *social model* strengthened. The social model emphasizes processes by which social institutions and practices create barriers to full participation in society. People are born with impairments, and disability is created or exacerbated by the exclusion, marginalization, and discrimination people with impairments experience throughout their lives (Priestley 2003; Verbrugge and Jette 1994; World Health Organization 2011). The problem is not that Arnie uses a wheelchair, it is that we, society, built a theater without a ramp. Thus, disability may shift with social and political changes. For example, the 1990 Americans with Disabilities Act guaranteed equal treatment in, and equal access to, employment and public accommodations. Yet while all businesses and service providers are required to provide reasonable accommodations to employees and consumers with disability, many do not. Ongoing disability rights activism has prompted increased inclusion of people with disability, but proponents of the social model of disability note that people with impairments often find such accommodations incomplete and inadequate (Araujo 2009; Dunn and

Andrews 2015; Harlon and Robert 1998; National Early Childhood Technical Assistance Center 2011; Priestley 2003).

Measuring disability rates is complex. The U.S. Census Bureau uses the American Community Survey (Bialik 2017) to measure disability for all ages, with six questions concerning whether the respondent has difficulty with hearing, vision, cognition, walking or climbing stairs, self- care or independent living. Using those measures, 13% of the civilian US population, or 40 million, report having a disability. Alternately, the Centers for Disease Control and Prevention (CDC) uses the Behavioral Risk Factor Surveillance System to measure disability in adults related to mobility, cognition, hearing, vision, independent living, and self-care. CDC reports 25% of adults, or 61 million, have a disability (Centers for Disease Control and Prevention 2018; Okoro et al. 2018). CDC uses the National Health Interview Survey (NHIS) to measure developmental disability, excluding attention-deficit hyperactivity disorder (ADHD) and learning disabilities, among children ages 3 to 17. They report that 7% of children have been diagnosed with developmental disability (Zablotsky, Lindsey, and Blumberg 2017). Using the NHIS, and a broader definition of developmental disability that includes ADHD and learning disabilities, Boyle et al. (2011) report that 15% of children have disability. Medicaid generally accepts people under age 65 who have had disabling conditions since birth or who have acquired disabling conditions through illness, injury, or trauma but deeming of disability varies dramatically by time and place.

However disability is measured, it rises markedly with age. The U.S. Census Bureau suggests that less than 1% of children under age five, 5% of children ages 5 to 17, 6% of adults ages 18-34,13% of those 35 to 64, and 25% of those ages 65 to 74 report disability. For those ages 75 and older, 50% report a disability (Bialik 2017). Alternately, CDC reports that 25% of all adults, and 40% of those age 65 and older, have a disability (Okoro et al. 2018).

Disability has increased somewhat over time. The U.S. Census Bureau reports that the percent of people of all ages with a disability has risen from 12.7% in 2008 to 13.2% in 2017 (Houtenville and Boege 2019). Zablotsky, Lindsey, and Blumberg (2017) report that among children, the incidence of developmental disability rose from just under 6% to 7% between 2014 and 2016, while Boyle et al. (2011) report that childhood developmental disability rates rose from 12.8% to 15% between 1997 and 2008. Childhood increases tend to be concentrated in just a few diagnoses: ADHD rates rose by 33%, and Autism by 400% over that time period (Boyle et al. 2011).

Disability rates also vary by sociodemographic factors including gender, race, income, education, and geographic location. Though the U.S. Census Bureau does not report gender differences in disability rates (Bialik 2017), CDC (2018) reports that for adults, for most types of disability, women have slightly higher disability rates than men (Okoro et al. 2018). But among children the patterns are reversed; by most measures boys have higher rates than girls (Zablotsky, Lindsey, and Blumberg 2017). Race matters as well. Among adults, Asians and Pacific Islanders report the lowest rates and blacks and Native Americans report the highest rates of disability (Bialik 2017; Ross and Bateman 2018). Among children, whites have the highest and Hispanics the lowest rates of developmental disability (Zablotsky, Linsey, and Blumberg 2017). Disability rates decrease as income rises. For example, mobility disability is five times more common among 45 to 64 year olds living below the poverty line compared to those whose income is twice the poverty level (Okoro et al. 2018). Disability rates vary markedly by education level. Adults with only a high school education have disability rates that are three times higher than those with a BA, 12% and 4% respectively (Okoro et al. 2018). Disability rates also vary by geographic region. Adults in West Virginia have the highest disability rates, over 19%, and in Utah have the lowest, just under 10% (Bialik 2017; Centers for Disease Control and Prevention 2018; Okoro et al. 2018; Ross and Bateman 2018). Among cities, adults in Flint, Michigan have one of the highest rates, 22%, while adults in Fishers, Indiana, less than 300 miles away, have one of the lowest, under 4% (Bialik 2017).

MEDICAID ELIGIBILITY FOR THOSE WITH DISABILITY

Though the US has been in an era of welfare state retrenchment and devolution since the 1980s, Medicaid is exceptional. Targeted by legislative efforts to end welfare as we know it, programs such as AFDC, TANF and SSI have been shrinking in recent decades (Estes 2001; Hacker 2004; Harrington Meyer and Herd 2007; Levy 2010; Zylan and Soule 2000). But since the creation of Medicaid in 1965, Congress has generally expanded coverage, eligibility, and funding (Rudowitz, Garfield, and Hinton 2019). Early legislation required all Medicaid recipients to be categorically eligible, meaning that they to receive either AFDC, TANFF or SSI. But since 1997, the Children's Health Insurance Program (CHIP) has allowed children in families with somewhat higher incomes to be eligible for Medicaid. The Kaiser Family Foundation suggests that these "expansions in Medicaid coverage of children marked the beginning of later reforms that recast Medicaid as an income-based health coverage program" (Rudowitz, Garfield, and Hinton 2019:3). That legislation also prompted many states to conduct outreach campaigns and simplify enrollment procedures. Participation in the program increased accordingly.

In 2010, the Affordable Care Act (ACA) continued to loosen the rule of categorical eligibility by creating an optional expansion of Medicaid eligibility to include nonelderly adults with higher incomes and assets (Kaiser Family Foundation 2017a). Medicaid enrollments have again risen steadily and uninsured rates have dropped in response. Much of the increase has been for people with disability. Between 1975 and 2012, 71% of the increase in Medicaid expenditures was due to growth in enrollment: 3% due to increased enrollments among people ages 65 and older, 15% due to increased enrollment among adults, 16% due to increased enrollment among children, and 38% was due to increased enrollment among persons with disability (MACPAC 2016). As Figure 1 shows, of the increase in Medicaid expenditures due to enrollment increases, those with disability accounted for 53%. In 2015, people with disability accounted for 15% of the enrollees and 42% of the expenditures on Medicaid (Musumeci and Foutz 2017). Per capita Medicaid spending is highest for those with disability. Average per capita expenses for those with disability are more than six times those for all children, and five times those of all adults without disability, and 1.2 times those of all people age 65 and older (Musumeci and Foutz 2017).

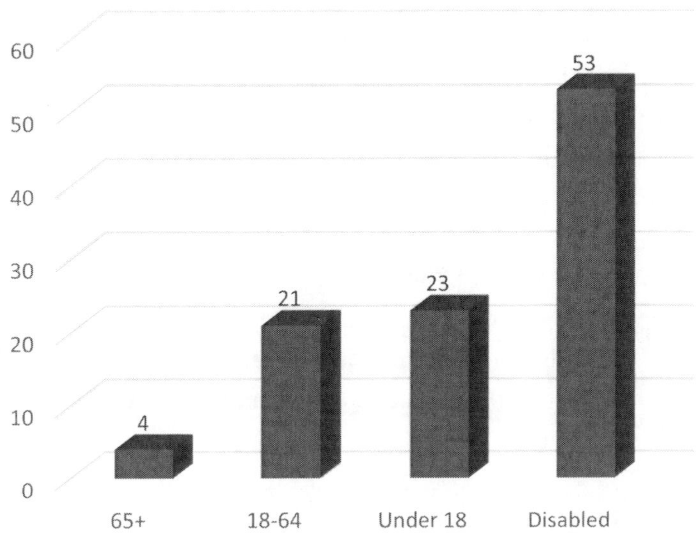

Source: MACPAC 2016.

Figure 1. Percent of the increase in Medicaid expenditures due to enrollment increases, 1975-2012, due to enrollment increases for each group.

Types of Benefits for People with Disability

In addition to needing medical care, people with disability may need long-term services and supports such as home nursing care assistance with feeding tubes and IV medications, attendant care to assist with bathing, dressing or eating; assistive technologies such as power wheelchairs or speech generating devices; medical equipment and supplies; mental health counseling; or other supportive services to maintain community-based housing or employment (Musumeci and Foutz 2017). Many of these services are not covered by private insurance (Shea 2016). Indeed, private health insurance is often less than desirable for those with disability because employer-based plans, and plans offered through the ACA exchanges, generally do not cover disability-related services. Medicaid offers a multitude of services tailored to people with a variety of disabilities, chronic health conditions, special health care needs, and disabling mental health conditions across all ages: (1) Long-term services and supports (LTSS), (2) Early and Periodic Screening Diagnostic and Treatment (EPSDT), and (3) behavioral health services comprise specialized services Medicaid enrollees with disability may access. Each provides services to distinct populations with specific needs, but states vary in who and what is covered.

(1) LTSS are provided through optional HCBS waivers, aimed at keeping people out of nursing homes. LTSS provide personal and technical assistance with activities of daily living and instrumental activities of daily living. Services include home nursing care, attendant care, assistive technologies and medical equipment, and many other services aimed at improving or maintaining the highest possible level of physical functioning and quality of life. LTSS accounted for 30% of Medicaid expenditures in 2016, and provides the most robust support for those with limited ability to perform self-care (Eiken et al. 2018; Harris-Kojetin et al. 2013; Lewis et al. 2018; Reaves and Musumeci 2015; Thach and Wiener 2018).

Ongoing efforts to decrease Medicaid's historic institutional bias are generally working. In 2012, two years after the implementation of the ACA, the U.S. began spending more money on HCBS than on institutional placements (Eiken et al. 2018). Currently, all 50 states and Washington, D.C. extend HCBS waivers to people with intellectual and developmental disability; 37 states offer HCBS to seniors and adults with physical disability; 22 states offer HCBS to those with traumatic brain or spinal cord injuries; 16 states offer HCBS to children who are medically needy; 12 states offer HCBS to those with mental health disability; and 7 states offer HCBS to those with HIV/AIDS (Musumeci, Chidambaram, and O'Malley Watts 2019a). Cumulatively, nearly 4.6 million enrollees used HCBS in 2017. However, because HCBS coverage of community-based LTSS are optional, many states have set caps on LTSS enrollments or services to contain expenditures (Eiken et al. 2018; Harris-Kojein et al. 2013; Lewis et al. 2018;

Thach and Wiener 2018). Currently over 707,000 are waiting for services due to the limited number of waivers available (Kaiser Family Foundation 2017b).

(2) EPSDT is mandatory for the states and provides extensive health-related services to children with special health care needs that extend beyond private insurance and school-based services (Musumeci and Foutz 2019). In 2017, over 13.3 million children with special health care needs qualified for EPSDT (Musumeci, and Chidambarm 2019). EPSDT provides regular medical, vision, hearing, and dental screenings, and it provides related interventions to improve conditions in early life. In addition to doctor visits, hospitalizations, x-rays, lab tests, and prescription drugs, EPSDT may include physical, occupational, and speech therapy, personal attendants, assistive technologies, private nursing, and medical transportation to appointments. Benefits are shaped by diagnosis: a child with autism may receive in-home therapy as well as speech and occupational therapy, while a child with cerebral palsy may receive personal care, case management, and assistive technology (Musumeci, and Chidambarm 2019). EPSDT expanded in 2014 when the Centers for Medicare and Medicaid Services outlined pathways through which children with autism, pervasive developmental disorder, and Asperger syndrome may qualify for extra specialized services such as other licensed practitioner services, preventive services, and more specific therapies (Mann 2015).

(3) Often overlooked in discussions about health care for those with disability, Medicaid provides the greatest amount of public funding in the treatment of mental health disability and substance use disorders in the U.S. (Mark et al. 2016; Smith et al., Chapter 10 of this volume). The ACA expanded mental health and substance use treatment services. In 2015, an estimated 43 million adults had mental health conditions while 19 million had substance use disorders (Kaiser Family Foundation 2017c, 2017d). In the same year, Medicaid funded 25% of all mental health spending and 21% of all addiction spending (Kaiser Family Foundation 2017c, 2017d; Mark et al. 2016). Medicaid covered 26% of adults with serious mental illness, 21% of those with any mental illness, and 17% of those with addiction (Kaiser Family Foundation 2017c, 2017d). Medicaid's behavioral health services

include psychiatric care, counseling, prescription medications, inpatient treatment, case management, and supportive housing. As Opioid Use Disorder (OUD) has increased, Medicaid has expanded and now covers 38% of non-elderly adults with OUD, 55% of low-income adults with OUD, and 21% of all spending on treatment for OUD (Orgera and Tolbert 2019).

Medicaid Eligibility: Age, State, Pathway Variation

People with disability are slightly more likely than those without disability to have health insurance, but the types of health insurance vary significantly. According to the American Community Survey, in 2017, 89% of adults age 18 to 64 with a disability, compared to 87% of those without a disability, had health insurance (Houtenville and Boege 2019). However, people with disability are only one-half as likely to be employed and less likely to work full time. In part because of this, adults ages 18 to 64 with disability are much less likely to be covered by private health insurance (Musumeci and Foutz 2017). As Figure 2 shows, in 2015, 31% of those with disability, compared to just 10% of those without, were on Medicaid; 41% of adults ages 18 to 64 with disability, compared to 74% of those without, were covered by private health insurance (Musumeci and Foutz 2017). Medicaid is a vital source of care for people with disability, but accessing Medicaid coverage varies dramatically by age of recipient and state of residence (Kaiser Family Foundation 2019a; Levy 2010; Musumeci, Chidambaram, and O'Malley Watts 2019b; Musumeci and Foutz 2019; Shea 2016). For example, in Louisiana, newborns and one year-olds on Medicaid funded programs are eligible with family incomes up to 142% of the federal poverty line. By comparison, in Iowa, newborns may have income up to 380% of the federal poverty line, but one year-olds are only eligible with incomes up to 172% (Kaiser Family Foundation 2019a). In New Mexico, children up through age 5 are eligible for Medicaid funded programs with incomes up to 245% of the federal poverty line, but once they celebrate their sixth birthday incomes must be below 190% (Kaiser Family Foundation 2019a). In Oregon, uninsured children up to age 18 on separate CHIP funded programs may have incomes up to the federal poverty line, while in New York they may have incomes up to 400% of the poverty line.

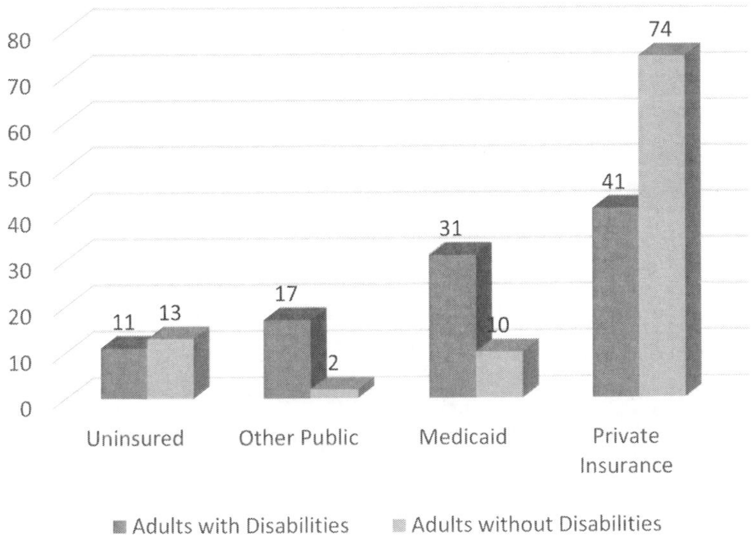

Source: Musumeci and Foutz 2017.

Figure 2. Percent with each type of insurance, among non-institutionalized adults with and without disabilities, ages 18-64, 2015.

For people with disability, becoming eligible for Medicaid is a complex process. Medicaid provides a set of pathways to eligibility, all of which vary by age, state, and other factors. In this section we describe several pathways to Medicaid eligibility for people with disability: (1) the SSI Disability Pathway, (2) the Optional ACA Expansion, (3) the Medically Needy Pathway, (4) HCBS Waivers and the Katie Beckett Rule, (5) Medicaid Buy-Ins, and (6) the Special Income Rule. Understanding and navigating these options is complex, burdensome, and at times insurmountable (Moynihan and Herd 2010).

(1) The SSI Disability Pathway

Federal policy requires all 50 states to provide Medicaid to all Supplemental Security Income (SSI) beneficiaries. SSI is a poverty-based program that, since 1972, has provided income to people who are poor, and who have disability, or are age 65 and older. Adult recipients must have impaired ability for gainful employment due to old age or significant disability. They must also be sufficiently poor. Federal income limits are equal to 74% of the federal poverty line, and asset limits, frozen since 1989, are equal to $2,000 per individual and $3,000 per couple. Some state rules are even stricter, while others are less restrictive (Musumeci, Chidambaram, and O'Malley Watts 2019b). States are permitted to offer Medicaid to older persons and persons with disability up to an income limit at 100% of the federal poverty line, and in 2018, 21 states did so. In addition, 11 states set the asset limit higher than the federal guideline (Musumeci, Chidambaram, and O'Malley Watts 2019b; Kaiser Family Foundation 2017d). Roughly one-third of persons with disability who qualify for Medicaid do so through the SSI pathway; the remainder qualify through the pathways described below (Musumeci, Chidambaram, and O'Malley Watts 2019b).

(2) The Optional ACA Expansion

The ACA created an optional expansion that allows states to set the income limit for Medicaid eligibility at 138% of the federal poverty line and remove the asset limit. As of 2019, 37 states and DC have adopted the expansion (Rudowitz, Orgera, and Hinton 2019). The expansion has been particularly important for those with disability who may receive Medicaid while they await their disability determination, or who may have a disability that does not meet the more strict SSI medical criteria, or who do not qualify for SSI (Musumeci and Foutz 2017).

(3) The Medically Needy Pathway

Some people with disability qualify for Medicaid on the medically needy pathway. This option extends Medicaid eligibility to individuals with high medical expenses whose income exceeds the maximum limit for other pathways. They become eligible when their income minus their health care expenses places them below state income limits. As of 2018, 34 states have a Medicaid medically needy program in place (Kaiser Family Foundation 2018). There is tremendous state variation in the income, asset, and spending guidelines. In 2018, the median medically needy income eligibility standard, after medical expenses, was just 48% of the federal poverty line (Musumeci, Chidambaram, and O'Malley Watts 2019b). Only nine states set the medically needy income standard, minus health care expenses, at or above the SSI level while 25 states set them below SSI standards. Asset limits tend to remain very strict under medically needy coverage. Of the states with medically needy coverage, 19 set the asset limits at the SSI levels, Connecticut has a lower asset limit, and 14 states have set a higher asset limit.

(4) HCBS Waivers and Katie Beckett Rule

Long criticized for having an institutional bias, Medicaid policies have, over time, eased eligibility in ways that encourage at-home, community-based care (MACPAC 2016; Musumeci, Chidambaram, and O'Malley Watts 2019a, 2019b, 2019c; Zylan and Soule 2000). Medicaid Home and Community-Based Services (HCBS) help people with disability who require institutional level care to instead receive that care in the community. Waivers cover people with cognitive, physical, and mental health disability, and people with chronic illnesses, by providing assistance with self-care and household activities. In 2017, 4.6 million Medicaid enrollees received HCBS at a combined federal and state cost of $83 billion. Medicaid HCBS per capita spending averaged nearly $18,000 in 2017, ranging from $5,000 for those with HIV/AIDS to $44,000 for those with intellectual or developmental disabilities (Musumeci, Cidambarm, and O'Malley Watts 2019a). Eligibility, coverage, and spending vary markedly by state.

Currently all states except Tennessee cover children with significant disability who would otherwise need institutional care but are living at home under the Katie Beckett pathway or a comparable waiver program (Kaiser Family Foundation 2019a; Musumeci, Chidambarm, and O'Malley Wats 2019b; Musumeci and Chidambaram 2019; Musumeci and Foutz 2017; Rudowitz, Garfield, and Hinton 2019). As with children living in institutions, the Katie Beckett pathway disregards parental income and assets when covering children with disability who are receiving care at home with their families. Only the child's own income, up to 300% of SSI limits, or 222% federal poverty line, and assets, usually up to $2,000, are counted. Some states cover Katie Beckett children as an optional state plan group, while other states use a Medicaid HCBS waiver. Using a waiver allows states to cap enrollment and has led to waiting lists (Musumeci, Chidambarm, and O'Malley Wats 2019c; Rudowitz, Orgera, and Hinton 2019). Six of the 50 states that provide Katie Beckett (or equivalent coverage) charge monthly premiums that vary by state. For example Maine charges all Katie Beckett enrollees a premium based on income and whether the child has private health insurance, while North Dakota charges premiums equal to 5% of gross countable income beginning at 83% of the federal poverty line (Musumeci, Chidambarm, and O'Malley Wats 2019b).

(5) Medicaid Buy-Ins

In 2018, 45 states offer a pathway for working people with disability (Musumeci, Chidambarm, and O'Malley Wats 2019b). In some cases Medicaid allows those who would not meet the income or asset limits to purchase Medicaid by paying a premium. The Ticket to Work and Work Incentives Improvement Act of 1999 allows states to create a Medicaid buy-in program for working people ages 18 to 64 with disability. Whether beneficiaries were born with disability or injured on or off the job, ticket to work is intended to incentivize employment and reduce reliance on cash assistance programs. It allows those who are receiving Social Security Disability Insurance (SSDI) or SSI due to disability to buy-in to Medicaid coverage if they have income or assets above their state guidelines, impairment-related work expenses, a plan to achieve self-support, publicly funded personal attendant expenses, or medical expenses above the state average (Medicaid.gov 2019; Shea 2016; Social Security Administration 2019). This option provides people with disability the opportunity to work and receive Medicaid coverage without having to choose between working and qualifying for Medicaid (Kaiser Family Foundation 2017a; Social Security Administration 2019). Income and asset limits vary markedly by state. Of the 45 states that offer this pathway, three have no income limits and eight have no asset limits (Musumeci, Chidambarm, and O'Malley Wats 2019b; Shea 2016; Social Security Administration 2019). Of the 45 states, 34 charge either sliding scale or flat premiums for the working people with disability on this pathway (Musumeci, Chidambarm, and O'Malley Wats 2019b).

Enrollment in Ticket to Work (TTW) has grown slowly but steadily (Shea 2016). Since the ACA was passed ten years ago, more than 400,000 individuals with disability have taken part (Medicaid.gov 2019; Social Security Administration 2019). Efforts to encourage earnings are generally successful; total earnings among all Medicaid buy-in participants in 2011 were about $1.15 billion (Shea 2016). Analysis of expenditures and services-used showed Medicaid buy-in participants incurred lower annual Medicaid costs than other adult Medicaid enrollees with disability (Shea 2016). Studies in Kansas and New York have demonstrated that Medicaid buy-in participants had a better quality of life while Medicaid expenditures were less (Medicaid.gov; Shea 2016). The difference was not likely due to selection bias wherein healthier people chose to enroll in Medicaid buy-in. In New York, for example, researchers used a variety of sociodemographic variables to create a matching quasi-random control group and found that those who participated in Medicaid buy-in had reduced health care utilization and Medicaid expenses (Shea 2016).

The Family Opportunity Act of 2005 allowed families to buy-in to Medicaid if their child has significant disability but does not need an institutional level care. Unlike the Katie Beckett pathway, which considers only the child's income, this pathway considers household income. In 2018, only five states offer this optional plan, and a sixth state does so through a waiver. This pathway extends Medicaid to children who have disability in families with incomes up to 300% of the federal poverty line, though some states limit it to just 150% (Musumeci, Chidambarm, and O'Malley Wats 2019b). There are no asset limits. Five of the six states that offer this pathway charge premiums, which vary significantly by state. For example, Iowa does not charge premiums, while Louisiana changes $15 per month beginning at

201% of the federal poverty line (Musumeci, Chidambarm, and O'Malley Wats 2019b).

(6) The Special Income Rule

The special income rule allows states to provide Medicaid coverage to those with functional needs that require institutional level care, whether they are receiving care in an institution or in the community (MACPAC 2016; Musumeci, Chidambarm, and O'Malley Wats 2019b; Rudowitz, Orgera, and Hinton 2019). Currently, 43 states offer this pathway to those with incomes up to 300% of the SSI income limit, or 222% federal poverty level. Though there is state variation in income and asset limits, most states set the asset rules at the SSI levels of $2,000 for an individual and $3,000 for a couple (Musumeci, Chidambarm, and O'Malley Wats 2019b).

In addition to multiple pathways for eligibility, Medicaid offers numerous programs that permit families to reconfigure resources as they attempt to qualify. For example, 48 states allow individuals to qualify for Medicaid using supplemental needs and pooled income trusts. These trusts allow any amounts remaining in the trusts upon death of the beneficiary to go to the state to help recover Medicaid expenditures (Musumeci, Chidambarm, and O'Malley Wats 2019b).

Per a 2014 federal law, all 50 states now offer Achieving a Better Life Experience (ABLE) accounts that allow people with disability occurring before age 26, and their families, to save money to fund disability-related expenses that are disregarded when determining Medicaid eligibility. ABLE accounts can be used to pay for education, housing, employment training, assistive technology, legal fees, and many other expenses. The maximum lifetime limit for accounts ranges from $235,000 in Mississippi to over $500,000 in Pennsylvania (Musumeci, Chidambarm, and O'Malley Wats 2019b).

Overall, despite an atmosphere of welfare retrenchment in the US, Medicaid has used an ever-expanding set of pathways and policies to expand coverage in recent decades. As a result, increasingly large shares of children and adults with disability now receive medical care through Medicaid.

Medicaid's Administrative Burden for People with Disability

Though Medicaid has expanded in recent decades, navigating the various pathways and policies can be overwhelming, particularly for those with disability. Like all poverty-based welfare programs, Medicaid is mired in red tape (Moynihan and Herd 2010). Medicaid red tape contributes to low uptake among eligible people (Elder and Powers 2006; Korpi and Palme 1998; Rudowtiz, Orgera, and Hinton 2019; Shore-Sheppard 2008; Whit et al. 2017); decreases civil and social rights (Moynihan and Herd 2010); increases stigma and negative psychological effects (Bagatell et al.2017; Whittle et al. 2017); and communicates how the state views its constituents (Campbell 2003; Soss 1999, 2005). Managing the extensive paper work, rules, and policies creates an administrative burden that may be especially challenging for those with disability. Administrative burdens that haunt those with disability in particular include (1) extensive paperwork surrounding disability determinations, (2) state variations in Medicaid policies, and (3) stigmatized treatment.

(1) Extensive Paperwork Surrounding Disability Determination

Proving that one is poor enough to qualify is an administrative hurdle all Medicaid applicants must surmount, but proving that one is disabled enough to qualify constitutes an additional burden only for those with disability. Both processes vary markedly by state. In New York, for example, all applicants must file the general 14-page Medicaid application (New York State Department of Health 2015). Then, those with disability must also complete Supplement A which includes eight more pages on work history for adults among other topics (New York State Department of Health 2010). As authors of this chapter, we each took nearly 20 minutes to simply read the NY application, and had difficulty understanding what documentation was required and how to obtain it. Hirschi and colleagues'

(2019) mixed-methods survey of 615 parents or caregivers of children with disability reported unclear eligibility criteria, burdensome paperwork, and drawn-out administrative procedures. Administrative burdens increased out-of-pocket expenses, usurped time and energy, and delayed care (Hirschi et al. 2019). Others have found strict eligibility criteria, complex application processes, and lengthy redetermination procedures deter benefit program uptake (Hogan 2012; Katch, Wagner, and Aron-Dine 2018). Some potential enrollees with disabling chronic health conditions report difficulty distinguishing the different social safety-net programs and their respective eligibility criteria (Whittle et al. 2017).

In addition to lengthy Medicaid application forms, those who apply for Medicaid based on disability status undergo a disability determination process. In New York, certification includes an interview and observation during which caseworkers are instructed to obtain an unofficial diagnosis (U.S. Government Accountability Office 2008). During the interview, applicants with disability are encouraged to supply full medical histories including clinical and laboratory findings, diagnostic statements, prescribed treatments, and functional capacity assessments from numerous medical sources. As part of the process, physicians must take full medical histories; assess severity, permanency, and type of impairment; determine psychosocial factors and psychiatric conditions; and compare impairment to physical and mental job demands (Hyman 2016). The process is often complicated because, as noted above, disability diagnoses are ever-changing, often ambiguous, and generally difficult to determine, thus the process tends to delay eligibility, especially for children (Hogan 2012). Moreover, many Medicaid doctors are "nonproductive," or refuse to provide consultative exams and requested documentation for applicants with disability. The United States Government Accountability Office (2008) notes that doctors are more likely to refuse to provide documents for patients with outstanding medical bills. More generally, however, many medical providers find it difficult to prioritize providing documentation because the process is time-consuming and expensive; they would prefer to devote time and resources to seeing additional patients (U.S. Government Accountability Office 2008).

After all the information has been collected and reviewed by a caseworker, the agency sends the application to the Disability Review Team for assessment (U.S. Government Accountability Office 2008). For applicants with disability, the review is allowed to take 90 days or more. While delays are not supposed to influence eligibility, delays have significant impacts on potential beneficiaries (Whittle et al. 2017; Candisky 2019). Among the 88,000 pending Medicaid applications in Ohio, many with disability have faced delays in services (Candisky 2019). One Ohio applicant with substance abuse disorder was able to locate a clinic for free addiction treatment, but had a heart attack while waiting for Medicaid determination (Candisky 2019). Determination delays may result in worsening illness, increased risk for complications, and longer future hospital stays. Moreover, hospitals, nursing homes, physicians and other health care providers often experience delays in receiving Medicaid reimbursements and, as a result, avoid accepting Medicaid patients (U.S. Government Accountability Office 2008; Cunningham and O'Malley 2008).

(2) State Variation in Medicaid Policies

State variation in Medicaid creates administrative burdens that have serious implications for people with disability and their families. Because of substantial state differences in Medicaid, people with disability are often locked into certain states. Grossman (2018a, 2018b) reveals that nonelderly adult Medicaid beneficiaries with disability who need personal care attendants may be limited in their ability to move for opportunities such as careers, job-training, and higher education. For example, Shawn Murinko (2014) had to pass on a career with the U.S. Department of Justice in Washington D.C. paying $124,000 because of state variation in Medicaid eligibility and coverage. In Washington State, Medicaid covered services that assisted Shawn with activities of daily living. In Maryland, Medicaid did not, and he would have to pay $114,000 annually out-of-pocket to cover those same services. Conversely, some people live in states with less generous Medicaid programs and would like to move to states with more comprehensive coverage but cannot because of personal or employment obligations. Circle of Moms, a blog for mothers of children with disability, includes many posts about wanting to move to states with more generous Medicaid benefits (PopSugar 2019). It is easy to imagine why the parents of a newborn with disability in Louisiana, which sets the income limit for eligibility at 142% of the federal poverty line, might want to move to Iowa, where the income limit is 380% (Kaiser Family Foundation 2019a).

(3) Stigmatized Treatment of Applicants with Disability

Interpersonal and institutional treatment of potential and actual Medicaid beneficiaries is often cited as a barrier to program participation. Welfare stigma, which is the felt or perceived prejudice against benefit recipients, can be particularly damaging for those who also grapple with the disability stigma (Hansen, Bourgois, and Drucker 2014). In one ethnography of people with disability, a participant diagnosed with depression and psychosis said he was going to commit suicide because he ended up on Medicaid and other benefit programs after being dishonorably discharged from the military, stating, "I'm to blame. Because I'm a loser. I'm a freaking addict" (Hansen, Bourgois, and Drucker 2014). Other studies have noted differences in welfare stigma based on disability type (Bagatell et al. 2017). For example, young adults with cerebral palsy entering the U.S. social welfare system for the first time as adults report stigmatizing encounters with caseworkers who assume they are incompetent and have intellectual disability (Bagatell et al. 2017). Focus group participants reported service providers did not take them seriously, treated them as inferiors, and gave them "dummied down" information (Bagatell et al. 2017). Other studies suggest low-income public insurance beneficiaries, many of whom have disability, experience stigma across intersectional identities of race, gender, immigration status, and illness status (Hansen, Bourgois, and Drucker 2014; Martinez-Hume et al. 2017). For example, Carrie a 38-year old white, unemployed, woman with HIV reported instances of significant stigma based on her gender and HIV status which limited the quality of care she received while covered by Medicaid (Martinez-Hume et al. 2017). While at the gynecologist, Carrie's doctor asked her to swab herself for a sexually transmitted disease test and other doctors wore multiple sets of gloves while interacting with her (Martinez-Hume et al. 2017). Those with disability who are receiving Medicaid may be subjected to multiple levels of stigmatization.

All Medicaid enrollees must overcome challenging administrative burdens, but those with disability tend to face even more challenges and often have fewer resources to address them. We are not able to estimate the numbers of people with disability that are effectively kept off the program by red tape, but we hope this issue will be addressed by future researchers.

PROGRAM EFFECTIVENESS

Effectiveness of Medicaid for people with disability is generally mixed. People with disability tend to have fewer resources and greater health care needs. For those who are eligible, Medicaid provides essential access to health care. Compared to people with disability who do not have health insurance, those with disability who have Medicaid coverage have better access to care and health outcomes. But compared more generally to people without disability, those with disability tend to have less access to care. This is particularly true for those who live in rural areas and in certain states.

People with disability tend to be poorer, have more functional limitations, and have greater health care needs. For those who are eligible, Medicaid provides essential care. Over half of Medicaid recipients ages 18 to 64 with disability have incomes below the federal poverty line, and nearly 85% have incomes below 200% of the federal poverty line (Musumeci and Foutz 2017). Those on Medicaid tend to have more health care needs than those who are privately insured. Nonelderly Medicaid adults with disability are four times more likely to receive nursing or other health care at home, 2.5 times more likely to have three or more functional limitations, and 1.5 times more likely to have ten or more health care visits a year, compared to nonelderly adults with disability who are privately insured (Musumeci and

Foutz 2017). Medicaid beneficiaries with intellectual and developmental disability experience higher prevalence of multiple chronic conditions and obesity, and make more insurance claims than those with private insurance (Philips, Houtenvile, and Reichard 2019; Reichard and Stozle 2011; Rimmer and Yamaki 2006). They often require a broad array of services (Musumeci and Foutz 2017). For example, Curtis, age 20, has been diagnosed with autism, intellectual disability, and sensory integration issues. He cannot be left alone and needs assistance with personal hygiene and taking medications. Medicaid helps to cover an attendant who accompanies him on errands and provides instruction for basic life skills while his mother is at work (Musumeci and Foutz 2017).

When compared to people with disability who have no insurance, people with disability on Medicaid have better access to health care, better health outcomes, and are less likely to postpone or go without needed care (Okoro et al. 2018). A nationwide survey of Medicaid beneficiaries with disability found 78% always or usually obtained needed care, and 82% received care quickly (Medicaid.gov 2017). Nearly 90% of Medicaid recipients with disability report usually or always having good doctor-patient communication, and 78% report having positive customer service interactions. However, variation in access is clear. For example, 81% of Medicaid recipients with disability who have established medical providers report the highest overall quality of care, but only 62% among Medicaid recipients with disability without established medical providers report the highest quality of care (Medicaid.gov 2017). Moreover, 38% of Medicaid recipients with disability report always having difficulty obtaining special medical equipment and other technologies. But most, like Nicholas, find Medicaid to be responsive. Currently age 33, Nicholas was diagnosed with multiple sclerosis and has impaired mobility, hearing, and vision, as well as a great deal of pain. Medicaid covers his medications, doctor visits, and power wheelchair (Musumeci and Foutz 2017). Medicaid also helped to make his home shower accessible and arranged home delivered meals.

When compared to people who do not have disability, those who have disability have more difficulties accessing needed health care. Among adults ages 18-44 who have any type of disability, one-third do not have a regular health care provider, one-third have an unmet health care need due to cost in the past year, and one-fourth did not have a routine check-up in the past year (Okoro et al. 2018). Even in the context of ACA expansions, people with a range of disabilities report higher rates of delaying and forgoing medical care, typically due to difficulties accessing or paying for care, than those without disability despite similar or slightly lower rates of uninsurance (Kaye 2019). Type of disability and age influences access to care. For example, almost one-quarter of 18-44 year olds with self-care disability did not have a usual health care provider while over one-third of those with cognitive disability did not (Okoro et al. 2018). Kaye (2019) finds people with mental health disability are three times more likely than those without disability to delay or forgo medical care. As Medicaid adults reach age 65 and qualify for Medicare coverage, many of the health care deficits among those with disability diminish due to overlapping coverage (Okoro et al. 2018).

Program effectiveness varies by rural versus urban settings (Beck, Page, and Buche 2018; Drainoni et al. 2006; Iezzoni, Killeen, and O'Day 2006; Medicaid.gov 2017; Santhanam 2018). Rural citizens with disability experience multiple barriers to care (Beck, Page, and Buche 2018; Drainoni et al. 2006; Iezzoni, Killeen, and O'Day 2006; Santhanam 2018). Among all Medicaid beneficiaries with disability, 12% report transportation barriers related to distance and accessibility, 9% report difficulty finding physicians who take Medicaid and serve populations with disability, 14% report delays in services, and 9% report inability to afford care (Medicaid.gov 2017). These problems are more pronounced for rural Medicaid recipients with disability since many rural communities lack health resources (Beck, Page, and Buche 2018; Drainoni et al. 2006; Iezzoni, Killeen, and O'Day 2006; Santhanam 2018). For example, 13% of rural counties have no behavioral health care providers while only 3% of urban counties lack these providers (Beck, Page, and Buche 2018). Toni, a focus group participant with disability receiving Medicaid services, was denied transportation to Boston, Massachusetts for specialist services after receiving inadequate care from doctors nearer her home in rural Massachusetts (Beck, Page, and Buche 2018). For Casey Britton and her son Seth, Medicaid recipients from

Tennessee, the lack of a pediatrician in their rural and impoverished county proved to be problematic (Santhanam 2018). When Seth entered elementary school and was identified as having developmental delays related to motor skills, Britton had to drive 60 miles to walk-in clinics to receive services for her son (Santhanam 2018).

Program effectiveness also varies by state. Using an overall performance score based on access to care, speed of care, doctor-patient communication, health plan information and customer service, and access to special medical equipment, a national survey of Medicaid recipients with disability reveals some states are outperforming others in administering Medicaid to those with disability (Medicaid.gov 2017). Minnesota was the only state where most Medicaid recipients with disability rated effectiveness high on all measures. In thirteen states, most Medicaid beneficiaries with disability reported never or sometimes having issues on between two and four measures of effectiveness. Five states were performing well in only one of the five indicators, and 20 states achieved zero markers of high performance. More state-level comparisons in program effectiveness are needed to determine what problems are most prevalent, where they are most prevalent, and how high-performing states differ from low-performing states.

DISCUSSION

Medicaid has expanded to meet the increasing demand for health insurance among those with lower incomes and less education who are seeing the most significant increases in disability rates. CHIP and the ACA have expanded eligibility criteria and extended more services to children and adults with disability, and more people with disability are able to access needed hospitals, doctors, diagnostic care, dentists, hospice services, prescription drugs, preventive medicine, telemedicine, LTSS, EPSDT, and behavioral health services. However, ongoing state variations are pronounced and problematic, the program's multiple eligibility pathways are mind-boggling in their complexity, and administrative delays interfere with timely receipt of much-needed services. Indeed, Medicaid recipients with disability report interruptions in coverage, service gaps, inability to use services, stigmatization, and significant administrative burden. Given the growing Medicaid budget and expanding eligibility criteria, policy experts and disability advocates have developed a variety of Medicaid proposals. Some policy proposals are generated by a spirit of retrenchment and aimed at reducing eligibility and program costs, such as introducing work requirements and expanding managed care. Other policy proposals are generated in the spirit of expansion, aimed at increasing eligibility and coverage, such as unfreezing the asset limit and expanding HCBS waivers. To the extent that any of these proposals are implemented, they will have substantive effects on the everyday lives of people with disability.

In an effort to reduce Medicaid enrollment and expenditures, some states are implementing or considering work requirements (see also Rocco, Chapter 5 of this volume). Medicaid work requirements force beneficiaries to prove that they have pursued or held employment by providing hours of work, job training, and job-seeking activities on a weekly or monthly basis. As of April 2019, fifteen states are entertaining work requirements for Medicaid recipients, and seven states have approved them (Kaiser Family Foundation 2019b; Musumeci, Garfield, and Rudowitz 2018). Work requirements generally exclude those with disability, although legislation recently passed in Kansas does not (Bailey and Solomon 2018; Wagner and Solomon 2018). Work requirements still influence Medicaid recipients with disability because many do not qualify for Medicaid through a disability-related pathway, thus they are subjected to work requirements (Wagner and Solomon 2018). Moreover, regardless of disability status, work requirements increase verification processes, adding to the already extensive and labor-intensive paperwork associated with Medicaid applications and re-verification (Bailey and Solomon 2018; Wagner and Solomon 2018;). Those with disability, specifically mental health conditions, physical disability, and substance use disorders, tend to be poorly situated to deal with these increases in administrative burden. The challenges of understanding how to provide documentation under tight deadlines cause some people with disability to be excluded from programs for which they are eligible (Wagner and Solomon 2018). Others who perform a great deal of care work for family members with disability and themselves rely on Medicaid struggle to juggle those duties with employment (Harrington Meyer 2014). For example, Casey Britton, a Medicaid recipient from Tennessee, is particularly concerned with implementation of work requirements (Santhanam 2018). Britton explains that, given the care work responsibilities associated with her son, full-time employment is nearly impossible. She fears she will be forced off Medicaid if work requirements are passed in Tennessee. To the extent that states implement work requirements, even if they exclude those with disability, they may adversely impact people with disability and the family members who care for them.

In an effort to contain costs, Medicaid is increasingly shifting to managed care. Of particular importance to those with disability, as of 2017, 21 states have adopted managed care programs for Medicaid LTSS. Many have seen mixed financial and individual results (Hall et al. 2015; Kaye 2012; Lewis et al. 2018; McCue and Bailit 2011; Musumeci, Chidambaram, and O'Malley Watts 2019a; Owen, Heller, and Bowers 2016). In these programs, Managed Care Organizations (MCOs) receive a fixed amount of money per person per month for services. While empirical studies across states are limited, some studies reveal most beneficiaries have received the same level and quality of care (Hall et al. 2015).

Managed care may seem like a simpler alternative to the complicated health delivery systems with which people with disability often wrestle because MCOs offer comprehensive services provided through a network of physicians as it consolidates care delivery and receipt (Tanenbaum and Hurley 1995). However, the complex needs of people with disability are often difficult to address via managed care, especially ancillary services such as in home care, personal attendants, and assistive technology (Tanenbaum and Hurley 1995). In a mixed-methods survey project on managed care transitions in LTSS for people with disability, 64% of the 105 Kansans with disability who participated reported satisfaction or high satisfaction with services post-transition (Hall et al. 2015). However, 25% reported inability to access needed medical services, 16% reported difficulty in obtaining waiver-based services, 22% reported limitations in covered benefits, and 13% reported limited provider networks among other difficulties such as difficulties paying for medicines and assistive technologies and transportation (Hall et al. 2015). Some respondents from a study of managed care recipients with disability in Kansas reported that they could no longer see their doctors, obtain needed medications, or obtain medical supplies (Hall et al. 2015).

Several unique cases have demonstrated problems with managed care. For example, Anna Landre, a Georgetown University student with type two spinal muscular atrophy, was notified by Horizon NJ Health, her MCO, that the 16 hours of daily care she received would be cut to 10 hours per day despite no changes in her day to day or health condition (Carino 2019; Wieffering 2019). Despite a judge siding with Landre, the MCO only offered to settle the dispute with Landre after her case caught national attention. The MCO then agreed to approve the original 112 hours per week if Landre agreed to drop her appeal (Carino 2019). Landre signed the agreement, but noted, "It's a big relief that I'm no longer in a state of crisis, but this only helps me, this agreement…There are plenty of people who have to keep dealing with this until we fix it" (Carino 2019). While these programs can increase autonomy in the type, timing, and source of care, managed care has pitfalls that must be addressed by accounting for the unique care needs of people with disability.

Conversely, in an effort to continue Medicaid expansion and make it more readily available to those with disability, some policy proposals are aimed at expansion. For example, some policy analysts want to unfreeze the asset limit for Medicaid eligibility (Rudowitz, Garfield, and Hinton, 2019; Harrington Meyer and Herd 2007; Harrington Meyer 2014). Though there is tremendous state and pathway variation, most Medicaid recipients are required to have assets of less than $2,000 for an individual and $3,000 for a couple. That asset limit, frozen since 1989, keeps many who would otherwise qualify from receiving Medicaid benefits. Policy experts note that had the asset limit been indexed to inflation it would now be $8,000 for an individual and $12,000 for a couple. Redefining the asset limit and indexing it to inflation would increase access to Medicaid for those with disability (Center on Budget and Policy Priorities 2017; Harrington Meyer and Herd 2007).

Another policy proposal aimed at program growth is expansion of HCBS waivers either by adding them to the federal mandate or by increasing funding. HCBS waivers support community living and participation for children and adults, and are one of the most important Medicaid services available to people with a variety of disability. However, states determine how many HCBS waivers are available to eligible state residents, hence enrollment caps and waiting lists often occur (Musumeci, Chidambaram, and O'Malley Watts 2019a, 2019c). Indeed, demand exceeds availability. Of the more than 707,000 eligible Medicaid beneficiaries on waitlists for HCBS in 2017, over two-thirds had intellectual or developmental disabilities and over one-fourth were seniors and adults with disability (Kaiser Family Foundation 2017b). Since 2016, this number has increased 8% (Musumeci, Chidambaram, and O'Malley Watts 2019c). Beneficiaries spend an average of 30 months on waiting lists (Musumeci, Chidambaram, and O'Malley Watts 2019c). States are able to opt into and out of offering HCBS to Medicaid beneficiaries, and this optional status leaves HCBS particularly susceptible to budget cuts. Based on the significant role HCBS plays in the lives of people with disability, policy experts advocate making HCBS part of the federal mandate of services provided by Medicaid. As an intermediate step, policy advocates support decreasing waiting lists by increasing funding for these services.

Any changes to Medicaid policy will most certainly have sizable impacts on people with disability and their families. Though researchers and policy makers are attentive to Medicaid's responsiveness to changes in poverty rate, there is little attention to Medicaid's responsiveness to changes in disability rates. People with disability are very diverse, thus assessments of impacts should consider age of beneficiaries, types and severity of impairments, types of services needed, and implications for families. Medicaid policy proposals must be informed by a social, rather than an individualistic, disability policy framework that is cognizant of the heterogeneity of the population served and the role that society plays in mitigating or exacerbating disability. Seemingly simple changes may lead to complex variations in eligibility, costs, administrative burdens, gaps in coverage, delays in health care, quality of care, and, most importantly, quality of life for people with disability.

REFERENCES

Albrecht, Gary. 2012. "Series Introduction to Disability through the Life Course." In *Disability through the Life Course*, edited by Tamar Heller, Sarah Parker Harris, and Gary Albrecht, vii-xviii. Thousand Oaks, CA: SAGE Publications.

Araujo, Blanca E. 2009. "Best Practices in Working with Linguistically Diverse Families." *Intervention in School and Clinic* 45(2): 116-123.

Bagatell, Nancy, Dara Chan, Kimberly Karrat Rauch, and Deborah Thorpe. 2017. "'Thrust Into Adulthood': Transition Experiences of Young Adults with Cerebral Palsy." *Disability & Health Journal* 10(1): 80-86. Accessed June 7, 2019. doi.org/10.1016/j.dhjo.2016.09.008.

Bailey, Anna, and Judith Solomon. 2018. "*Medicaid Work Requirements Don't Protect People with Disabilities*." Center on Budget and Policy Priorities. Accessed June 7, 2019. https://www.cbpp.org/sites/default/files/atoms/files/11-14-18health.pdf.

Beck, Angela J., Cory Page, and Jessica Buche. 2018. "*Characteristics of the Rural Behavioral Health Workforce: A Survey of Medicaid/Medicare Reimbursed Providers*." Ann Arbor, MI: UMSPH. Accessed June 4, 2019. http://www.behavioralhealthworkforce.org/wp-content/uploads/2019/01/Y3-FA2-P1-Rural-Pop_Full-Report.pdf.

Bialik, Kristen. 2017. "*7 Facts About Americans with Disabilities*." Pew Research Center. Accessed June 7, 2019. https://www.pewresearch.org/fact-tank/2017/07/27/7-facts-about-americans-with-disabilities/.

Boyle, Coleen A., Sheree Boulet, Laura A. Schieve, Robin A. Cohen, Stephen J. Blumberg, Marshalyn Yeargin-Allsopp, Susanna Visser, and Michael D. Kogan. 2011. "Trends in the Prevalence of Developmental Disabilities in US Children, 1997-2008." *Pediatrics* 127(6): 1034-1042. doi:10.1542/peds.2010-2989.

Brien, Michael J., and Christopher A. Swann. 2001. "*Prenatal WIC Participation and Infant Health: Selection and Material Fixed Effects*." Charlottesville, VA: Department of Economics, University of Virginia.

Campbell, Andrea L. 2003. *How Policies Make Citizens: Senior Political Activism and the American Welfare State*. Princeton, NJ: Princeton University Press.

Candisky, Catherine. 2019. "Medicaid Backlog Delaying Care for Needy and Payments for Health Providers." *Akron Beacon Journal*. Accessed June 19, 2019. https://www.ohio.com/news/20190304/medicaid-backlog-delaying-care-for-needy-and-payments-for-health-providers/1.

Carino, Jerry, and Dustin Racioppi. 2019. "*Disabled Student Wins Battle Vs. NJ Medicaid; Won't have to Drop Out of Georgetown*." Asbury Park Press. Accessed June 19, 2019. https://www.app.com/story/news/health/2019/06/17/nj-medicaid-anna-landre-georgetown/1475982001/.

Center on Budget and Policy Priorities. 2017. *Policy Basics: Supplemental Security Income (SSI) Program*. Accessed June 21, 2019. https://www.cbpp.org/research/social-security/policy-basics-supplemental-security-income.

Centers for Disease Control and Prevention. 2018. "*1 in 4 US Adults Live With a Disability*." Accessed June 7, 2019. https://www.cdc.gov/media/releases/2018/p0816-disability.html.

Cunningham, Peter J., and Ann S. O'Malley. 2008. "Do Reimbursement Delays Discourage Medicaid Participation by Physicians?" *Health Affairs* (Web Content). Accessed June 7, 2019. Doi.org/10.1377/hlthaff.28.1.w17.

Drainoni, Mari-Lynn, Elizabeth Lee-Hood, Carol Tobias, Sara S. Bachman, Jennifer Andrews, and Lisa Maisels. 2006. "Cross-Disability Experiences of Barriers to Health-Care Access." *Journal of Disability Policy Studies* 17(2): 101-115.

Dunn, Dana S., and Erin E. Andrews. 2015. "Person-First and Identity-First Language: Developing Psychologists' Cultural Competence Using Disability Language." *American Psychologist* 70(3): 255-264.

Eiken, Steve, Kate Sredl, Brian Burwell, and Angie Amos. 2018. *Medicaid Expenditures for Long-Term Services and Supports in FY 2016.*

Baltimore, MD: Medicaid.Gov. Accessed June 7, 2019. https://www.medicaid.gov/medicaid/ltss/downloads/reports-and-evaluations/ltssexpenditures2016.pdf.

Elder, Todd E., and Elizabeth T. Powers. 2006. "The Incredible Shrinking Program: Trends in SSI Participation of the Aged." *Research on Aging* 28(3): 341-358. Accessed June 7, 2019. doi.org/10.1177/0164027505285918.

Estes, Carroll L. 2001. *Social Policy & Aging: A Critical Perspective*. Thousand Oaks, CA: Sage Publications.

Grossman, Brian R. 2018a. "Disability and Corporeal (Im)Mobility: How Interstate Variation in Medicaid Impacts the Cross-State Plans and Pursuits of Personal Care Attendant Service Users." *Disability and Rehabilitation*. Accessed June 7, 2019. Doi.org/10.1080/09638288.2018.1483436.

Grossman, Brian R. 2018b. "Barriers to Cross-State Movement for Disabled People and Their Families: A Social Problem." *Disability Studies Quarterly* 38(2). Accessed June 7, 2019. http://dsq-sds.org/article/view/6097/4913#top.

Hacker, Jacob S. 2004. "Privatizing Risk without Privatizing the Welfare State: The Hidden Politics of Social Policy Retrenchment in the United States." *The American Political Science Review* 98(2): 243-260. Accesed June 19, 2019. https://www.jstor.org/stable/414530.

Hall, Jean P. Noelle K. Kurth, Shawna L.C. Chapman, and Theresa Shireman. 2015. "Medicaid Managed Care: Issues for Beneficiaries with Disabilities." *Disability and Health Journal* 8: 130-135. Accessed June 4, 2019. doi.org/10.1016/j.dhjo.2014.08.010.

Hansen, Helena, Philippe Bourgois, and Ernest Drucker. 2014. "Pathologizing Poverty: New Forms of Diagnosis, Disability, and Structural Stigma Under Welfare Reform." *Social Science & Medicine* 103: 76-83. Accessed June 19, 2019. doi.org/10.1016/j.socscimed.2013.06.033.

Harlan, Sharon L., and Pamela M. Robert. 1998. "The Social Construction of Disability in Organizations: Why Employers Resist Reasonable Accommodation." *Work and Occupations* 25(4): 397-435.

Harrington Meyer, Madonna, and Pamela Herd. 2007. *Market Friendly or Family Friendly? The State and Gender Inequality in Old Age*. New York: Russell Sage Foundation.

Harrington Meyer, Madonna. 2014. *Grandmothers at Work: Juggling Families and Jobs*. New York, NY: NYU Press.

Harris-Kojetin, L., M. Sengupta, E. Park-Lee, and R. Valverde. 2013. "Long-term Care Services in the United States: 2013 Overview." *Vital Health Statistics* 3(37). Accessed June 7, 2019. https://www.cdc.gov/nchs/data/series/sr_03/sr03_037.pdf.

Hirschi, Melissa, Angela Wangari Walter, Kasey Wilson, Kate Jankovsky, Beth Dworetzky, Meg Comeau, and Sara S. Bachman. 2019. "Access to Care Among Children with Disabilities Enrolled in the MassHealth CommonHealth Buy-In Program." *Journal of Child Health Care* 23(1): 6-19. Accessed June 7, 2019. Doi.org/10.1177/1367493518777310.

Hogan, Dennis. 2012. *Family Consequences of Children's Disabilities*. New York: Russel Sage Foundation.

Houtenville, A and S. Boege. 2019. *Annual Report on people with Disabilities in America: 2018*. Durham, NH: University of New Hampshire, Institute on Disability. Accessed June 7, 2019. https://disabilitycompendium.org/sites/default/files/user-uploads/Annual_Report_2018_Accessible_AdobeReaderFriendly.pdf.

Hyman, Mark H. 2016. "Work Ability and Return to Work." In *AMA Guides to Navigating Disability Benefit Systems*, edited by Les Kertay, Marjorie Eskay-Auerbach, and Mark H. Hyman, 30-41. Chicago, IL: American Medical Association.

Iezzoni, Lisa I., Mary B. Killeen, and Bonnie L. O'Day. 2006. "Rural Residents with Disabilities Confront Substantial Barriers to Obtaining Primary Care." *Health Research and Educational Trust* 41(4): 1258-1275. Accessed June 4, 2019. Doi.org/10.1111/j.1475-6773.2006.00534.x.

Kaiser Family Foundation. 2017a. "*Medicaid Eligibility through the Aged, Blind, Disabled Pathway*." Accessed June 7, 2019. https://www.kff.org/medicaid/state-indicator/medicaid-eligibility-through-the-aged-blind-disabled-pathway/?currentTimeframe=0&sortModel=%7B%22colId%22:%22Location%22,%22sort%22:%22asc%22%7D.

Kaiser Family Foundation. 2017b. "*Waiting List Enrollment for Medicaid Section 1915(c) Home and Community Based Services Waivers*." Accessed June 21, 2019. https://www.kff.org/health-reform/state-indicator/waiting-lists-for-hcbs-waivers/?currentTimeframe=0&sortModel=%7B%22colId%22:%22Location%22,%22sort%22:%22asc%22%7D.

Kaiser Family Foundation. 2017c. "*Medicaid's Role in Behavioral Health*." Accessed June 28, 2019. https://www.kff.org/infographic/medicaids-role-in-behavioral-health/.

Kaiser Family Foundation. 2017d. "*Facilitating Access to Mental Health Services: A look at Medicaid, Private Insurance, and the Uninsured*" Accessed June 7, 2019. https://www.kff.org/medicaid/fact-sheet/facilitating-access-to-mental-health-services-a-look-at-medicaid-private-insurance-and-the-uninsured/.

Kaiser Family Foundation. 2018. "*Medicaid Eligibility through the Medically Needy Pathway*." Accessed August 21, 2019. https://www.kff.org/other/state-indicator/medicaid-eligibility-through-the-medically-needy-pathway/?currentTimeframe=0&sortModel=%7B%22colId%22:%22Location%22,%22sort%22:%22asc%22%7D.

Kaiser Family Foundation. 2019a. "*Medicaid and CHIP Income Eligibility Limits for Children as a Percent of the Federal Poverty Level*." Accessed June 7, 2019. https://www.kff.org/health-reform/state-indicator/medicaid-and-chip-income-eligibility-limits-for-children-as-a-percent-of-the-federal-poverty-level/?currentTimeframe=0&sortModel=%7B%22colId%22:%22Location%22,%22sort%22:%22asc%22%7D.

Kaiser Family Foundation. 2019b. "*Medicaid Waiver Tracker: Approved and Pending Section 1115 Waivers by State*." Accessed June 7, 2019. https://www.kff.org/medicaid/issue-brief/medicaid-waiver-tracker-approved-and-pending-section-1115-waivers-by-state/#Table2.

Katch, Hannah, Jennifer Wagner, and Aviva Aron-Dine. 2018. "*Medicaid Work Requirements Will Reduce Low-Income Families' Access to Care and Worsen Health Outcomes*." Center on Budget and Policy Priorities. Accessed June 7, 2019. https://nationaldisabilitynavigator.org/wp-content/uploads/news-items/CBPP_Work-Reqs-Low-Income_Feb-2018.pdf.

Kaye, H. Stephen. 2012. "Gradual Rebalancing of Medicaid Long-Term Services and Supports Saves Money and Serves More People, Statistical Model Shows." *Health Affairs* 31(6):1195-1203. Accessed June 4, 2019. 10.1377/hlthaff.2011.1237.

Kaye, H. Stephen. 2019. "Disability-Related Disparities in Access to Health Care Before (2008-2010) and After (2015-2017) the Affordable Care Act." *American Journal of Public Health*, Policy 109(7): 1015-1021. Accessed June 7, 2019. 10.2105/AJPH.2019.305056.

Korpi, Walter, and Joakim Palme. 1998. "The Paradox of Redistribution and Strategies of Equality: Welfare State Institutions, Inequality, and Poverty in the Western Countries." *American Sociological Review* 63(5): 661-687. Accessed June 7, 2019. 10.2307/2657333.

Levy, Jonah D. 2010. "Welfare Retrenchment." In *The Oxford Handbook of the Welfare State*, edited by Francis G. Castles, Stephan Leibfried, Jane Lewis, Herbert Obinger, and Christopher Pierson, 1-14. Oxford, UK: Oxford University Press.

Lewis, Elizabeth, Steve Eiken, Angela Amos, and Paul Saucier. 2018. *The Growth of Managed Long-Term Services and Supports Programs: 2017 Update*. Princeton, NJ: Mathematica.

Mann, Cindy. 2015. "*Clarification of Medicaid Coverage of Services to Children with Autism*." Baltimore, MD: Department of Health and Human Services. Accessed June 7, 2019. https://www.medicaid.gov/federal-policy-guidance/downloads/cib-07-07-14.pdf.

Mark, Tami L., Tracy Yee, Katherine R. Levit, Jessica Camacho-Cook, Eli Cutler, and Christopher D. Carroll. 2016. "Insurance Financing Increased for Mental health Conditions but Not for Substance Use Disorders, 1986-2014." *Health Affairs* 35(6). Accessed June 7, 2019. https://doi.org/10.1377/hlthaff.2016.0002.

Martinez-Hume, Anna C., Allison M. Baker, Hannah S. Bell, Isabel Montemayor, Kristan Elwell, and Linda M. Hunt. 2017. "'They Treat

You a Different Way:' Public Insurance, Stigma, and the Challenge to Quality Health Care." *Cultural Medical Psychiatry* 41: 161-180. Accessed June 7, 2019. 10.1007/s11013-016-9513-8.

McCue, Michael J., and Michael H. Bailit. 2011. "Assessing the Financial Health of Medicaid Managed Care Plans and the Quality of Patient Care They Provide." *The Common Wealth Fund* 1511(11). Accessed June 7, 2019. https://www.commonwealthfund.org/sites/default/files/documents/___media_files_publications_issue_brief_2011_jun_1511_mccue_assessing_financial_hlt_medicaid_managed_care_plans_ib_final.pdf.

Medicaid and CHIP Payment and Access Commission (MACPAC). 2016. *Trends in Medicaid Spending*. Accessed June 28, 2019. https://www.macpac.gov/wp-content/uploads/2016/06/Trends-in-Medicaid-Spending.pdf.

Medicaid.gov. 2017. "*Health Care Experiences of Adults with Disabilities Enrolled in Medicaid Only: Findings from a 2014-2015 Nationwide Survey of Medicaid Beneficiaries*." Accessed June 4, 2019. https://www.medicaid.gov/medicaid/quality-of-care/downloads/performance-measurement/namcahpsdisabilitybrief.pdf.

Medicaid.gov. 2019. "*Ticket to Work*." Accessed June 7, 2019. https://www.medicaid.gov/medicaid/ltss/employment/ticket-to-work/index.html.

Moynihan, Donald and Pamela Herd. 2010. "Red Tape and Democracy: How Rules Affect Citizenship Rights." *The American Review of Public Administration* 40(6): 654-670.

Moynihan, Donald P., Pamela Herd, and Elizabeth Ribgy. 2016. "Policymaking by other means: Do States Use Administrative Barriers to Limit Access to Medicaid?" *Administration & Society* 48(4): 497-524. Accessed June 7, 2019. 10.1177/0095399713503540.

Murinko, Shawn. 2014. "Held Down by Red Tape, Not Disability." *The Hill*. Accessed June 7, 2019. https://thehill.com/blogs/congress-blog/civil-rights/208381-held-down-by-red-tape-not-disability.

Musumeci, MaryBeth, Priya Chidambaram, and Molly O'Malley Watts. 2019a. "*Medicaid Home and Community Based Services Enrollment and Spending*." Kaiser Family Foundation. Accessed June 21, 2019.

https://www.kff.org/medicaid/issue-brief/medicaid-home-and-community-based-services-enrollment-and-spending/.

Musumeci, Mary Beth, Priya Chidambaram, and Molly O'Malley Watts. 2019b. "*Medicaid Financial Eligiblity for Seniors and People with Disabilities: Findings from a 50-State Survey*." Kaiser Family Foundation. Accessed June 20, 2019. https://www.kff.org/ medicaid/ issue-brief/medicaid-financial-eligibility-for-seniors-and-people-with-disabilities-findings-from-a-50-state-survey/.

Musumeci, MaryBeth, Priya Chidambaram, and Molly O'Malley Watts. 2019c. "*Key Questions About Medicaid Home and Community-Based Services Waiver Waiting Lists*." Kaiser Family Foundation. Accessed June 21, 2019. https://www.kff.org/medicaid/issue-brief/key-questions-about-medicaid-home-and-community-based-services-waiver-waiting-lists/.

Musumeci, MaryBeth and Priya Chidambarm. 2019. "*Medicaid's Role for Children with Special Health Care Needs: A Look at Eligibility, Services, and Spending*." Kaiser Family Foundation. Accessed June 7, 2019. https://www.kff.org/medicaid/issue-brief/medicaids-role-for-children-with-special-health-care-needs-a-look-at-eligibility-services-and-spending/.

Musumeci, MaryBeth, and Julia Foutz. 2017. "*Medicaid Restructuring Under the American Health Care Act and Nonelderly Adults with Disabilities*." Kaiser Family Foundation. Accessed June 7, 2019. https://www.kff.org/medicaid/issue-brief/medicaid-restructuring-under-the-american-health-care-act-and-nonelderly-adults-with-disabilities/.

Musumeci, MaryBeth, Rachel Garfield, and Robin Rudowitz. 2018. "*Medicaid and Work Requirements: New Guidance, State Waiver Details and Key Issues*." Kaiser Family Foundation. Accessed June 7, 2019. https://www.kff.org/medicaid/issue-brief/medicaid-and-work-requirements-new-guidance-state-waiver-details-and-key-issues/.

New York State Department of Health. 2015. "*Access New York: Health Insurance Application for Children, Adults and Families*." Accessed June 28, 2019. https://www.health.ny.gov/forms/doh-4220.pdf.

New York State Department of Health. 2019. "*Access NY Supplement A*." Accessed June 7, 2019. https://www.health.ny.gov/forms/doh-4495a.pdf.

Okoro, Catherine A., NaTasha D. Hollis, Alissa C. Cyrus, and Shannon Griffin-Blake. 2018. "Prevalence of Disabilities and Health Care Access by Disability Status and Type Among Adults – United States, 2016." *Morbidity and Mortality Weekly Report* 67(32): 882-887. Accessed June 7, 2019. http://dx.doi.org/10.15585/mmwr.mm6732a3.

Orgera, Kendal and Jennifer Tolbert. 2019. "*The Opioid Epidemic and Medicaid's Role in facilitating Access to Treatment*." Kaiser Family Foundation. https://www.kff.org/medicaid/issue-brief/the-opioid-epidemic-and-medicaids-role-in-facilitating-access-to-treatment/.

Owen, Randall, Tamar Heller, and Anne Bowers. 2016. "Health Services Appraisal and the Transition to Medicaid Managed Care from Fee For Service." *Disability and Health Journal* 9(2): 239-247. Accessed June 7, 2019. doi.org/10.1016/j.dhjo.2015.10.004.

Phillips, Kimberly G., Andrew J. Houtenville, and Amanda Reichard. 2019. "Using All-payer Claims Data for Health Surveillance of People with Intellectual and Developmental Disabilities." *Journal of Intellectual Disability Research* 63(4):327-337. Doi.org/10.1111/jir.12578.

PopSugar. 2019. "Better State for Disability Services?" *Circle of Mom's*. Accessed June 21, 2019. https://www.circleofmoms.com/mothers-of-special-needs-children/better-state-for-disability-services-630193.

Priestley, Mark. 2003. *Disability: A Life Course Approach*. Cambridge, UK: Polity Press.

Reaves, Erica and MaryBeth Musumeci. 2015. "*Medicaid and Long-Term Services and Supports: A Primer*." Kaiser Family Foundation. Accessed June 4, 2019. https://www.kff.org/medicaid/report/medicaid-and-long-term-services-and-supports-a-primer/.

Reichard, Amanda, and Hayley Stozle. 2011. "Diabetes Among Adults with Cognitive Limitations Compared to Individuals with no Cognitive Disabilities." *Intellectual and Developmental Disabilities* 49: 141-154. doi.org/10.1352/1934-9556-49.2.141.

Rimmer, James H. and Kiyoshi Yamaki. 2006. "Obesity and Intellectual Disability." *Mental Retardation and Developmental Disabilities* 12: 22-27. https://doi.org/10.1002/mrdd.20091.

Ross, Martha, and Nicole Bateman. 2018. "*Disability Rates among Working-Age Adults are Shaped by Race, Place, and Education*." Brookings Institute. Accessed June 7, 2019. https://www.brookings.edu/blog/the-avenue/2018/05/15/disability-rates-among-working-age-adults-are-shaped-by-race-place-and-education/.

Rudowitz, Robin, Kendall Orgera, and Elizabeth Hinton. 2019. "*Medicaid Financing: The Basics*." Kaiser Family Foundation. Accessed June 7, 2019. https://www.kff.org/report-section/medicaid-financing-the-basics-issue-brief/.

Rudowitz, Robin, Rachel Garfield, and Elizabeth Hinton. 2019. "*10 Things to Know about Medicaid: Setting the Facts Straight*." Kaiser Family Foundation. Accessed June 7, 2019. https://www.kff.org/medicaid/issue-brief/10-things-to-know-about-medicaid-setting-the-facts-straight/.

Santhanam, Laura. 2018. "In Rural America, Tightened Access to Medicaid Means Tough Choices." *PBS News Hour*. Accessed June 19, 2019. https://www.pbs.org/newshour/health/in-rural-america-tightened-access-to-medicaid-means-tough-choices.

Schalock, Robert L., Ruth A. Luckasson, and Karrie A. Shogren. 2007. "The Renaming of Mental Retardation: Understanding the Change to the Term Intellectual Disability." *Intellectual and Developmental Disabilities* 45(2):116-124.

Shea, Annette. 2016. "Ticket to Work and Health Care: Incentivizing Employment with Medicaid and Medicare." *Administration for Community Living*. Accessed June 7, 2019. https://acl.gov/news-and-events/acl-blog/ticket-work-and-healthcare-incentivizing-employment-medicaid-and-medicare.

Shore-Sheppard, Lara D. 2008. "Stemming the Tide? The Effect of Expanding Medicaid Eligibility On Health Insurance Coverage." *The B.E. Journal of Economic Analysis & Policy* 8(2). Accessed June 7,

2019. https://econ.williams.edu/files/Shore-Sheppard_Stemming_BEJEAP.pdf.

Social Security Administration. 2019. "*Ticket to Work*." Accessed June 7, 2019. https://choosework.ssa.gov/.

Soss, Joe. 1999. "Lessons of Welfare: Policy Design, Political Learning, and Political Action." *American Political Science Review* 93(2): 363-380. Accessed June 7, 2019. doi.org/10.2307/2585401.

Soss, Joe. 2005. "Making Clients and Citizens: Welfare Policy as a Source of Status, Belief, and Action." In *Deserving and Entitled: Social Constructions and Public Policy*, edited by Anne L. Schneider and Helen M. Ingram, 291-328. Albany, NY: State University of New York Press.

Tanenbaum, Sandra J., and Robert E. Hurley. 1995. "Disability and The Managed Care Frenzy: A Cautionary Note." *Health Affairs* 14(4): 213-219. Accessed June 19, 2019. doi.org/10.1377/hlthaff.14.4.213.

Thach, Nga T., and Joshua M. Wiener. 2018. *An Overview of Long-Term Services and Supports and Medicaid*. Washington, D.C.: US Department of Health and Human Services. Accessed June 7, 2019. https://aspe.hhs.gov/system/files/pdf/259521/LTSSMedicaid.pdf.

The National Early Childhood Technical Assistance Center. 2011. "*The Importance of Early Intervention for Infants and Toddlers with Disabilities and Their Families*." Accessed June 7, 2019. http://www.nectac.org/~pdfs/pubs/importanceofearlyintervention.pdf.

U.S. Government Accountability Office. 2008. "*Social Security Disability: Collection of Medical Evidence Could be improved with Evaluations to Identify Promising Collection Practices*." Accessed June 7, 2019. https://www.gao.gov/assets/290/284422.pdf.

Verbrugge, Lois M., and Alan M. Jette. 1994. "The Disablement Process." *Social Science and Medicine* 38(1):1-14.

Wagner, Jennifer, and Judith Solomon. 2018. "*States' Complex Medicaid Waivers Will Create Costly Bureaucracy and Harm Eligible Beneficiaries*." Center on Budget and Policy Priorities. Accessed June 7, 2019. https://www.cbpp.org/research/health/states-complex-medicaid-waivers-will-create-costly-bureaucracy-and-harm-eligible#_ftnref30.

Whittle, Henry J., Kartika Palar, Nikhil A. Ranadive, Janet M. Turan, Margot Kushel, and Sheri D. Weiser. 2017. "'The Land of the sick and the land of the healthy': Disability, Bureaucracy, and Stigma among People Living with Poverty and Chronic Illness in the United States." *Social Science & Medicine* 190: 181-189. Accessed June 7, 2019. doi.org/10.1016/j.socscimed.2017.08.031.

Wieffering, Helen. 2019. "Georgetown Student and ANC Commissioner May Not Be Able to Return to School after 'Unexpected' Insurance Decision." *The DCist*. Accessed June 7, 2019. https://dcist.com/story/19/05/31/georgetown-student-and-anc-commissioner-may-not-be-able-to-return-to-school-after-unexpected-insurance-decision/.

World Health Organization. 2011. "*World Report on Disability*." Accessed June 7, 2019. https://www.who.int/disabilities/world_report/2011/report.pdf.

Zablotsky, Benjamin, Lindsey I. Black, and Stephen J. Blumberg. 2017. "Estimated Prevalence of Children with Diagnosed Developmental Disabilities in the United States, 2014-2016." *NCHS Data Brief* 291: 1-7. Accessed June 7, 2019. https://www.cdc.gov/nchs/data/databriefs/db291.pdf.

Zylan, Yvonne, and Sarah A. Soule. 2000. "Ending Welfare As We Know It (Again): Welfare State Retrenchment, 1989-1995." *Social Forces* 79(2):623-652.

In: Medicaid: Politics, Policy, and Key Issues ISBN: 978-1-53618-133-3
Editor: Daniel Lanford

Chapter 10

MEDICAID'S CONSUMER PARADOX: THE CASE OF SUBSTANCE USE DISORDER

Bikki Tran Smith[1,*], Colleen M. Grogan[1], PhD, Christina M. Andrews[2], PhD, Amanda J. Abraham[3], PhD, Melissa A. Westlake[2] and Samantha J. Harris[3]

[1]School of Social Service Administration,
University of Chicago, Chicago, IL, US
[2]College of Social Work, University of South Carolina,
Columbia, SC, US
[3]School of Public and International Affairs,
University of Georgia, Athens, GA, US

ABSTRACT

The ACA Medicaid-related reforms have significantly improved substance use disorder (SUD) treatment coverage and accessibility. However, for these improvements to be fully realized, expanded coverage

[*] Corresponding Author's Email: bikki@uchicago.edu.

must be implemented along with a clear information strategy that assures that eligible individuals *understand* (1) that SUD treatment services are covered under state Medicaid programs, (2) what specific SUD treatment services are covered, and (3) the specific benefits and restrictions for those services. We examined the process of locating information about SUD benefits on Medicaid websites for all 50 states and the District of Columbia as well as publicly available sources of information on SUD coverage from all 281 Medicaid managed care organizations. Our analysis revealed limited information on behavioral health coverage on both Medicaid and MCO websites, in conjunction with difficult and confusing language and a focus on providers rather than consumers. This presents a major barrier to accessing coverage information and, consequently, accessing treatment services. As Medicaid currently pays for the majority of SUD treatment services, behavioral health benefits information needs to be more accessible and comprehensible to ensure that current and potential Medicaid enrollees know what SUD treatment services and medications are covered and to what extent.

Keywords: substance use disorder coverage, Medicaid, affordable care act, consumer knowledge, health literacy, readability, Medicaid managed care benefits

INTRODUCTION

The Affordable Care Act (ACA) introduced a breakthrough in the Medicaid program. It gave states the option—with very generous federal financing—to provide coverage to *all* low-income Americans. People who were considered undeserving in the vast majority of states in the past—especially single adults with a substance use disorder (SUD), criminal justice-involved populations, and the homeless—were, after nearly fifty years of the Medicaid program, allowed access to Medicaid coverage. Between 2013 and 2018, enrollment in Medicaid expansion states increased by 36 percent (a total of 13.6 million enrollees) (Medicaid and CHIP Payment and Access Commission 2019). This growth was driven primarily by adults qualifying under the ACA's new Medicaid eligibility option. For example, as of 2017, Medicaid enrollees that fell into this new adult category made up 20% of total enrollment across the expansion states (Centers for Medicare and Medicaid Services 2016).

When Medicaid expansion began in 2014, an estimated 19% of the newly eligible were adults with an SUD (Mark 2019). Some states witnessed a dramatic increase in enrollment as a result of Medicaid expansion. For example, Kentucky experienced a 700-percent increase in the number of Medicaid enrollees using SUD treatment services after the expansion of Medicaid in 2014 (Center on Budget and Policy Priorities [CBPP] 2018). Indeed, Medicaid is now the single largest insurance payer for SUD treatment services in the United States, providing nearly $12 billion for SUD treatment annually—more than all private health insurers combined. National estimates suggest that expanding Medicaid reduced the unmet need for SUD treatment by 18 percent (Kaiser Family Foundation [KFF] 2019a).

As a result of this coverage, Medicaid has played a crucial role in the nation's response to the opioid epidemic. In 2017, approximately two million nonelderly adults in the United States had an opioid use disorder (OUD). Medicaid provides health insurance coverage for nearly 40% of Americans with OUD. Among low-income adults, Medicaid covers more than half of those with OUD across all states (KFF 2019b).

In addition to the Medicaid eligibility expansions, the ACA also required states to include SUD treatment services as part of the essential health benefits package. Moreover, the ACA required states to apply the parity provisions established in 2008 by the Mental Health Parity and Addiction Equity Act (MHPAEA) to their Medicaid programs. The MHPAEA provisions prohibit private insurers from applying more restrictive coverage for behavioral health treatments than they would for medical or surgical services to Medicaid managed care plans (Buck 2011).

The ACA Medicaid-related reforms have significantly improved SUD treatment coverage and accessibility. However, for these improvements to be fully realized, expanded coverage must be implemented along with a clear information strategy that assures that eligible individuals *understand* (1) that SUD treatment services are covered under state Medicaid programs, (2) what specific SUD treatment services are covered, and (3) the specific benefits and restrictions for those services (Figure 1).

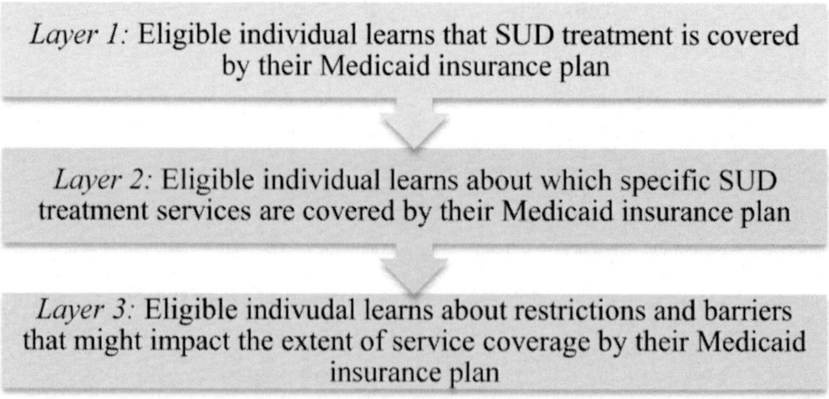

Figure 1. Knowledge layers of SUD treatment coverage and accessibility.

We sought to replicate how Medicaid enrollees with SUD attempt to locate information about SUD treatment benefits by reviewing the Medicaid websites for all 50 states and the District of Columbia, as well as publicly-available sources of information on SUD treatment coverage for all 281 Medicaid managed care organizations (MCO) (KFF 2019c). These sources included online enrollee handbooks, provider manuals, state formularies/preferred drug lists, and other supporting documents for those 38 states and the District of Columbia that contract with MCOs. These sources of information are important for Medicaid enrollees with SUD. For a person with SUD who needs a daily regimen of medication combined with outpatient SUD treatment services, knowing whether the state covers methadone treatment or limits the number of outpatient therapy visits per month might determine whether they move towards recovery. In essence, we ask: How easy (or difficult) is it for enrollees to find information on SUD treatment services offered through Medicaid?

Before we describe our methods for assessing the process of obtaining benefit information, we first provide brief historical and current overview of SUD treatment coverage under the Medicaid program. Next, we present our findings, starting with our assessment of Medicaid websites, followed by an examination of publicly available Medicaid MCO coverage information. Finally, we conclude the chapter with a discussion on the implications of these findings for Medicaid enrollees seeking treatment for SUD.

BACKGROUND

Medicaid has historically played a modest role in financing SUD treatment. National spending for SUD treatment increased by roughly $15 billion between 1986 and 2009, representing an average annual rate of growth in nominal dollars of 4.4 percent (Levit et al. 2013). Medicaid spending on SUD treatment services also grew substantially during this period, from less than $1 billion to $5 billion. However, because other funding sources for SUD treatment also increased during this time (namely the state block grant funds for SUD treatment), Medicaid's share of spending remained steady at approximately 20 percent of total outlays (Substance Abuse and Mental Health Services Administration [SAMHSA] 2016a).

Although the ACA has expanded coverage for SUD treatment, there are still large geographic disparities in coverage gains. Originally, all states were mandated to expand Medicaid. However, this was struck down by the Supreme Court and ruled as unconstitutional (Rosenbaum & Westmoreland 2012). Consequently, states were given the choice of whether or not to opt into the Medicaid expansion. As of May 2019, 36 states and the District of Columbia have done so (KFF 2019d).

Furthermore, while federal essential health benefits provisions and extension of the parity regulations have enabled expansion of SUD coverage requirements under Medicaid, they do not stipulate the types of treatment and medication services that must be covered, or what type of utilization management procedures can be applied to the coverage of particular services or medications (e.g., prior authorization, annual maximums, copayments and deductibles). This gives states the authority to designate the types of SUD treatment benefits that their Medicaid program will offer.

At the start of Medicaid expansion in 2014, only a little more than a quarter of states (n=13) required comprehensive SUD treatment coverage under their Medicaid programs – i.e., SUD treatment services that span the continuum of care, as recommended by the American Society of Addiction Medicine (ASAM) (Grogan et al. 2016). While overdose deaths due to the opioid epidemic were continuing to rise, only 18 states required comprehensive coverage across the ASAM levels of care, along with OUD treatment medications that are considered essential for recovery. Even when states provided comprehensive coverage, they often imposed limitations on covered services. Preauthorization was the most common service utilization limitation, followed by the use of annual maximums. Such limitations varied dramatically across states, as did treatment services and medication coverage.

The three years after implementation of Medicaid expansion in 2014 saw an increase in comprehensive SUD coverage (Andrews et al. 2018). The most significant gains were seen in coverage for residential treatment, which increased from 31 to 36 states for short-term residential and from 22 to 26 states for long-term residential treatment. Although preauthorization continued to be the most frequently employed service utilization limitation, its use declined. There was also a drastic decrease in the imposition of annual limits across SUD treatment services and medication types. There was an increase, however, in the use of copayments. This increase occurred primarily for newly eligible adults under state's alternative benefit plans attached to the Medicaid expansion programs, not in standard Medicaid plans. Ironically, during the same period, there was a dramatic drop in the percent of states with preauthorization requirements applied to OUD medications, buprenorphine and naltrexone, and many states implemented copayments for these same medications. This may be related to the relatively high cost of some of these medications (Gifford et al. 2018).

As the above description of state coverage policy makes clear, there continues to be wide variation across the states in terms of what SUD services are covered and administrative limitations on their use.

Medicaid Managed Care and SUD Treatment

Medicaid managed care plans have proliferated since the early 1980s when Medicaid first started contracting with MCOs (Garfield et al. 2018). Although MCO contracting has existed for several decades, the role of managed care in providing coverage for behavioral health has been a more recent development. Over the past three decades, an increasing number of states have shifted responsibility of Medicaid-funded behavioral health services to MCOs. This process, in which states integrate behavioral health with physical health benefits under contractual arrangements with MCOs, is commonly referred to as a "carve-in." In contrast, when states contract with MCOs for physical health benefits and keep behavioral health separate under their fee-for-service (typically state-run) program, that structure is called a "carve-out." Some states have opted to have mental health and SUD treatment services carved-in to their MCO plans for the standard population while continuing to contract with a fee-for-service plan for behavioral health services for "mandatory categorically needy" populations (e.g., pregnant women and children, individuals receiving supplemental security income (SSI), individuals receiving mandatory state supplements) (KFF n.d.). While it is clear there is substantial variability across the states with regard to the use of carve-ins, relatively little information has been available regarding the details of how states have used carve-ins to administer SUD treatment within Medicaid.

Not surprisingly, there is also considerable variation with regard to the type and extent of SUD treatment benefits covered by Medicaid MCOs. More than half the states contract with MCOs to provide Medicaid services (KFF 2019c). Although states set minimum thresholds in terms of what SUD services must be covered, states allow MCOs to exercise wide descretion on whether and how they set limits on access to SUD treatment services for Medicaid enrollees. For example, while a state may specify that MCOs must cover intensive outpatient SUD treatment for Medicaid enrollees, MCO plans may be allowed to limit the frequency or duration of such coverage by imposing an annual maximum on the number of intensive oupatient treatment sessions covered (Grogan et al. 2016).

Because there is such wide variation in coverage across states—with regard to what services are covered and to what extent utilization management procedures are used—there is no way for a Medicaid enrollee with SUD to know *a priori* what SUD services are covered and to what extent. Especially because many states use the argument that Medicaid enrollees should act like "responsible consumers," (Grogan, Singer, & Jones

2017) it is important to know whether comprehensible information is available to enrollees to *enable* such behavior. Consider that Seema Verma, now the Director of the federal government agency that oversees Medicaid (Centers for Medicare and Medicaid Services—CMS) and the architect of Indiana's Medicaid reforms, argued that the structure (e.g., co-payments, savings accounts, and a lockout period) was designed to "promote the notion of consumerism" and that it "transforms Medicaid beneficiaries into consumers" (Roob & Verma 2008). At the root of these design mechanisms is an assumption that Medicaid offers enrollees the information necessary to become knowledgeable consumers and choose the plan that best fits their needs.

As the number of Medicaid MCOs administering behavioral health benefits on behalf of states grows, information about their plans and the specific benefits they provide should be readily accessible to consumers. Just as www.healthcare.gov plays a crucial role in providing consumer information within the ACA's Marketplaces, state Medicaid websites are similarly important to a state's communication strategy regarding health insurance benefits. Information on health, health care, and health insurance have continued to flourish online, concomitant with growth in the number of people who use the internet as their primary source for health information (Schmeida & McNeal 2007). With the pervasiveness of information technology and reliance on technology to educate consumers, Medicaid websites could reasonably be expected to provide information on eligibility, benefits, and enrollment. How these sites are configured, and the information they display, likely has a considerable impact on individuals' ability to understand the application process and what treatment benefits are covered once enrolled. This is particularly important as the nation continues to battle the opioid epidemic.

However, communicating information regarding Medicaid benefits is hindered by the program's tremendous complexity, resulting from the availabilty of multiple, differing plans in most states, and varying carve-in or carve-out plan structures. Without information specific to local programs and beneficiaries of different types, this complexity may contribute to considerable confusion and difficulty in determining what benefits are available among program beneficiaries. Therefore, we extend our examination of the availability of SUD treatment benefits information on Medicaid websites to also explore the process of locating this information on MCO websites. Essentially, we ask: If Medicaid enrollees are expected to act as informed consumers, how easy (or difficult) is it for them to access information? In this paper, we focus particularly on persons with SUD. Given the opioid epidemic and the fact that Medicaid is the largest health care payer addressing the crisis (KFF 2019b), the question of how enrollees with OUD might access needed information is especially pressing.

METHODS

We begin our examination by documenting how state Medicaid programs convey information about their behavioral health treatment coverage. We use this broader phrase rather than SUD treatment, because most states utilize this phrase to include all mental health and SUD treatment services. Thus, we would expect to find any information about SUD treatment under the heading of behavioral health benefits.

Second, because of the prominence of states contracting with MCOs and because Medicaid websites are often linked to the state's contracted MCO website (which we discuss in more detail in the findings section), we also examine Medicaid MCO websites, looking specifically at their enrollee (a.k.a. "member") handbooks and provider manuals, as well as the state's formulary/preferred drug list. These handbooks provide information regarding Medicaid MCO plan benefits and service utilization limitations. We discuss the methods for these two data collection processes in turn below.

Medicaid Websites

We examined Medicaid websites for all 50 states and the District of Columbia. The URLs for official Medicaid websites were obtained from the links provided by the primary Medicaid government website.[1] We limited our analysis to the homepage of each Medicaid website and any subsequent pages regarding behavioral healthcare coverage as found through links from the homepage or via searches conducted within the site. Homepages have been found to be an acceptable unit of analysis. Ha and James (1998) contend that it is through the homepage that users decide whether or not to continue perusing the site. Inclusion of subsequent pages for analysis follows Mason and Wright's (2011) suggestion to examine an additional layer of a website as they found that homepages alone provide insufficient information. All data collection occurred between February and April of 2016.

To determine whether information regarding behavioral health treatment was available and accessible, we examine the following three research questions: (1) Do Medicaid program websites provide information about behavioral health coverage? (2) How accessible is the information to visitors of the websites? (3) What type of information is offered on behavioral health treatment on the websites?

When behavioral health information was absent on the homepage, we first searched for behavioral health coverage information within the sections detailing programs and services. If behavioral health coverage content was not listed among the programs and services offered, we conducted searches using the terms "behavioral health," "mental illness/health," "substance use/use disorder/abuse/dependence," "alcohol," and "addiction" via the search function of each Medicaid website. We excluded the terms "psychiatry/psychiatric" from our searches, as these terms are primarily referred to in billing code information for designated providers. Given that websites are periodically updated or changed, we collected screenshots of the webpages to ensure consistent and stable data for our analysis. Screenshots were captured for each Medicaid homepage and any pages that emerged from the search on terms related to behavioral health treatment coverage.

---

[1] www.medicaid.gov.

Content analysis was used to assess the type of information available about behavioral health coverage on Medicaid websites. To ascertain the availability of content on behavioral health, we assessed the presence and quality of information on behavioral health treatment benefits on each Medicaid program homepage, including eligibility details (e.g., citizenship status, age), available benefits, enrollment instructions, and access to information for assistance (e.g., a contact number). These items were targeted because they provide information that a consumer typically looks for when applying for Medicaid and selecting a Medicaid managed care plan, if applicable.

Two authors independently coded a stratified random sample of 10 Medicaid websites and then reconvened to compare the codes applied, discuss discrepancies, and establish consensus. There was initial confusion, in some instances, over which page was the official Medicaid homepage for the state, as some of the links from www.medicaid.gov did not direct to the state's official site. For a handful of states, the link directed us to the homepage for a managed care company contracted by the Medicaid program instead of the Medicaid program website itself. After clarifying the source of our discrepancy, we were able to obtain uniform results.

Additionally, textual data from relevant screenshots were analyzed using Microsoft Word's readability function to obtain the Flesch Reading Ease score and Flesch-Kincaid Grade Level (Flesch 1948; Kincaid et al. 1975). These two tests for evaluating health-related websites were used because of their ease of administration and high correlation with other readability tests (Friedman & Hoffman-Goetz 2006). The Flesch Reading Ease score rates content using a scale from 0 to 100, with higher scores indicating greater ease of reading. The Flesch-Kincaid Grade Level measures textual data in terms of reading grade level from 0 to 12 and number of years of education for scores of 13 and higher. The formulas for calculating both the Flesch Reading Ease score and the Flesch-Kincaid Grade Level are based on the average length of sentences and the average number of syllables per word. Given that the amount of text that appears varies across the Medicaid websites, we limited the amount of text assessed to the first five complete sentences to get enough variability in the composition of sentences and for consistency across sites. Analysis was limited to the Medicaid homepage regardless of whether it contained information on behavioral health, as the readability of this first page may determine how consumers proceed in navigating the website as a whole. When the homepage contained no complete sentences, we used text from the "behavioral health page" if available. This was the case for three states (Mississippi, Pennsylvania, and Washington). Textual analysis excluded five states (Arizona, Georgia, Kansas, Louisiana, and Virginia) because the homepages or behavioral health page did not have a sufficient amount of text to analyze.

Medicaid MCO Documents, Websites, and State Formularies

As of September 2018, 38 states and the District of Columbia contracted with comprehensive MCO plans with a total of 281 plans nationwide (KFF 2019c) for an average of about seven plans per state (Figure 2). States range in the number of MCO plans with which they contract— from one such plan in a less populous state like North Dakota to 24 plans in California. Data from 2018 MCO enrollee handbooks, collected between January and December of 2018, were saved and the process of accessing information on MCO websites was extensively documented. The following documents on MCO websites were analyzed for behavioral health benefits information: member handbooks, provider manuals, and state formularies/preferred drug lists for all state Medicaid programs contracting with an MCO plan for the 2018 contract year. When there were multiple products available for different enrollee groups, we selected the largest standard plan for adults, as this benefit information applies to the majority of Medicaid enrollees with SUD.

To address the main question of information availability, we used an approach similar to that employed for state Medicaid websites by focusing on the following two research questions: (1) What SUD treatment benefits coverage information is available in the MCO plan member handbook? and (2) What is the process of identifying SUD treatment benefits coverage and service utilization limitations? A flow chart outlining our inclusion criteria and review process can be found in Figure 2 below.

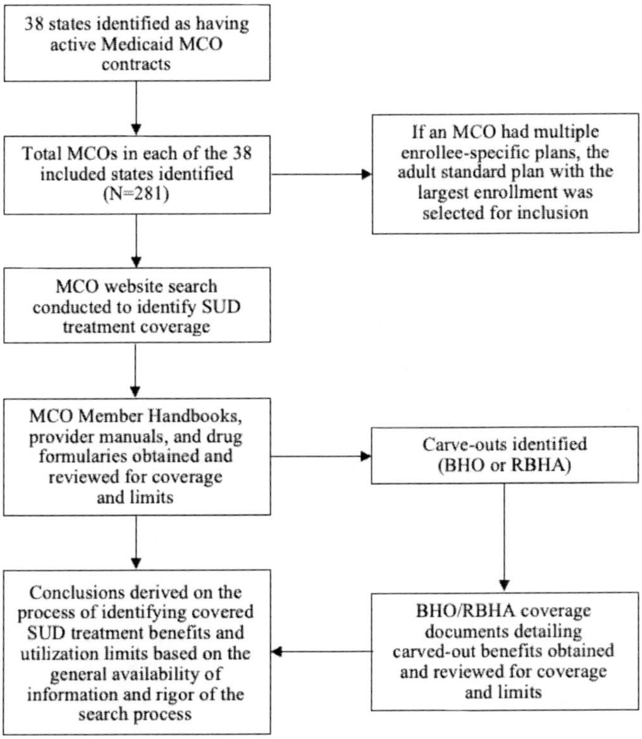

Figure 2. Medicaid MCO SUD treatment coverage review process.

Table 1 lists the key search terms used to determine behavioral health treatment benefits covered by each plan. We conducted our search in three phases, moving from the most general key terms to the most specific. The first set of key terms attempted to reflect those likely to be used by the average consumer to identify benefits. The second and third sets are specific terms for types of treatment and medication services and benefits restrictions. Although we acknowledge that the majority of consumers might not be fully aware of more targeted treatment modalities, medication types, or the full range of restrictions that may be imposed, we included these key terms in our search in order to comprehensively assess the difficulty of identifying such information.

Table 1. Keywords used in behavioral health treatment benefits search

First Set of Search Terms:
substance use
alcohol (use/abuse)
drug (use/abuse)
addiction
behavioral health
mental health
psychiatric
Second Set of Search Terms:
intensive outpatient
residential/residential treatment
formulary/preferred drug list
prescription/medication
opioid treatment/opioid/opiate
methadone/dolophine/methadone diskets
naltrexone/oral naltrexone/ injectable naltrexone/Revia/Vivitrol
buprenorphine/Subutex/Suboxone
detox/detoxification
counseling
Third Set of Search Terms:
preauthorization/pre-authorization/prior approval
fee-for-service/FFS
managed care
reimbursement/payment/carve-out
maximum
limit

RESULTS

Information on State Medicaid Homepage

Information on behavioral health treatment benefits was often limited, vague, and difficult to find on Medicaid homepages. Information about behavioral health treatment benefits appeared on the homepage on only 15 (29.4%) Medicaid websites (see Table 2). Fourteen (27.5%) of the 15 websites indicated eligibility criteria specific to behavioral health coverage. Only seven (13.7%) of all Medicaid websites listed detailed eligibility requirements (e.g., income, citizenship status, age). While sixteen state websites (31.4%) listed mental health services under covered benefits, only 11 states (68.8%) included SUD treatment among the list of covered services. All states provide some SUD treatment benefits to their Medicaid enrollees, but only 11 states made clear on the website that SUD treatment is covered. Among these 11 states, only 10 (19.5%) provided more detailed information about what specific SUD treatment services are covered. However, even the detail can be quite limited and misleading. For example, tobacco cessation is the only treatment listed as a covered SUD treatment benefit in three (27.2%) states. Twenty-one states (41.2%) provided a contact number on their homepage to provide additional assistance related to behavioral health services.

Readability assessments of Medicaid website homepages (N=45) indicated, on average, a high level of difficulty, with a Flesch Reading Ease score of 33.94 (SD = 16.01) and a Flesch-Kincaid Grade Level of 13.13 (SD = 0.49). These scores indicate college-level reading proficiency. In addition to a difficult reading level, text from the Medicaid websites was often filled with technical jargon.

Information on Designated Behavioral Health Pages

While only 14 states and the District of Columbia provided information regarding behavioral health treatment benefits on the homepage, 36 (71%) states hosted a webpage focused on behavioral health treatment benefits that could be located either through programs and services tabs on the website (26 states) or by using the website's search function (10 states). Searching for behavioral health treatment benefits information for these 36 states that did not provide treatment coverage information on their homepage proved to be a multistep process. When clicking on a service or program tab, it frequently required a long search— clicking through at least five links before finding the appropriate page. In a handful of instances, links supposedly leading to the behavioral health page were directed instead to the website of the state's contracted MCO. Louisiana's Medicaid homepage (see Figure 3) was one of the few instances where behavioral health treatment benefits offered by Medicaid were explicitly listed in the main tabs on the homepage. The tab, however, led to a page with a link indicating that behavioral health care is provided through an MCO. This link led to a webpage on "Provider and Plan Resources" which required selection of another tab entitled "Behavioral Health" to reach the "Behavioral Health Managed Care" webpage. This webpage did not include behavioral health coverage information but, instead, contained links directing users to other MCO websites.

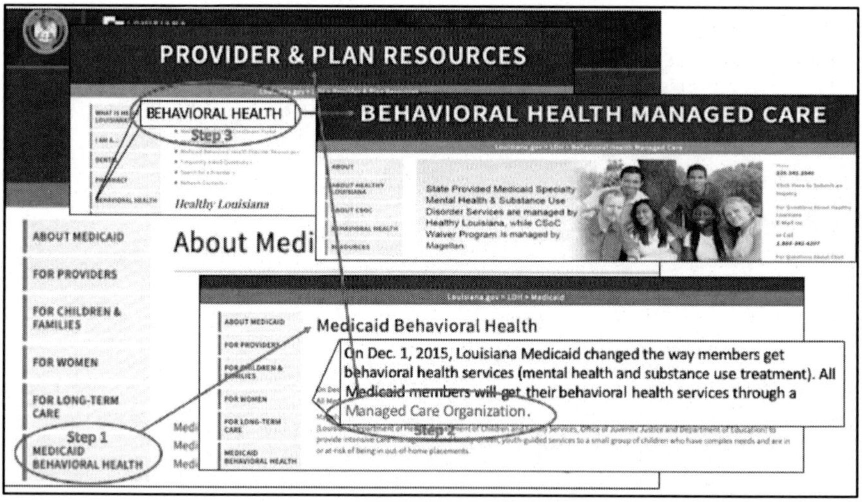

Figure 3. Louisiana Medicaid website: An example of unhelpful links.

Of the designated behavioral health website pages, only five (13.8%) made any reference to eligibility and only three of the five noted specific eligibility criteria. Six (16.7%) of the webpages contained content describing benefits and three (8.3%) displayed enrollment information.

Using the Search Function to Locate Behavioral Health Information

Overall, results obtained using the search function on Medicaid websites to locate behavioral health content were irrelevant.[2] In all eight cases when the search function was conducted using key terms, the top five results were primarily geared towards providers—e.g., links to manuals, fee schedules, regulations (see Figure 4 for an example from Maine's Medicaid website using the key term, "behavioral health" for illustrative purposes). None of the key search terms resulted in useful consumer information on behavioral health care coverage. Ironically, for those consumers who know that behavioral health treatment (and SUD treatment in particular) are covered under Medicaid, and therefore logically search directly on these terms, the website results suggested that this information is intended for providers—not consumers.

Content Analysis Criteria Met by Each State

Table 2 provides a breakdown of each state and the District of Columbia by Medicaid expansion status,[3] region, and the extent to which their respective Medicaid website met each of the six criteria for our content analysis. Twenty-one states met none of the six criteria of which 12 of them were expansion states and nine were non-expansion states. Fourteen states and the District of Columbia met at least 50% of the criteria. Of those, only three states were non-expansion states, all meeting 50% of the criteria. There appeared to be no regional pattern for the percent of criteria met by states.

---

[2] The Medicaid websites for Hawaii and Delaware did not contain an internal search function.

[3] Medicaid expansion status for 2016 was used to align with the data collection period.

You searched for **behavioral health site:www.maine.gov/dhhs/oms/**

Web results by bing

Questions and Answers about Behavioral Health Home ...
Questions and Answers about Behavioral Health ... Behavioral Health Home providers are required to follow Maineâ€™s Rights of Recipients. Each mental
http://www.maine.gov/dhhs/oms/pdfs_doc/vbp/HH/Behavorial%20HH/Behavioral-Health-Homes-FAQ-Adults.pdf

Behavioral Health Homes (Stage B) Website - Maine.gov
Behavioral Health Homes (Stage B) Behavioral Health Homes are an important component of Maine's Value Based Purchasing strategy, a multi-pronged MaineCare initiative ...
http://www.maine.gov/dhhs/oms/vbp/health-homes/stageb.html

MaineCare Behavioral Health Homes Quality Strategy
MaineCare Behavioral Health Homes â€" Quality Strategy November 21, 2013 3 conditions were: 1) matching diagnostic codes of conditions seen frequently both in hospital
https://www1.maine.gov/dhhs/oms/pdfs_doc/vbp/HH/Behavorial%20HH/BHH_quality_measures.pdf

Behavioral Health Homesâ‚¬Application - Maine.gov
Page 1 Behavioral Health Homesâ‚¬Application The objective of this application is to identify qualified and interested behavioral health providers to deliver ...
http://www.maine.gov/dhhs/oms/pdfs_doc/vbp/HH/BHH_Application_for_reference_only.pdf

MaineCare Behavioral Health Homes
MaineCare Behavioral Health Homes Managing your or your childâ€™s Mental and Physical Health Needs For a list of Behavioral Health Home providers
https://www1.maine.gov/dhhs/oms/pdfs_doc/vbp/HH/Behavorial%20HH/BHHInformationalPage.pdf

Figure 4. Maine's Medicaid website key terms search: Provider-centric results.

Table 2. Content analysis of behavioral health coverage information available on official Medicaid websites

			Content Analysis Categories						
State	Medicaid Expansion Status	Region	1. Any info. at all re: beh. health care on the official Medicaid homepage	2. Eligibility	2a. Eligibility description	3. Benefits	4. Enrollment	5. Assistance service/contact #	% Criteria Met
Arizona	1	W	0	0	0	0	0	0	0%
California	1	W	0	0	0	0	0	0	0%
Delaware	1	NE	0	0	0	0	0	0	0%
Georgia	0	S	0	0	0	0	0	0	0%
Hawaii	1	W	0	0	0	0	0	0	0%
Illinois	1	MW	0	0	0	0	0	0	0%
Indiana	1	MW	0	0	0	0	0	0	0%
Kansas	0	MW	0	0	0	0	0	0	0%
Kentucky	1	S	0	0	0	0	0	0	0%
Maine	0	NE	0	0	0	0	0	0	0%
Maryland	1	S	0	0	0	0	0	0	0%
Michigan	1	MW	0	0	0	0	0	0	0%
Nevada	1	W	0	0	0	0	0	0	0%
Ohio	1	MW	0	0	0	0	0	0	0%
Rhode Island	1	NE	0	0	0	0	0	0	0%
South Carolina	0	S	0	0	0	0	0	0	0%
South Dakota	0	MW	0	0	0	0	0	0	0%
Tennessee	0	S	0	0	0	0	0	0	0%
Texas	0	S	0	0	0	0	0	0	0%
Utah	0	W	0	0	0	0	0	0	0%
Wyoming	0	W	0	0	0	0	0	0	0%
Alabama	0	S	0	1	0	0	0	0	17%
Alaska	1	W	1	0	0	0	0	0	17%
Massachusetts	1	NE	0	0	0	0	0	1	17%
Mississippi	0	S	0	0	0	1	0	0	17%
Nebraska	0	MW	0	0	0	1	0	0	17%
North Carolina	0	S	0	0	0	0	0	1	17%
Oregon	1	W	0	0	0	0	0	1	17%
Virginia	0	S	0	0	0	0	0	1	17%
Washington	1	W	0	0	0	0	1	0	17%
Wisconsin	0	MW	0	0	0	0	0	1	17%
Arkansas	1	S	0	0	0	1	0	1	33%
North Dakota	1	MW	0	1	0	0	1	0	33%

Table 2. (Continued)

			Content Analysis Categories						
State	Medicaid Expansion Status	Region	1. Any info. at all re: beh. health care on the official Medicaid homepage	2. Eligibility	2a. Eligibility description	3. Benefits	4. Enrollment	5. Assistance service/contact #	% Criteria Met
Oklahoma	0	S	0	0	0	1	0	1	33%
Pennsylvania	1	NE	1	0	0	0	0	1	33%
West Virginia	1	S	1	0	0	1	0	0	33%
Florida	0	S	0	1	1	1	0	0	50%
Idaho	0	W	1	1	0	0	0	1	50%
Iowa	1	MW	0	0	0	1	1	1	50%
Missouri	0	MW	1	0	0	1	1	0	50%
New Jersey	1	NE	0	1	1	0	0	1	50%
Colorado	1	W	1	1	0	1	0	1	67%
Connecticut	1	NE	1	0	0	1	1	1	67%
Louisiana	1	S	1	1	0	0	1	1	67%
New Hampshire	1	NE	1	1	0	1	0	1	67%
District of Columbia	1	S	1	1	0	1	1	1	83%
Minnesota	1	MW	1	1	1	1	0	1	83%
Montana	1	W	1	1	0	1	1	1	83%
New Mexico	1	W	1	1	1	0	1	1	83%
New York	1	NE	1	1	1	1	1	1	100%
Vermont	1	NE	1	1	1	1	1	1	100%

Medicaid MCO Benefits Information

Tracking down MCO plan information also proved to be very difficult. For example, on Iowa's Medicaid website, it was necessary to click on four different links to locate relevant information on behavioral health treatment benefits (see Figure 5). On the state's Medicaid homepage, "Medicaid Services" was selected, and from there "Medicaid Programs" was chosen. This brought up a long list of programs, including a link to the "Iowa Health

Link"[4] managed care program that mentioned behavioral health treatment and appeared toward the bottom of the list. Clicking on this link then directed users to either reference the member handbook or contact the MCO directly.

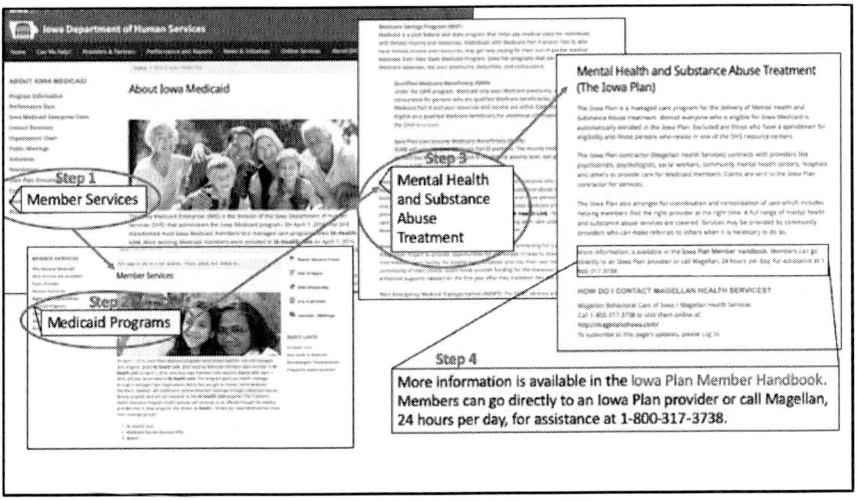

Figure 5. Iowa Medicaid website: Locating MCO benefits information for behavioral health treatment.

The webpage noted that the benefits the consumer will receive varies by the type of coverage the consumer qualifies for and goes on to encourage consumers to work with their health care provider to determine if their needed services are covered. Because the behavioral health treatment benefits information from the "Iowa Health Link" list is only for members on an MCO plan, users unsure of the type of Medicaid plan they will choose—those trying to be a proactive consumer gathering information before choosing a plan—would have to go back to the "Member Services" page and select "Medicaid Fee-for-Service (FFS)" from the list of three coverage groups in order to view the covered benefits under this plan. The Medicaid Fee-for-Service page included a list of programs, none of which were related to behavioral health treatment benefits. To find information

[4] https://dhs.iowa.gov/iahealthlink/benefits.

related to behavioral health, users would have to self-elect to search for a linked guidebook.

Navigation of Multiple MCO Plans

Medicaid programs in 38 states and the District of Columbia contracted with MCOs to administer 281 plans in total, with an average of 7 MCOs in each state (KFF 2019c). As mentioned above in the "Iowa Health Link" example, information about behavioral health treatment benefits was rarely featured on the homepage of the MCO website. More frequently, it took several clicks through the MCO website to find information about behavioral health treatment benefits. As noted above, SUD treatment benefits were often lumped together with other mental health treatment benefits under the more general term, "behavioral health treatment." Thus, someone searching for SUD treatment benefits would be unable to locate them without prior knowledge of what "behavioral health" encompasses and how behavioral health is defined in their state. Even when behavioral health treatment benefits, including SUD treatment services, were clearly defined, benefits were described using vague language, which made it difficult to determine what SUD services the MCO actually covered. Moreover, and as discussed further below, it was not uncommon to have to search the websites of organizations the state carved behavioral health treatment services out to in order to gain more detailed information about coverage. This process often required repeating the steps described above to access information regarding behavioral health treatment benefits on other Medicaid plan websites.

Use of Carve Outs in Medicaid MCO Plans

Of the 38 states and the District of Columbia that have at least one Medicaid MCO, 26 states carved in inpatient or outpatient SUD treatment services, while eight states carved out outpatient SUD treatment and seven states carved out inpatient SUD treatment (Gifford et al. 2017). For the remaining states, the carve-in of SUD treatment services varied by geographic areas or enrollment group (e.g., enrollees with SUD may be put into a separate behavioral health speciality plan).

It was common for states to carve out behavioral health services from their contracts with MCOs. In some cases, behavioral health treatment was carved out to a separate specialty behavioral health organization contracted to administer these benefits. For example, Michigan's MCO plans do not cover SUD treatment. Instead, outpatient SUD treatment is carved out to ten regional Prepaid Inpatient Health Plan organizations and more intensive behavioral health treatments are further carved out to local treatment facilities (i.e., community health centers) with which the state has specialized contracts. These multiple layers of administration and carve outs increase the complexity of navigating MCO plans to determine what types of SUD treatment benefits are covered and how. When services are carved out to another organization, this requires consumers to go to yet another website to locate information about benefits coverage. This is not easy.

In cases such as this, consumers are required to engage in an intensive, multi-stage investigation in order to understand the details of their behavioral health treatment benefits. In California, like in Michigan, searches for comprehensive coverage information regularly involved multiple websites, external links, and coverage handbook downloads due to the complex arrangements involving multiple management entities in the coverage of behavioral health treatment. For example, in California, MCO plans only cover behavioral health treatment offered by their primary care provider (i.e., assessment, referral). Benefits for outpatient behavioral health treatment are carved out to a behavioral health organization (i.e., Cenpatico, Beacon). Treatment benefits for behavioral health disorders deemed "severe" are carved out yet again— this time, to the regional behavioral health authority, which administers payment for services financed by the state's fee-for-service plan. To illustrate, the typical process for a consumer in California looking for detailed information about behavioral health treatment for a severe OUD would likely involve the following:

1) Select a Medicaid MCO plan from a list of X plans;
2) Locate the Medicaid MCO plan's website;
3) Locate the link on the MCO plan's webpage to behavioral health information;
4) Follow 1-3 additional links;
5) Download and search the member coverage handbook, possibly to find out that SUD is carved out to a behavioral health organization
6) Locate the behavioral health organization's website;
7) Repeat steps 4-5, possibly to learn that treatment for severe OUD is again carved out to a regional or county behavioral health authority;
8) Determine which regional or county behavioral health authority has jurisdiction over your community;
9) Locate the regional/county behavioral health authority website; and
10) Repeat step 4 and possibly 5.

In failing to provide explicit information about carve-outs upfront, MCOs often burden consumers with time consuming and complex searches that, in some cases, likely deter them from accessing the information they need in order to make informed choices among possible Medicaid MCO plans. State Medicaid programs require consumers to be technologically savvy and become intimately familiar with the structure and financing of health care in their state.

Even in situations in which a Medicaid MCO plan's website explains that behavioral health services are carved out, the carve-out organization is not always named, thus making it impossible to locate information online about benefits under the carve-out. This is exemplified in the case of Mississippi's Medicaid Magnolia Health, for which neither member nor provider handbooks mention that behavioral health services are carved out to Cenpatico. The phone number for Cenpatico is listed as the source to call for behavioral health treatment authorization under a section of the website providing information about prior authorization. However, it was only through conducting a Google search of the telephone number that we were able to identify the carve-out organization. Although billing documents would sometimes list the carve-out organization, billing documents would not be the most intuitive place to look when searching for benefits coverage information.

Once one actually gets to the right MCO website, or when accessing multiple sites, the use of technical language and the lack of specificity can make it very difficult or even impossible for consumers to determine what is actually covered. The use of vague and technical language was a common occurrence across all the MCO plans making the definitive determination of benefits coverage challenging. To illustrate, an excerpt from an MCO plan through Fidelis in Washington, D.C. indicated that, "*all inpatient and most non-routine outpatient services require prior authorization by the Behavioral Health Department. Routine outpatient services do not require prior authorization.*" It is unclear, though, what constitutes "routine services," as this term was neither defined nor elaborated on.

In order to understand what is covered by an MCO, a Medicaid enrollee would also need to know what specialized terms such as "specialty treatment services" or "care management and coordination" mean to accurately determine the type of coverage. To further complicate matters, and similar to what is described above when navigating a carve-out, a consumer must conduct a new online search to locate the Public Behavioral Health System (the system to which all Maryland MCO plans carve out behavioral health treatment) Participant Handbook for detailed descriptions of covered services they could receive if they are successful in obtaining a referral for specialty behavioral health treatment.

As noted above, benefits were often lumped together under the umbrella of behavioral health without specifying if the coverage is for mental health, SUD, or both. For example, Maryland Physician's Care MCO website reads *"Behavioral health services include but are not limited to case management, emergency crisis/mobile crisis services, inpatient psychiatric services, outpatient mental health centers, residential treatment centers,"* without further detail to establish if these services are covered for both mental health and SUD.

Moreover, benefits listed on some plan websites were accompanied by disclaimers stating that benefits are subject to change or that services covered are not the same across all plans, without further information about how they differ. In situations where a link to the designated behavioral health webpage was available on the Medicaid homepage, the link sometimes led to the state's department of mental health page.

Lack of detail was also evident when looking at coverage for specific SUD medications. The preferred drug list does not always specify what medications are classified as approved for what types of treatment. For example, because methadone is indicated for both pain management and SUD treatment, without explicit classification, one cannot be sure whether this medication is covered for SUD treatment or only for pain management.

While there are medications that are FDA-approved only for SUD treatment (e.g., disulfiram, acamprosate, naltrexone), it requires knowledge of these medication's names (both generic and brand name) and their use. Furthermore, even with such understanding of medications, MCOs often list medications with similar labels that are not in fact the same medication. One example is "methylnaltrexone bromide injectable." Although this medication includes the name naltrexone, which is a medication for OUD, it is not FDA-approved for OUD. The only FDA approved formulation of injectable naltrexone for OUD treatment is Vivitrol. An MCO plan in Missouri provides another illustration of the confusion that these medication names can cause. Buprenorphine-naloxone, which is buprenorphine and not naloxone, has the brand name Suboxone. In Missouri, as in many other states, Suboxone does not require prior authorization, but mono-buprenorphine does. However, the mono buprenorphine product is not widely used and is generally used to treat pregnant women (American Society of Addiction Medicine 2015). Without knowing this distinction, one might assume the need for prior authorization for coverage, which can delay access to care.

To further add to the confusion, there were cases in which outdated medications are listed as covered services. Hawaii's MCO plans, for example, include levomethadyl acetate (LAAM), which is an opioid agonist that was introduced as an alternative to methadone. Although still FDA-approved, it was taken off the market in 2003 in the U.S. due to evidence of life-threatening side-effects (e.g., cardiac disorder) (Ghodse & Galea 2012).

Discussion

Our findings suggest that online information regarding Medicaid behavioral health treatment benefits is limited, difficult to access, and hard to comprehend when it is available. There was great variability between states in terms of their website design, with some being more straightforward than others. The college-level reading proficiency required by the text on Medicaid websites is rather concerning as it exceeds the education level of almost two-thirds of the Medicaid eligible population. In 2016, only 15.2% of uninsured individuals had a high school education (Berchick, Hood, & Barnett 2018). The recommended reading level of content in order to meet the needs of the average person in the U.S. is an eighth-grade reading level or below (Kutner, Greenberg, & Baer 2006). According to the U.S. Department of Health and Human Services' guidelines for reading ease, any content beyond a ninth-grade level is considered "difficult" (Walsh & Volsko 2008).

In addition to poor readability, many of the websites required clicking through multiple links. Even then, the information retrieved was vague or uncertain. In some instances, Medicaid websites linked to an MCO plan website for more information regarding behavioral health treatment benefits, requiring consumers to contact the MCO directly instead of the Medicaid office. Basic information about enrollment, eligibility, and benefits ought to be easily available as consumers will not likely linger on a website for an extended period of time if the information they are seeking is not readily accessible (Koiso-Kanttila 2005). It is problematic that the search function to track down behavioral health coverage content often resulted in irrelevant material or provider-related content. This finding raises important issues regarding how Medicaid websites communicate with their intended audience. If state Medicaid programs are seeking to reach both consumers and providers, then separate platforms should be developed for these two audiences, and platforms for consumers need to be more user-friendly and written at a more appropriate literacy level.

Each of the 281 MCOs has a separate benefits package. Although some of the benefits across the different plans are the same, a consumer would not be aware of this without searching through each benefits package. Consequently, a consumer would have to read through several provider handbooks or browse MCO websites to determine each plan's behavioral health benefits. Based on our study of MCO SUD treatment coverage, locating benefits information was an onerous and time-consuming task. Tracking down documents and conducting exhaustive searches for information took a significant amount of time. The first plan in a state took upwards of 3 hours to interpret, due to wide variation in the structure of and coverage offered by MCOs across states. Remaining plans in the state often followed a similar pattern, but would still require well over an hour to review. Like the Medicaid websites, the use of vague and technical language regarding coverage made it difficult to correctly determine benefits.

Overall, MCO websites provided limited information about benefits, thus requiring consumers to dig deeper into multiple documents. Even as health policy researchers with specialized expertise in SUD treatment modalities and medication treatments, we had difficulty finding complete benefits information. The average consumer with more general knowledge would certainly find this task frustrating and unfruitful. Consumers may become overwhelmed by the information presented and the time necessary to sort through it, or may try to gather information by contacting the MCO by phone. However, some MCOs will not provide customer service to individuals who are not enrolled members, creating an additional barrier to accessing benefits information.

Some consumers may turn to health care providers directly to try to access information about what benefits are covered under their health care plan. This increases burden on both consumers and providers, especially for providers with less administrative capacity or high demand. Perhaps more importantly, by failing to provide consumers with a comprehensive and up-to-date version of covered services, organizations diminish consumers' ability to act as their own health advocates by increasing their dependency on providers for accurate and current information on available services.

Finally, our findings raise concerns about consumers' understanding of who defines what SUD treatment benefits must be covered. By law, states must specify the minimum level of SUD treatment benefits covered under the state Medicaid plan it submits to the federal government. MCOs can cover more treatments, but not less. If a Medicaid enrollee wanted to learn about services that should be covered by all the MCOs (under the state plan), these websites do not provide this basic information. Instead, when the websites direct the enrollee to specific MCO plans, it conveys a misunderstanding that the state does not set the minimum level of SUD treatment benefits.

Limitations

By reviewing State Medicaid and MCO websites, we essentially simulated the consumer experience of attempting to locate information about what SUD treatments are covered. While we systematically followed a series of logical steps to reflect the experience of an average user and to ensure consistency in locating behavioral health information across all Medicaid and MCO websites, we acknowledge that not all users would follow this same navigation path. Additionally, since the analysis was completed, changes have occurred to www.medicaid.gov as well as some MCO websites. Our study reflects a snapshot in time.

Although this method allowed us to test the multiple ways a consumer might approach gathering information on the Medicaid website, it would be helpful to talk directly with Medicaid consumers with SUD to determine whether they attempted to gather information about coverage and if so, how. This would be a fruitful endeavor for future research.

We also did not survey those responsible for updating and maintaining the content on the Medicaid and MCO websites to better understand their objectives and challenges. States are operating under different budgetary constraints and may not have the necessary resources to invest in design and technological improvements so that websites can more adequately act as effective tools for informing consumers of behavioral health care coverage.

The use of word processing programs to assess reading ease and level vary based on their formulas, and thus, literacy scores based on Medicaid website content are not definitive and should merely be used as a general guide (Friedman & Hoffman-Goetz 2006).

Finally, reliance on computer and internet accessibility alone inherently presents a problem. Not all consumers will rely on this form of technology to seek out information about Medicaid benefits coverage. However, the health care navigators that consumers may seek for assistance often rely on Medicaid and insurance plan websites to provide consumers with needed information. Thus, the ease in locating behavioral health content and understanding behavioral health coverage on Medicaid and MCO websites is nonetheless relevant.

Implications for Substance Use Disorder Treatment Access

Medicaid and MCO website configurations, and the information displayed on the websites, may have a considerable impact on beneficiary knowledge about SUD treatment benefits. Difficulty in locating information on SUD treatment coverage in general, presents an obstacle to understanding coverage and, likely, accessing care. Despite improvements in SUD treatment coverage and access made possible by the ACA's Medicaid expansion, only about 4.0 million Americans received any type of SUD treatment in 2017 (Bose et al. 2018). Of those Americans who felt they needed SUD treatment but did not receive it, about 1 in 10 reported that they did not know where to go for treatment (Bose et al. 2018). Further, several studies support this finding— identifying patient lack of knowledge as a barrier to receiving SUD treatment, particularly medications (e.g., Oliva et al. 2011; Roman, Abraham, & Roman 2011). Thus, even with legislative efforts such as Medicaid expansion and federal parity provisions to increase SUD treatment coverage, the positive contributions of such efforts will be limited in scope and reach if not accompanied by enhanced access to such information, whether through improvements in website design, increased transparency of benefits information, or increased educational supports to enhance consumer health and health insurance literacy.

CONCLUSION

People with SUD need treatment to effectively manage their condition and maintain health. For example, with the current opioid epidemic, many parents are seeking Medicaid coverage for their children with OUD (Moore 2018). States vary in their coverage of important OUD medications such as buprenorphine, naltrexone, and methadone (Grogan et al. 2016; Andrews et al. 2018). Given the growing death toll resulting from the opioid epidemic, those personally affected by this crisis will want to know whether these potentially life-saving medications are covered. Yet, nowhere on Medicaid websites—in any state—is this information available. As for MCO websites, this information, when available, was difficult to locate and included many caveats to coverage (e.g., prior authorization, if the medication is specified for SUD versus pain management).

Medicaid enrollees are told by policymakers that they should act as "responsible consumers" (Grogan, Singer, & Jones 2017). However, states and their contracted MCOs have made that option nearly impossible. The limited information on behavioral health coverage on both Medicaid and MCO websites, in conjunction with the difficult and confusing language used and the focus on providers rather than consumers, presents a barrier to accessing coverage information and, consequently, accessing treatment services. As Medicaid currently pays for the majority of SUD treatment services, behavioral health benefits information needs to be more accessible and comprehensible to ensure that current and potential enrollees know what SUD treatment services and medications are covered and to what extent.

References

American Society of Addiction Medicine. "The ASAM National Practice Guideline for the Use of Medications in the Treatment of Addiction Involving Opioid Use." *Rockville, MD: ASAM* (2015). https://www.asam.org/docs/default-source/practice-support/guidelines-and-consensus-docs/asam-national-practice-guideline-supplement.pdf?sfvrsn=24.

Andrews, Christina M., Colleen M. Grogan, Bikki Tran Smith, Amanda J. Abraham, Harold A. Pollack, Keith Humphreys, Melissa A. Westlake, and Peter D. Friedmann. "Medicaid Benefits for Addiction Treatment Expanded After Implementation of the Affordable Care Act." *Health Affairs* 37, no. 8 (2018): 1216-1222, doi:10.1377/hlthaff.2018.0272.

Barber, S. L. "Supplemental Security Income Recipients for Whom the Alcoholism and Drug Addiction Provisions Apply (DA&A Recipients)." *Washington, DC: Office of Program Benefits Policy,* Social Security Administration (1995).

Berchick, Edward R., Emily Hood, and Jessica C. Barnett. "Health Insurance Coverage in the United States: 2017." *Current Population Reports. Washington, DC: US Government Printing Office* (2018): 60-264. https://www.census.gov/content/dam/Census/library/publications/2018/demo/p60- 264.pdf.

Bose, Jonaki, Hedden, Sarra L., Lipari, Rachel N., and Park-Lee, Eunice. "*Key Substance Use and Mental Health Indicators in the United States: Results from the 2017 National Survey on Drug Use and Health.*" Rockville, MD: US Department of Health and Human Services (2018). https://www.samhsa.gov/data/report/2017-nsduh-annual-national-report.

Buck, Jeffrey A. "The Looming Expansion and Transformation of Public Substance Abuse Treatment under the Affordable Care Act." *Health Affairs* 30, no. 8 (2011): 1402-1410, doi:10.1377/hlthaff.2011.0480.

Centers for Medicare & Medicaid Services (CMS). "Total Medicaid Enrollees—VIII Group Break Out Report." *Baltimore, MD: US Department of Health and Human Services* (2016). https://www.

medicaid.gov/medicaid/program-information/downloads/cms-64-enrollment-report-oct-dec-2016.pdf.

Center on Budget and Policy Priorities (CBPP). "*Medicaid Works for People with Substance Use Disorders*." Washington, DC: CBPP (2018). https://www.cbpp.org/research/health/medicaid-works-for-people-with-substance-use-disorders.

Center on Budget and Policy Priorities (CBPP). "*Taking Away Medicaid for Not Meeting Work Requirements Harms People with Substance Use Disorders*." Washington, DC: CBPP (2019). https://www.cbpp.org/research/health/taking-away-medicaid-for-not-meeting-work-requirements-harms-people-with-substance.

Flesch, Rudolph. "A New Readability Yardstick." *Journal of Applied Psychology* 32, no. 3 (1948): 221, doi:10.1037/h0057532.

Friedman, Daniela B., and Laurie Hoffman-Goetz. "A Systematic Review of Readability and Comprehension Instruments Used for Print and Web-based Cancer Information." *Health Education & Behavior* 33, no. 3 (2006): 352-373, doi: 10.1177/1090198105277329.

Garfield, Rachel, Elizabeth Hinton, Elizabeth Cornachione, and Cornelia Hall. "*Medicaid Manage Care Plans and Access to Care*." Washington, DC: KFF (2018). http://files.kff.org/attachment/Report-Medicaid-Managed-Care-March-Plans-and-Access-to-Care.

Ghodse, A. H., and S. Galea. "Opioid Analgesics and Narcotic Antagonists." *Side Effects of Drugs Annual* 34 (2012): 145-180, doi:10.1016/B978-0-444-59499-0.00008-8.

Gifford, Kathleen, E. Ellis, B. Coulter Edwards, A. Lashbrook, E. Hinton, L. Antonisse, and R. Rudowitz. "*Medicaid moving ahead in uncertain times: Results from a 50-state Medicaid budget survey for state fiscal years 2017 and 2018.*" San Francisco, CA: KFF (2018). www. kff.org/medicaid/report/medicaid-moving-ahead-in-uncertain-times-results-from-a-50-state-medicaid-budget-survey-for-state-fiscal-years-2017-and-2018/.

Gresenz, Carole Roan, Katherine Watkins, and Deborah Podus. "Supplemental Security Income (SSI), Disability Insurance (DI), and Substance Abusers." *Community Mental Health Journal* 34, no. 4

(1998): 337-350, https://link.springer.com/content/pdf/10.1023/A:1018779805833.pdf.

Grogan, Colleen M., Christina Andrews, Amanda Abraham, Keith Humphreys, Harold A. Pollack, Bikki Tran Smith, and Peter D. Friedmann. "Survey highlights differences in Medicaid coverage for substance use treatment and opioid use disorder medications." *Health Affairs* 35, no. 12 (2016): 2289-2296, doi:10.1377/hlthaff.2016.0623.

Grogan, Colleen M., Phillip M. Singer, and David K. Jones. "Rhetoric and Reform in Waiver States." *Journal of Health Politics, Policy and Law* 42, no. 2 (2017): 247-284, doi:10.1215/03616878-3766719.

Ha, Louisa, and E. Lincoln James. "Interactivity Reexamined: A Baseline Analysis of Early Business Web Sites." *Journal of Broadcasting & Electronic Media* 42, no. 4 (1998): 457-474, doi:10.1080/08838159809364462.

Kaiser Family Foundation. "*Medicaid Behavioral Health Services Database*." San Francisco, CA: KFF (n.d.). https://www.kff.org/data-collection/medicaid-behavioral-health-services-database/.

Kaiser Family Foundation. "*Medicaid's Role in Addressing the Opioid Epidemic*." San Francisco, CA: KFF (2019a). https://www.kff.org/infographic/medicaids-role-in-addressing-opioid-epidemic/.

Kaiser Family Foundation. "*The Opioid Epidemic and Medicaid's Role in Facilitating Access to Treatment*." San Francisco, CA: KFF (2019b). https://www.kff.org/medicaid/issue-brief/the-opioid-epidemic-and-medicaids-role-in-facilitating-access-to-treatment/.

Kaiser Family Foundation. "*Total Medicaid MCOs*." San Francisco, CA: KFF (2019c). https://www.kff.org/medicaid/state-indicator/total-medicaid-mcos/?activeTab=graph&currentTimeframe=0&startTimeframe=3&sortModel=%7B%22colId%22:%22Location%22,%22sort%22:%22asc%22%7D.

Kaiser Family Foundation. "*Status of State Action on the Medicaid Expansion Decision*." San Francisco, CA: KFF (2019d). https://www.kff.org/health-reform/state-indicator/state-activity-around-expanding-medicaid-under-the-affordable-care-act/?current

Timeframe=0&sortModel=%7B%22colId%22:%22Location%22,%22sort%22:%22asc%22%7D.

Kincaid, J. Peter, Robert P. Fishburne Jr, Richard L. Rogers, and Brad S. Chissom. "*Derivation of New Readability Formulas (Automated Readability Index, Fog Count and Flesch Reading Ease Formula) for Navy Enlisted Personnel.*" Institute for Simulation and Training (1975), https://stars.library.ucf.edu/istlibrary/56.

Koiso-Kanttila, Nina. "Time, Attention, Authenticity and Consumer Benefits of the Web." *Business Horizons* 48, no. 1 (2005): 63-70, doi: 10.1016/j.bushor.2004.10.004.

Kutner, Mark, Elizabeth Greenberg, and Justin Baer. "*A First Look at the Literacy of America's Adults in the 21st Century. NCES 2006-470.*" Washington, DC: National Center for Education Statistics US Department of Education (2006). http://nces.ed.gov/naal/pdf/2006470.pdf.

Levit, Katharine R., Tami L. Mark, Rosanna M. Coffey, Sasha Frankel, Patricia Santora, Rita Vandivort-Warren, and Kevin Malone. "Federal spending on behavioral health accelerated during recession as individuals lost employer insurance." *Health Affairs* 32, no. 5 (2013): 952-962, doi:10.1377/hlthaff.2012.1065.

Mark, Tami L. "*The Effect of the Affordable Care Act on Uninsured Rates Among Individuals with Mental and Substance Use Disorders*." *Psychiatric Services* (2019): appi-ps, doi:10.1176/appi.ps.201800437.

Mason, Alicia, and Kevin B. Wright. "Framing Medical Tourism: An Examination of Appeal, Risk, Convalescence, Accreditation, and Interactivity in Medical Tourism Web Sites." *Journal of Health Communication* 16, no. 2 (2011): 163-177, doi:10.1080/10810730.2010.535105.

Medicaid and CHIP Payment and Access Commission (MACPAC). "*Medicaid Enrollment Changes Following the ACA*." Washington, DC: MACPAC (2019). https://www.macpac.gov/subtopic/medicaid-enrollment-changes-following-the-aca/#_ftn1.

Moore, Lela. "Clean, Sober, and $41,000 Deep in Out-of-Pocket Addiction Recovery Costs: People Recovering from Opioid Addiction and their

Families Discuss the Financial and Emotional Costs of Treatment. *New York, NY: NY Times* (2018). https://www.nytimes.com/2018/07/26/reader-center/costs-of-drug-rehab.html.

Roob, Mitchell, and Seema Verma. "Indiana: Health Care Reform Amidst Colliding Values." *Health Affairs Blog, May* 1 (2008), doi:10.1377/hblog20080501.000383.

Rosenbaum, Sara, and Timothy M. Westmoreland. "The Supreme Court's Surprising Decision on the Medicaid Expansion: How Will the Federal Government and States Proceed?" *Health Affairs* 31, no. 8 (2012): 1663-1672, doi:10.1377/hlthaff.2012.0766.

Schmeida, Mary, and Ramona S. McNeal. "The Telehealth Divide: Disparities in Searching Public Health Information Online." *Journal of Health Care for the Poor and Underserved* 18, no. 3 (2007): 637-647, doi:10.1353/hpu.2007.0068.

Substance Abuse and Mental Health Services Administration (SAMHSA). "*Behavioral Health Spending and Use Accounts, 1986-2014*." Rockville, MD: US Department of Health and Human Services (2016). https://store.samhsa.gov/system/files/sma16-4975.pdf.

Substance Abuse and Mental Health Services Administration (SAMHSA). "*The TEDS Report: Health Insurance Status of Adult Substance Abuse Treatment Admissions Aged 26 or Older: 2011*." *Rockville, MD: US Department of Health and Human Services* (2016). https://www.samhsa.gov/data/sites/default/files/sr134-health-insurance-2014/sr134-health-insurance-2014/sr134-health-insurance-2014.htm.

Walsh, Tiffany M., and Teresa A. Volsko. "Readability Assessment of Internet-based Consumer Health Information." *Respiratory Care* 53, no. 10 (2008): 1310-1315. http://rc.rcjournal.com/content/respcare/53/10/1310.full.pdf.

In: Medicaid: Politics, Policy, and Key Issues ISBN: 978-1-53618-133-3
Editor: Daniel Lanford

Chapter 11

RESTRUCTURING MEDICAID'S LONG TERM CARE BENEFIT: SHIFTING SERVICES FROM INSTITUTIONS TO COMMUNITIES

Jill Quadagno*
Pepper Institute on Aging and Public Policy,
Florida State University, Tallahassee, FL, US

ABSTRACT

When Medicaid was created in 1965, it became the primary source of funding for long term care (LTC) for the frail and elderly poor, provided almost exclusively in nursing homes. In response to rising costs and quality concerns, policymakers sought ways to shift care toward home-and-community based services (HCBS). This chapter examines the factors that influenced the use of Medicaid to transform the delivery of LTC and asks whether these efforts have succeeded. Overall, success has been limited due to a number of obstacles. These include the joint federal-state structure of Medicaid; the lack of an infrastructure in communities in terms of personnel, service provider organizations, and housing; the policy legacy of institutional care; and the complexity of the HCBS delivery system.

* Corresponding Author's Email: jquadagno@fsu.edu.

Although the states may be "laboratories of democracy," HCBS operates at the level of cities, towns, and even neighborhoods and involves not only health policy experts, policymakers and practitioners but a wider array of stakeholders.

Keywords: long term care, home-and-community based services, nursing homes, assisted living facilities

INTRODUCTION

In the U.S., approximately one-third of people over age 65 have some type of disability. Although some people with disabilities experience minor inconveniences, others require assistance with basic activities of daily living (ADLs). They may need help with such basic functions as eating, bathing, getting dressed, and walking as well as managing finances, taking medications on time, and doing household chores. The term long-term care (LTC) refers to a range of services designed to help people with chronic conditions compensate for limits in their ability to function independently.

Although most informal care for the frail elderly is provided by family members, the primary source of payment for formal services is Medicaid. The program pays for nearly 70 percent of nursing home residents and an increasing amount of home-and-community-based services (HCBS) (Rudowitz and Garfield 2018). Because Medicaid is the single largest source of payment for LTC, the program has had a significant impact in determining how services are delivered and the type of care received. Historically, care was mainly delivered in nursing homes, but since the 1980s Medicaid has experimented with alternatives to institutionalization by covering services in community settings. This chapter asks whether efforts to use Medicaid to shift the delivery of LTC from nursing homes to HCBS have succeeded and if not, why.

THE ORIGINS OF MEDICAID'S LONG TERM CARE BENEFIT

In the post-World War II era, most people did not have the resources to pay for nursing home care. Due to the lack of a market, few facilities were available. Those that did exist were small board-and-care homes or nursing homes run by religious groups and labor unions. In the 1950s the nursing home industry began to expand due to three factors. The first was the Hill-Burton Act of 1946, which provided public funds for the construction of non-profit nursing homes. The second was the Federal Housing Administration's guarantee of mortgage loans to proprietary nursing homes. Third was the deinstitutionalization of mental hospital residents, which increased the supply of older people who were candidates for admission to nursing homes (Uhlenberg 1997).

The legislation that created both Medicare and Medicaid, the Social Security Act Amendments of 1965, established the institutional structure for long term care. It prohibited Medicare from covering "custodial care," ignoring the fact that many medical conditions create long term care needs. Medicare was allowed to pay for some services in extended care facilities, which were typically units in hospitals for convalescing patients, but not for chronically ill patients who were unlikely to recover. As Medicare costs grew, in 1969 eligibility for extended care was further curtailed (Smith 1999). Since then, Medicare has maintained rigid restrictions to avoid paying for LTC (Feder 2015). Under current rules, Medicare can pay for some nursing home and home-based care, but only for a short duration following a hospitalization. The exception is when a Medicare beneficiary is released to a skilled nursing facility (SNF) directly from an inpatient hospital stay of at least three days, not including the day of discharge. Even then, only the first 20 days in an SNF are fully covered, plus a portion of the cost up to 100 days.

Medicare's failure to cover LTC has made Medicaid the default payer for the chronically ill and as a consequence shifted a large share of responsibility to the states. The 1965 legislation extended Medicaid to people who were "categorically eligible" for the cash assistance programs for the poor - Old Age Assistance, Aid to the Blind, and Aid to Families with Dependent Children. The only exception was a rule that allowed states to create "medically needy" programs for people whose income was too high to qualify for cash assistance but too low to pay their medical expenses, mostly nursing home residents (Quadagno 2015). The caveat was that medical expenses would only be covered if they were provided in a nursing home.

Once Medicaid payment was guaranteed, nursing homes became profitable entities, and the number of new nursing homes grew exponentially. Between 1963 and 1977 more than one million new nursing home beds were created. By 1983, long term care facilities represented 43 percent of the Medicaid budget (Buchanan 1983). The rapid growth in nursing home beds created an upward inflationary spiral because there was no competition. However many beds were occupied, Medicaid would pay the full price. As a result, costs rose at an annual rate of 17.4 percent, higher than any other health expenditure (Smith 1999, 243). Unlike the nursing homes that operated before Medicaid, many of the new nursing homes were owned by national proprietary chains and treated sicker patients needing more medical care. Thus, Medicaid had multiple consequences for long term care. It greatly increased the for-profit nursing home industry, it made the nursing home the alternative to hospitals for recovering patients, and it limited living arrangements for the chronically ill elderly.

DETERMINING MEDICAID ELIGIBILITY

Medicaid eligibility rules for access to LTC services have changed dramatically since the program's inception. What began as a means-tested benefit for the elderly poor has evolved into a broader program that serves the middle class as well (Grogan and Patachnik 2003). Although rules remain quite restrictive, there is great variation across states. In determining Medicaid eligibility, states differ in what is counted as income but usually include Social Security benefits, Veterans benefits, employment wages, pension income, dividends from stocks and bonds, interest payments, IRA distributions, and estate income. The medically needy option also varies widely. Where it is operating, higher income individuals may qualify once the cost of nursing home care is deducted. Yet in 2019 only 32 states had the medically needy option, and in these states monthly income limits after health care costs were taken into account ranged from $114 in Arkansas to $1,134 in Vermont (American Council on Aging 2019).

Medicaid applicants not only have to meet income eligibility rules but also have to satisfy an asset test. In 2019 the asset limit for a single individual in most states was $2,000 excluding one's home and furnishings (American Council on Aging 2019). Individuals with assets over the federal limit are ineligible for Medicaid until they have "spent down" their resources. Given the high cost of nursing home care, which averaged $89,297 in 2019, few individuals can afford to pay for more than a few months (seniorliving.org). As a result, about 60 percent of nursing home residents enter as private payers and then deplete, i.e., spend down, their resources to become Medicaid eligible (Olson 2010,137). During this process, Medicaid applicants are allowed to spend their money on anything, not just on their care, but they cannot give resources away for less than fair market value.

Rules regarding the "spend down" process have become increasingly restrictive. In 1993 Congress instituted a "look back" period. Under the new regulations assets had to be transferred at least three years prior before an individual could apply for Medicaid. The objective was to prevent people from giving away assets that could be used to pay for their care. The Deficit Reduction Act (DRA) of 2005 increased the "look back" period to five years with the penalty period beginning when the individual applied for Medicaid, not when funds or assets were transferred. The DRA also required states to recover from the estate after death the amount Medicaid spent on an individual's care. Although state probate laws vary, they generally include as part of an estate all real and personal property such as a home and other assets. In addition, individuals must name the state as the sole beneficiary of any annuities they hold equal to the amount of the Medicaid funded assistance (Olson 2010).

A second route to Medicaid LTC eligibility is through a special income rule called the "300 percent rule." This rule requires states to provide Medicaid to people who receive federal Supplemental Security Income (SSI) benefits. To be eligible for SSI, beneficiaries must have low incomes, limited assets, and an impaired ability to work at a substantial gainful level as a result of old age or significant disability. The SSI federal benefit rate in 2018 was $750 per month for an individual and $1,125 per month for a couple, which is about 75% of the federal poverty level (FPL) (Social Security Administration 2019). SSI beneficiaries also are subject to an asset limit of $2,000 for an individual and $3,000 for a couple (Kaiser Family Foundation 2015).

One caveat is that if one spouse requires long-term care services, Medicaid will not require the other spouse to give up all assets and income. Every state has its own "spousal protection" rules to let the healthy spouse remain in the community. The rules allow the community dwelling spouse to keep anywhere from $22,000 to $110,000 in assets. In some states Medicaid applicants can put excess income above the Medicaid limit into a trust. If the community dwelling spouse is still alive when the Medicaid beneficiary dies, the estate may be exempt from recovery, but in these cases, states may seek recovery from the spouse's estate after death.

Medicaid recipients are required to contribute most of their income toward their long term care but may keep a small "personal needs allowance" to pay for uncovered medical expenses. The amount of the monthly allowance depends on the state's rules and varies according to the individual's living arrangements. Nursing home residents generally have a lower personal needs allowance than residents of an assisted living facility or recipient of home health care services. The important point is that the process of qualifying for Medicaid is complex with rules varying substantially across states. The rules generally require applicants to deplete their income and assets and to subsist on meager allowances.

THE LIMITS OF NURSING HOME CARE

Because Medicaid pays such a large share of care for the frail elderly, it has had an outsize influence on how care is delivered and on the quality of care received.

Quality Concerns

As noted above, historically, Medicaid resources have been devoted to institutional care, which fueled the growth of the nursing home industry and a powerful lobby. The current voice of the industry is the American Health Care Association, an organization with more than 13,000 members that represents nursing homes and other long term care providers. For more than two decades, lobbyists opposed efforts to enact regulations governing nursing home quality and ensured that the standards that were in place were minimal and largely unenforceable. Yet there was growing criticism that nursing homes were merely warehouses for the elderly and numerous reports of abuse, fraud, and neglect. Following a series of exposés, in 1987 Congress established an elaborate system of regulations and report cards requiring all facilities participating in Medicare and Medicaid to meet 18 standards of adequacy. To ensure that these standards are being met, states are required to conduct regular inspections and post all nursing home deficiencies on a website run by the federal government. Although this rating system initially appeared to improve the quality of care, it left many unresolved issues. Many nursing homes continue to have deficiencies, especially those with a high percentage of Medicaid residents (Thompson 2012). Yet even facilities with numerous deficiencies often do not close because patients have nowhere else to go (Feder 2015).

Most facilities that receive citations for deficiencies are owned by for-profit chains. Chains spend less on nursing care and support services and have lower staff to patient ratios (Lloyd et al. 2014; Harrington, Ross and Kang 2015). They also have a different patient mix than high quality facilities, with higher proportions of African Americans and other minorities. (Grabowski, Angellini and Mor 2004). Thus, minorities are much more likely than whites to be concentrated in nursing homes that have serious deficiencies, lower staffing ratios, and financial vulnerabilities (Smith et al. 2007).

Efforts to ensure quality of nursing home care face an ongoing battle with the nursing home industry. At both the state and federal level, the industry lobbyists have continued efforts to water down regulations and limit enforcement. In 2019 lobbyists for Kentucky's nursing home industry wrote two bills that would place new restrictions on state inspections of nursing homes and limit wrongful death and personal injury lawsuits filed against facility owners (Cheves 2019). At the federal level, the Centers for Medicare and Medicaid Services under the Trump administration has become increasingly responsive to lobbyists requests to eliminate, delay, and reduce enforcement of key regulations (Cohens 2018).

Limitations on Access

Another issue of concern is access. In many states, nursing homes have attempted to maximize revenues by saving beds for Medicare patients because Medicare pays almost three times as much as Medicaid (Street et al. 2003). States also engage in a variety of strategies to keep Medicaid costs down by limiting the number of new nursing home beds or freezing reimbursement rates. For example, in the 1990s, state officials in Illinois concerned about the rising cost of Medicaid halted nursing home reimbursement rate increases for three years. In response, many nursing homes limited the number of Medicaid patients they would accept and some stopped taking any Medicaid patients (Harrington-Meyer and Kesterke-Storbakken 2000). As a result, Medicaid patients had longer waits to gain admission and ended up in less desirable homes. Thus, Medicaid funding for care in nursing homes is not only expensive but also inefficient, as efforts to reduce costs have also tended to limit access.

RESTRUCTURING LONG TERM CARE

Over the past three decades Medicaid has sought to shift funding from institutional care to HCBS. To a large degree, the transition was spurred by cost considerations. LTC accounts for six percent of Medicaid enrollees but 40 percent of Medicaid spending with a disproportionate share of those costs going to nursing homes (Rudowitz and Garfield 2018). As noted above, in 2019 the average yearly cost of a semi-private room in a nursing home care was $89, 297 (senior living.org). By contrast, the median annual cost of home health care was $48,800 and adult day care for five days a week was $28,000 (senior living.org; Reeves and Musumeci 2015). Another incentive to shift to HCBS was the Olmstead Supreme Court decision, which held that under the Americans with Disabilities Act, individuals with mental disabilities have the right to live in the community rather than in institutions. Despite the legal and financial incentives, the effort to transition to HCBS has faced numerous challenges because of a lack of infrastructure, institutional obstacles, policy legacies, and the complexity of HCBS delivery systems.

The Waiver Alternative

In the mid-1980s nursing homes began to lose their dominance in the face of a shift to community-based care. The transition began in the private sector as older people, largely middle class white women who were able to pay for their own care, chose less institutional settings, either hiring home care providers or moving into assisted living facilities (ALFs). As private sector options became available, Medicaid too began exploring non-institutional delivery methods.

The Medicaid transition began modestly with an option that allowed states to apply for waivers to experiment with offering services outside of a nursing home. Services provided under waivers could be directed to a variety of settings including an individual's home, a senior living complex, or an ALF. Initially, states were cautious in expanding options for LTC outside of nursing homes, and just a few applied for waivers. In the 1990s the shift to HCBS gained steam as new Medicaid statutes gave states additional flexibility to offer community care, putting HCBS and institutional care on a more equal footing. The Home and Community Based Waiver Services program allows states to provide low income and disabled individuals a variety of services to help them avoid institutional care. Among the services offered through waivers are personal care, homemaker services, day care, and case management. From 1988 to 1999, Medicaid spending on HCBS grew from 10 percent to 28 percent. By 2005 all 50 states had HCBS waivers (CMS 2006).

PACE

In 1990 an ambitious waiver option, the Program of All-Inclusive Care for the Elderly (PACE), received federal funding. What began modestly with 21 PACE programs operating in 15 states in 1996 expanded considerably (https://www.npaonline.org/). By 2015 there were 126 PACE programs operating in 260 PACE centers in 31 states serving 49,000 participants.

PACE is an optional benefit under both Medicare and Medicaid for older people who meet their state's standards for nursing home care. Services include meals, nutrition counseling, personal care, and adult day care with nursing, physical, recreational, and occupational therapy. PACE also offers prescription drugs, respite care, and medical services as needed. Most PACE enrollees are able to remain in their own homes while receiving services rather than be forced to move into a nursing home.

PACE was primarily designed for low-income people. In 2018 the annual income limit to qualify for PACE was $14,500 for an individual and $17,700 for a couple (Medicaid.gov 2019). The target population of PACE is "dual-eligibles," the nine million people who are eligible for both Medicare and Medicaid. Many dual eligibles have high rates of chronic illness, social risk factors, and mental health problems. As a result, they are among the highest-cost and most vulnerable individuals in the health care system and account for a disproportionately large share of both Medicare and Medicaid expenditures (CMS 2019). In 2006, PACE eligibility was extended to Medicare beneficiaries who do not qualify for Medicaid, if they paid a monthly premium (Medicaid.gov 2019). Despite high ambitions for the program, many states that had applied for funding failed to get their programs operating, and those that were in operation were never state-wide. The heaviest concentration was in the northeast with just one or two programs available in many less urban states.

Money Follows the Person

The Deficit Reduction Act (DRA) of 2006 gave states new authority to provide HCBS as an optional Medicaid benefit. It differed from previous policy where HCBS could be offered only through waivers. The key program created by the DRA was called Money Follows the Person (MFP), the largest demonstration program in the history of Medicaid. Its objective is to give people needing LTC services more choice about where they live and increase the capacity of the state to serve people in community settings. MFP offers states matching funds to move Medicaid beneficiaries who reside in nursing homes back to their own homes or to alternative community housing. Case workers evaluate each nursing home resident and their potential support system to determine whether that individual can safely leave the nursing home and move into the community. Once transitioned, participants are eligible for services through MFP for one year (HHS 2017)

By 2012 46 states and the District of Columbia had joined the demonstration. Of the 47 grants awarded, Florida and New Mexico dropped out before implementing a program, followed by Oregon in 2014 (HHS 2017). Most states cautiously planned for a slow start, but the number of individuals transitioned quickly fell below even those conservative projections. One state, Texas, accounted for one-third of all transitions (Rahman 2018).

Why has MFP largely failed to achieve its objectives when surveys of older people consistently show that the nursing home is the least preferred living arrangement? One reason is that over the past several decades more alternatives have become available. This means that those who do end up in nursing homes typically have multiple chronic conditions and are quite frail. A majority suffers from dementia, few can perform ADLs without assistance, and many are incontinent (Uhlenberg 1997). Further, these conditions are usually progressive and likely to worsen. Thus, most elderly individuals that the MFP hoped to target are simply incapable of making the transition from the nursing home to the community. For those who do make the transition, the prognosis is not good. Research has shown that relocation is among the most stressful life events for older adults, leading to feelings of loneliness and isolation. Both mental and physical health may decline among elders moved from familiar to unfamiliar environs (Street et al. 2007). Not surprisingly, most successful MFP beneficiaries were younger individuals with mental health problems and/or physical disabilities. The program had little impact on older nursing home residents (Rahman 2018).

Other factors have limited state ability or willingness to implement the MFP. These include a paucity of appropriate housing in the community, an insufficient pool of trained workers to provide services to individuals leaving nursing facilities, and an inadequate network of HCBS to serve those transitioning out of nursing homes (Feder 2015).

ACA Innovations

The Patient Protection and Affordable Care Act (ACA) of 2010 gave states new opportunities to enhance access to Medicaid LTC services and smooth transitions between care settings. It created the Center for Medicare and Medicaid Innovation and gave CMS the authority to test new payment and service delivery models that would reduce hospitalizations, lower costs, and improve patients' outcomes. Ideally, these goals would be achieved not only by assisting individuals with activities of daily living and health-related tasks but also by helping them acquire the skills to accomplish these tasks (Kaiser Commission on Medicaid and the Uninsured 2013).

One priority was increasing funding for state demonstrations to integrate care for dual eligibles by aligning the financing of Medicare and Medicaid under the Financial Alignment Initiative (FAI). The impetus for the FIA stemmed from the concern that dual eligibles had to navigate disconnected delivery and payment systems. Some were first enrolled in Medicare due to age or disability and then later qualified for Medicaid based on income or vice versa. These demonstration programs would provide the full array of Medicare and Medicaid services for enrollees, with savings coming from paying a single capitated rate set up front (CMS 2019). In 2012 26 states submitted proposals to CMS to test a capitated and/or managed fee-for-service model for this group.

Under the capitated model, a state, CMS, and a health plan would enter into a three-way contract, and the plan would receive a prospective blended payment to provide comprehensive, coordinated care. In the Managed Fee-for-Service model, a state and CMS would enter into an agreement that would make the state eligible to benefit from savings resulting from initiatives that improved quality and reduced costs for both Medicare and Medicaid. One way cost savings would be achieved was by preventing hospitalizations, which often lead to nursing home entry. The key to prevention was through the appropriate delivery of HCBS in partnership with primary care physicians to ensure that participants received proper nutrition, hydration, fall prevention, skin care, medication management, and incontinence management.

Nine states initially were granted funds for demonstration projects and others were added later. Initial evaluations identified a number of issues that made implementing these demonstrations challenging. Implementation requires integrating multiple systems and sometimes conflicting Medicare and Medicaid policies, involving major investments of time and resources by the states and CMS. As the demonstrations proceeded, differences in Medicare and Medicaid policies and processes continue to emerge but in many cases were resolved (Clark, Lehman and Brangan 2015). By 2019 two states had completed the demonstrations while others were still operating.

The overall assessment of the effectiveness of these efforts appears positive but guarded due to the complexity involved.

Another complementary ACA innovation was a new Medicaid option that established "health homes" for beneficiaries with chronic conditions coupled with additional federal funds to support these homes for two years (Reinhard, Kassner and Houser 2011). Health homes were intended to integrate and coordinate all primary, acute, behavioral health, and long term care services for individuals with two or more chronic conditions. Washington and Colorado tested a managed fee-for-service model under the FAI, leveraging their Medicaid health homes to coordinate care for high risk beneficiaries (CMS 2019).

The ACA also increased federal funding and expanded eligibility for the MFP demonstration to move Medicaid beneficiaries out of institutions. As part of the expansion, the ACA created a new optional Medicaid eligibility group that allows people not otherwise eligible for full Medicaid benefits to receive services (based on diagnosis, age, disability or coverage group). A 2017 report by the Secretary of Health and Human Services assessed whether state grantees had met the MFP numerical benchmarks. HHS found that efforts to transition nursing home residents to communities had continued and that by 2015 63,337 Medicaid beneficiaries had been moved out of nursing homes and into the community. The report concluded that the MFP had improved quality of life for beneficiaries and was sustainable (HHS 2017).

Despite this optimistic assessment, crucial concerns remain unaddressed. States are supposed to have used all their grant funds by 2020. By that time the program is supposed to put itself out of business by reversing avoidable institutional placements and increasing the capacity to prevent them in the first place. Given the need for continued resources, Congress has made several attempts to reauthorize the program or lock in more permanent funding. Even though the House of Representatives authorized an additional $20 million in 2019 to keep MFP operating, as yet there is no long term commitment in the federal budget (congress.gov).

The MFP has given states incentives for moving patients from nursing homes to the community, but this option has worked best for younger people with disabilities. It appears thus far to have had little impact on frail elders. The problem is that federal funding for services is guaranteed for just one year after an individual makes the transition to the community with state Medicaid programs assuming responsibility after that. Presumably, frail elderly people will need HCBS for the rest of their lives and further, their needs will increase as they age. Placing the burden of continuing care on state budgets limits the likelihood of success in the long term.

Is the sticky policy legacy of nursing home care reversible? Although the ACA laid out a series of ambitious options to reduce institutionalization and expand home care, progress has been scattered. A key issue is that adoption of new programs remains optional. Because states have no mandate to respond, they are hesitant to make long term commitments with uncertain budgetary consequences.

External Obstacles to HCBS

Even if Medicaid totally shifted gears and provided substantially greater resources for HCBS on a nationwide basis, a number of obstacles remain. A critical problem is the lack of resources, both in terms of housing options and care personnel. As noted above, since the 1990s the most significant trend in housing for the elderly has been the growth in ALFs. This growth was a response to the demand for an intermediate level of care, higher than care provided at home but less than that provided in a nursing home. Since then the number of ALFs has continued to increase with the majority catering to single, white women who pay privately. Although Medicaid will pay for services within an ALF setting, the bias toward private pay residents has created a scarcity of ALF's that accept Medicaid-eligible residents.

Another issue is the cost to family caregivers. The implicit assumption behind the shift to HCBS is that a family member, usually a wife or daughter, will provide much of the care. Family caregivers help with bathing, dressing, managing finances, preparing special diets, and managing incontinence. They also frequently have responsibility for the emotional and practical burden of managing pain (AARP 2019) as well as performing complex medical procedures such as wound care and monitoring specialized medical equipment, often without instruction (Reinhard, Levine and Samis 2012). Many caregivers perform these services willingly, but in doing so they suffer from emotional strains, disrupted plans, stress, physical exhaustion, and deterioration of their own health (Coe and Van Houtven 2009).

Caregivers also pay an economic price in the form of lost income from employment. Many reduce the number of hours at work, diminishing their earnings, while approximately one-third leave their jobs entirely. Caregivers who are taking care of a spouse are most likely to retire permanently, while caregivers of elderly parents are more likely to return to work after a period out of the labor market (Gonzales, Lee and Brown 2017). The former are likely to be older women who have fewer skills and more competing roles (Wakabayashi and Donato 2005). Those who stop working completely are at greater risk than non-caregivers of similar ages to be living in poverty (Wakabayashi and Donato 2006). Thus, the hidden cost of shifting care from nursing homes to home care increases the burden on women.

Often familial care is supplemented or largely replaced by formal HCBS by paid caregivers. As was once true of nursing home care, there is little regulation of these services. Currently, training requirements for long term care workers vary widely by state and by setting. One survey of licensed board and care homes found that only 20 percent required any staff training at all (Wellin 2018). Most paid caregivers, regardless of setting, are minority women receiving minimum wage, and more than one-fourth are foreign born. They work long hours and drive from home to home with no reimbursement for travel. Low wages coupled with poor working conditions create high turnover, which in turn jeopardizes the quality of care. HCBS could be improved by employing better trained people, but this would require paying higher wages. When Medicaid funds these services, there are strong pressures to limit costs by keeping wages low (Wellin 2018).

There are also environmental obstacles that make it difficult for frail older people to remain in their communities, even with HCBS funded by Medicaid or paid-for privately. The majority of people 65 and older own their homes, and their preference tends to be for aging-in-place (Connidis and Barnett 2019). The problem is that many homes owned by the elderly are old and in need of costly repairs. Some are located in aging neighborhoods that are no longer safe or convenient. Many also have architectural barriers such as steep stairs or deep bathtubs (Clarke 2014). For those older people who do not own their own homes, the option to remain in the community and receive services may be limited by housing affordability (Miller and Kirk 2016).

Another issue is that in most rural communities HCBS is simply unavailable. One study in Maine found that rural Medicaid long term care users were less likely than their urban counterparts to receive HCBS and more likely to reside in nursing homes. Further, in Maine, spending for nursing facility services was significantly higher for rural than urban residents while expenditures for personal care, home health, hospice, adult day care, and rehabilitation were all significantly lower for rural residents (Coburn et al. 2016).

Beyond the immediate household, other environmental barriers exist. Over many decades, America's cities and towns have developed in ways that poorly serve an aging population. Many buildings cannot be entered without using stairs, and bathrooms may be inaccessible. Access to basic services can also be limited by lack of adequate transportation (Scharlach and Lehning 2016). The larger issue that extends beyond a simple transition in Medicaid funding patterns is to improve the environment of older people within their own homes and in the community so they can remain independent as long as possible.

The Private Insurance Alternative

Medicaid is likely to remain the primary payer for LTC, but private individuals will provide more of the financing in the future. Given that most of the frail elderly have insufficient income to pay a significant amount for either nursing home care or home care services, an unanswered question is: who will provide the funds? In the 1980s, private insurance companies sought to fill the gap in LTC payment options by offering a new product - long term care insurance (Brown and Finkelstein 2011). Most policies initially only covered care in a nursing home but gradually expanded to include care in an ALF or home care. The idea was that people would pay premiums while they were relatively young and then receive benefits when they were no longer able to care for themselves. Many individuals purchased these policies, believing that long term care insurance would keep them from draining their savings, relying on their children, or applying for Medicaid. Sales of long term care insurance policies rose during the 1990s and peaked in 2002 with about 750,000 sold (Scism 2018). Since then sales have declined and by 2018 only a dozen insurance companies offered these policies (Cohen 2014).

One reason for the failure of private LTC coverage was that insurance companies underestimated their costs and found they were unable to pay for the services they had promised. Having no experience with this market, they failed to accurately predict how many people might file claims and how long people would live. As a result, the premiums people had paid for years did not cover the actual cost of the benefits. In response insurers raised their rates substantially. Since insurance companies have no limit on how much they can raise their rates in most states, many long-term policyholders were forced drop their coverage when they most needed care (Feder 2015). Other insurers tried to reduce their risk by refusing to cover some illnesses like diabetes or strokes. Some even denied legitimate claims. For example, the Senior Health Insurance Company was sued for breach of contract when it rejected a woman's claim for benefits. Even though the claimant suffered from memory loss, the company questioned whether she was sufficiently incapacitated to draw benefits (Scism 2018). The court decided in her favor and she eventually received $77,000. Another problem involved some widely-publicized scandals where unscrupulous sales people misrepresented the benefits of the plans they sold to vulnerable older people. Thus, the practices of insurance companies undermined public faith in the product.

There was one moment where it appeared that private LTC insurance might succeed. Embedded in the ACA was a provision called the Community Living Assistance Services and Supports Act (CLASS). The objective of the CLASS Act was to provide "a national voluntary insurance program for purchasing community living assistance services and support" (Frankford 2011, 534). The CLASS Act would have offered guaranteed-issue LTC insurance with established premiums, not based on individual underwriting, coupled with automatic enrollment of employees whose employer chose to participate. Enrollees would pay a monthly premium through payroll deduction and would be eligible for benefits after five years. Once they met the eligibility criteria based on level of impairment, they would have received a lifetime cash benefit. In 2011 the Obama administration announced it was unworkable and would be dropped. The CLASS Act was repealed in 2013.

Although industry critics argued that Medicaid coverage for long term care prevented a private insurance alternative from succeeding, the more likely culprit is the private insurance industry's failure to adequately assess its own costs or to develop products that were trustworthy. Currently, long term care insurance does pay benefits for some people, but it is expensive and thus unaffordable for most. Most purchasers have relatively high incomes, leaving the vast majority of Americans without coverage. It seems clear that the private insurance industry will not solve the dilemma of how to pay for the needs of an aging population and that Medicaid will remain the primary source of payment.

Discussion

Surveys show that the vast majority of older people would prefer to remain in their own homes and community, and efforts have been made to reverse the course set over half a century ago. Although the percentage of Medicaid funding for HCBS relative to nursing home care has steadily increased, institutional care still predominates. The expansion of HCBS has been piecemeal and not universally available. Even when HCBS program are in operation, applicants can become confused by variations in state eligibility rules under waivers. Some states apply more restrictive income eligibility criteria to waiver recipients than nursing home residents, some states only provide the medically needy and spend-down options to nursing home residents, and many states do not provide the same level of income and asset spousal protection to waiver recipients compared to nursing home residents (Kassner and Shirey 2000).

Funding remains an issue as well. Initially HCBS proponents believed that states could cut Medicaid expenditures by reducing institutional care. What policymakers failed to recognize was that savings from lower costs in an institutional setting could be offset by greater demand for community care (James, Gellad and Hughes 2017). Fear of rising and unpredictable costs have made states reluctant to expand HCBS. Even where states have responded to federal incentives, services are only available to some individuals and are never universally offered on a statewide basis. These obstacles have prevented Medicaid from expanding care in a less restrictive setting.

There are also institutional obstacles to widespread adoption of HCBS. One factor that has impeded the transition is the joint federal-state structure of Medicaid. States may receive incentives from the federal government in the form of funds for waivers or demonstration programs but they are not obliged to do so. In all states Medicaid long term care funds not only have to compete with other items in state budgets such as education but also with other Medicaid benefits for children and low income families. This conflict makes states reluctant to adopt innovations where future costs are unknown. Another institutional obstacle is the nursing home industry itself. Nursing homes have received the largest share of the Medicaid budget in most states for nearly 60 years, and there are vested interests in place that oppose reductions in funding. These interests include the nursing home corporations, lawyers that advise families on how to gain eligibility for Medicaid, and families seeking care for frail elders. The American Health Care Association is vigilant in lobbying against changes to Medicaid or Medicare that might adversely impact the nursing home industry. Finally, HCBS involves a complex delivery system compared to care in a nursing home. Rather than a single site for the delivery of services, HCBS is delivered in a variety of physical locations, meaning that care workers must move between locations. Not only is there less possibility for oversight, but the logistical complexity of delivering high quality care in a timely and consistent fashion is considerable.

CONCLUSION

Over the past half century, there has been a significant improvement in the U.S. in life expectancy at birth and in life expectancy after age 65. Several factors have contributed to this increase including modern technology, better health care, and life style changes. Although people are living longer than in the past, a growing number of older people are living with multiple chronic health problems. This trend has increased the demand for long term care, and this demand is likely to continue to expand in the future. The problem is that the current organization of care, divided between families, the federal government, the states, and private insurance companies is poorly organized to serve an aging population.

Thus far, the main response to increasing demand has been to look to the states. Historically, the states have been viewed as the laboratories of democracy, and many programs that eventually were adopted at the national level began as state experiments (Kail, Quadagno and Dixon 2009). In regard to an issue such as expanding Medicaid to new population groups, the states do face challenges, but the central task is comparatively simple. In contrast, the job of reducing reliance on nursing homes and expanding access to HCBS is vastly more complex. One obstacle is the experiments themselves. When states experiment with new options, they also discover the challenges of a given plan. HCBS demonstrations, in some cases, have hindered progress because they revealed unanticipated demand and thus unpredictable costs.

Another obstacle is the theoretical framework that organizes the response to the task. It is time to think beyond the idea that the states are laboratories of democracy to include cities, towns, and even neighborhoods. While demonstration initiatives may come from the federal government and be implemented by the states, the actual target of these programs is the local community. This suggests an approach that extends the discussion beyond the silos of health policy experts, policymakers, and practitioners to involve a wider array of stakeholders. These would include, first, city and county commissions whose task is to approve new developments. Although these organizations often take into account such factors as the environmental impact of a proposed project or the effect on traffic flows, they rarely consider access for frail older people and the disabled, not only within the development, but also to the wider community. Urban planners are also stakeholders who have greater expertise in regard to transportation and accessibility in the built environment but typically don't have input into local politics when it comes to approving developments. At the bottom of the ladder in regard to political power and influence are the paid and unpaid caregivers, even though they are responsible for delivering the services and it is on their shoulders that many of the burdens rests.

What, then, can be done to enhance delivery of HCBS? One solution would be to eliminate the state option and instead mandate that states adopt one of the experimental programs such as PACE. Yet such a solution could be difficult to implement due to the issues noted above, specifically the lack of an infrastructure of services, transportation, and personnel. Another possibility is to allow Medicare to cover HCBS, a measure that would bypass the states. There are already programs in operation that align Medicaid and Medicare LTC financing, but only for the elderly poor. A pilot program has been proposed (but not enacted) that would expand Medicare to offer HCBS to all beneficiaries (James, Gellad and Hughes 2017). The advantage of expanding Medicare LTC coverage is that it would help build a political constituency for HCBS by giving the middle class stake in the outcome. The current emphasis on dual eligibles, while laudable as this group is the neediest, nonetheless leaves HCBS without political support in the community. A constituency of middle class people and frail elders and their family members would demand better services. Demand would then expand HCBS, improve quality, and help create an infrastructure. Yet the policy legacy that has created the current long term care system presents an imposing political barrier, one that offers no simple solution.

REFERENCES

AARP. 2019. *Home Alone Revisited: Family Caregivers Providing Complex Care*. https://www.aarp.org/content/dam/aarp/ppi/2019/04/home-alone-revisited-family-caregivers-providing-complex-care.pdf.

American Council on Aging. 2019. *Medicaid Eligibility: 2019 Income, Asset and Care Requirements for Nursing Homes and Long Term Care*. https://www.medicaidplanningassistance.org/medicaid-eligibility.

Brown, Jeffrey and Amy Finkelstein. 2011. "Insuring Long-term Care in the United States." *Journal of Economic Perspectives* 25 (4): 119-142.

Buchanan, R.J. 1983. "Medicaid Cost Containment: Prospective Reimbursement for Long Term Care." *Inquiry* 20(4): 334-342.

Cheves, John. 2019. "Nursing Home Lobbyists Write Bills to Restrict Inspections, Lawsuits against Owners." *Lexington Herald Leader*, Feb. 11, 2019. https://www.kentucky.com/news/politics-government/article 226084360.html.

Clark, William, Daniel Lehman and Normandy Brangan. 2015. *Report on Early Implementation of Demonstrations under the Financial Alignment Initiative*. CMS, October 15, 2015. https://innovation.cms.gov/Files/reports/fai-implementationrpt.pdf.

Clarke, Philippa. 2014. "The Role of the Built Environment and Assistive Devices for Outdoor Mobility in Later Life." *Journal of Gerontology* 69B: 8-15.

Coburn, Andrew, Eileen Griffin, Deborah Thayer, Zachariah Croll and Erika Ziller. 2016. "Are Rural Older Adults Benefitting from Increased State Spending on Medicaid Home-and-Community-Based Services?" Maine Rural Health Research Center, *Research and Policy Brief PB 65*, June 2016. http://muskie.usm.maine.edu/Publications/rural/Medicaid-Home-Community-Based-Services-Rural.pdf.

Coe, Norma and Courtney Van Houtven. 2009. "Caring for Mom and Neglecting Yourself? The Health Effects of Caring for an Aging Parent." *Health Economics* 18(9): 991-1010.

Cohen, Philip. 2018. *The Family: Diversity, Inequality and Social Change*. W.W. Norton & Company.

Cohens, Katrina. 2018. "*Nursing Home Residents at Risk as CMS Prioritizes Industry Lobbyists Over Residents*." www.JusticeinAging.org.

CMS. 2006. *State Waiver and Demonstration Programs*. Centers for Medicare and Medicaid Services, Baltimore, MD: CMS.

____. 2019. Three New Opportunities to Test Innovative Models of Integrated Care for Individuals Dually Eligible for Medicaid and Medicare. *Letter from HHS to State Medicaid Directors*, April 24, 2019. www.medicaid.gov/federal-policy-guidance.

Connidis, Ingrid and Amanda Barnett. 2019. *Family Ties and Aging*. Thousand Oaks, California: Sage.

Feder, Judith. 2015. "The Missing Piece: Medicare, Medicaid and Long Term Care." In *Medicare and Medicaid at 50*, edited by Alan Cohen, David Colby, Keith Wailoo and Julian Zelizer, 255-272. New York: Oxford University Press.

Frankford, David. 2011. "At Least We're Still Free to Choose to Die at Home: A CLASS Act." *Journal of Health Politics, Policy and Law* 36 (3): 533-538.

Gonzales, Ernest, Yeonjung Lee and Celeste Brown. 2017. "Back to Work? Not Everyone: Examining the Longitudinal Relationship between Informal Caregiving and Paid Work after Formal Retire-ment." *Journal of Gerontology* 72(3):532-539.

Grogan, Colleen and Eric Patashnic. 2003. "Universalism within Targeting: Nursing Home Care, the Middle Class and the Politics of the Medicaid Program." *Social Service Review* 7 (1):51-71.

Grabowski, David, Joseph Angelelli and Vincent Mor. 2004. "The Relationship of Medicaid Payment Rates, Bed Constraint Policies, and Risk-Adjusted Pressure Ulcers." *Health Services Research* 39:793-812.

Harrington, Charlene, Leslie Ross and Taewoon Kang. 2015. "Hidden Owners, Hidden Profits and Poor Nursing Home Care." *International Journal of Health Services* 45: 779-800.

Harrington-Meyer, Madonna and Michelle Kesterke-Storbakken. 2000. "Shifting the Burden Back to Families." In *Care Work*, edited by Madonna Harrington Meyer, 217-228. New York: Routledge.

HHS. 2017. Report to the President and Congress The Money Follows the Person Rebalancing Demonstration. Department of Health and Human Services. https://www.macpac.gov/wp-content/uploads/2018/03/ MAC PAC-Comment-Letter-on-HHS-MFP-Report-to-Congress.pdf.

James, Everett, Walid Gellad and Meredith Hughes. 2017. "In This Next Phase of Health Reform, We Cannot Overlook Long Term Care." *Health Affairs Blog*, March 16, 2107. https://www.healthaffairs.org/ do/10.1377/hblog20170316.059218/full/

Kail, Ben, Jill Quadagno and Marc Dixon. 2009. "Can States Lead the Way to Universal Coverage? The Effect of Health Care Reform on the Uninsured." *Social Science Quarterly* 90 (5):1-20.

Kaiser Commission on Medicaid and the Uninsured. 2013. "*How is the Affordable Care Act Leading to Changes in Medicaid Long-Term Services and Supports (LTSS) Today? State Adoption of Six LTSS Options*." Washington, D.C.: The Kaiser Family Foundation. https://kaiserfamilyfoundation.files.wordpress.com/2013/04/8079-02.pdf

Kaiser Family Foundation. 2015. *Medicaid Eligibility through the Medically Needy Pathway*. https://www.kff.org/other/state-indicator/medicaid-eligibility-through-the-medically-needy-pathway/

Kassner, Enid and Lee Shirey. 2000. "*Medicaid Financial Eligibility for Older People: State Variations in Access to Home and Community Based Waiver and Nursing Home Services*." AARP Public Policy Institute. http://assets.aarp.org/rgcenter/health/2000_06_medicaid.pdf.

Lloyd, Liz, Albert Banerjee, Charlene Harrington, Frode Jacobsen and Marta Szebehely. 2014. "It is a Scandal!: Comparing the Causes and Consequences of Nursing Home Media Scandals in Five Countries." *International Journal of Sociology and Social Policy*, 34:2-18.

Medicaid.gov. 2019. "*Long Term Services and Support*." http://www.medicaid.gov/Medicaid-CHIP-Program-Information/By-Topics/Long-

Term-Services-and-Support/Integrating-Care/Program-of-All-Inclusive-Care-for-the-Elderly-PACE/PACE-Benefits.html.

Miller, Nancy and Adele Kirk. 2016. "Predicting State Investment in Medicaid Home-and-Community-Based Services, 2000-2011." *Journal of Aging and Social Policy* 28(1): 29-64.

Olson, Laura Katz. 2010. *The Politics of Medicaid*. New York: Columbia University Press.

Quadagno, Jill. 2015. "The Transformation of Medicaid from Poor Law Legacy to Middle Class Entitlement." In *Medicare and Medicaid at 50*, edited by Keith Wailoo, Julian Zelizer, and Alan Cohen, 77-94. Oxford University Press.

Rahman, Anna. 2019. *Money Follows the Person: Are We Getting Our Money's Worth?* American Society on Aging. Asaaging.org.

Reeves and Musumeci. 2015. *Medicaid and Long Term Services and Supports: A Primer*. Kaiser Family Foundation, Dec. 15, 2105. https://www.kff.org/medicaid/report/medicaid-and-long-term-services-and-supports-a-primer/

Reinhard, Susan, Enid Kassner and Art Houser. 2011. "How the Affordable Care Act Can Help Move States toward a High Performing System of Long-term Services and Supports." *Health Affairs* 30: 447-453.

Reinhard, Susan, Carol Levine and Sarah Samis. 2012. *Home Alone: Family Caregivers Providing Complex Chronic Care*. AARP Public Policy Institute. http://www.aarp.org/home-family/caregiving/info-10-2012/home-alone-family-caregivers-providing-complex-chronic-care.html.

Rudowitz, Robin and Rachel Garfield. 2018. "*Ten Things to Know about Medicaid: Setting the Facts Straight*." Issue Brief, April 12, 2018. Washington, D.C.: The Kaiser Family Foundation.

Scharlach, Andrew E. and Amanda J. Lehning. 2016. *Creating Age-Friendly Communities*. New York: Oxford University Press.

Scism, Leslie. 2018. "Safety Net Frays for Millions of Retirees." *Wall Street Journal*, January 18.

Seniorliving.org. https://www.seniorliving.org/nursing-homes/costs/.

Smith, David. 1999. *Health Care Divided*. Ann Arbor: University of Michigan Press.

Smith, David, Zhanlian Feng, Mary Fennel, Jacqueline Zinn and Vincent Mor. 2007. "Separate and Unequal: Racial Segregation and Disparities in Quality Across U.S. Nursing Homes." *Health Affairs* 26:1448-58.

Social Security Administration. 2019. *Understanding Supplemental Security Income, 2019 Edition*. https://www.ssa.gov/ssi/text-income-ussi.htm

Street, Debra, Stephanie Burge, Jill Quadagno, and Anne Barrett. 2007. "The Salience of Social Relationships on Resident Wellbeing in Assisted Living." *Journal of Gerontology* 62B (2):S129-134.

Thompson, Frank. 2012. *Medicaid Politics*. Washington, D.C.: Georgetown University Press.

Uhlenberg, Peter. 1997. "Replacing the Nursing Home." *Public Interest* 128:73.

Wakabayashi, Natalie and Katherine Donato. 2005. "The Consequences of Caregiving Effects on Women's Employment and Earnings." *Population Research and Policy Review* 24:467-488.

Wakabayashi, Natalie and Katherine Donato. 2006. "Does Caregiving Increase Poverty among Women in Later Life? Evidence from the Health and Retirement Survey." *Journal of Health and Social Behavior* 47: 258-274.

Wellin, Christopher. 2018. "Paid Caregiving for Older Adults with Serious and Chronic Illness: Ethnographic Perspectives, Evidence and Implications for Training." In *Critical Gerontology Comes of Age*, edited by Christopher Wellin, 112-133. New York: Routledge.

About the Editor

Daniel Lanford, PhD

Dr. Lanford is a researcher at the Georgia Health Policy Center in the Andrew Young School of Policy Studies at Georgia State University in Atlanta, Georgia. His work focuses on Medicaid policy, racial and ethnic politics, and cross-sector collaboration. His most recent publications address the expansion of Medicaid and recent attempts to repeal the Affordable Care Act.

About the Contributors

Amanda J. Abraham, PhD

Dr. Abraham is an Associate Professor of Public Administration and Policy in the School of Public and International Affairs at the University of Georgia. Her research focuses on the impact of federal and state policy on the accessibility and quality of substance use disorder treatment; the adoption, diffusion and implementation of evidence-based practices for the treatment of substance use disorder; organizational change; and workforce development. Dr. Abraham currently serves as principal investigator and co-investigator on numerous federal grants funded by the National Institute on Drug Abuse, the Substance Abuse and Mental Health Services Administration, and the U.S. Department of Agriculture.

Heidi Allen, PhD

Dr. Allen is an associate professor at Columbia University School of Social Work. She studies the impact of social policies, like Medicaid—America's health insurance for the poor—on health and financial well-being. She is a former emergency department social worker and spent several years in state health policy, where she focused on health system redesign and public health insurance expansions. Dr. Allen is currently involved in a variety of research projects focused on social policy at the intersection of health and poverty.

Christina M. Andrews, PhD

Dr. Andrews is an Associate Professor in the College of Social Work at the University of South Carolina. Her research focuses on the organization and financing of substance use disorder treatment on service access and quality. She is principal investigator for a five-year Mentored Research Scientist Development award from the National Institute on Drug Abuse examining the effects of Medicaid health homes identification and treatment of addiction.

Katherine Baicker, PhD

Dr. Baicker is the Dean and the Emmett Dedmon Professor at the Harris School of Public Policy at the University of Chicago. She is an elected member of the National Academy of Medicine, the National Academy of Social Insurance, the Council on Foreign Relations, and the American Academy of Arts and Sciences. She serves on the Congressional Budget Office's Panel of Health Advisers and as a Director of Eli Lilly and HMS. She is a member of the Advisory Board for the National Institute for Health Care Management; a Trustee of NORC; and a Trustee of the Mayo Clinic. She received her BA in economics from Yale and her PhD in economics from Harvard.

Sarah C. Blake, PhD

Dr. Blake is an assistant professor in the Department of Health Policy & Management at the Emory University Rollins School of Public Health in

Atlanta, Georgia. Her work focuses on Medicaid, reproductive health, and maternal and child health care policies. She leads several current projects that evaluate the policy implications of health disparities on women's health in Georgia.

Charles Courtemanche, PhD

Dr. Courtemanche is an Associate Professor of Economics and Director of the Institute for the Study of Free Enterprise at the University of Kentucky, as well as a Research Associate with the National Bureau of Economic Research and a Research Affiliate with the Institute for the Study of Labor. He is a health economist and applied microeconomist with particular research interests in the economics of obesity, public policies to expand insurance coverage, big box retailers, and the COVID-19 pandemic. He has published over 40 peer-reviewed articles and received funding from the National Institutes of Health, United States Department of Agriculture, and Food and Drug Administration. Dr. Courtemanche is Editor-in-Chief of the *Southern Economic Journal* and on the editorial boards of the *Journal of Policy Analysis and Management* and *Economics and Human Biology*.

Ishtiaque Fazlul, MS

Mr. Fazlul is a PhD candidate in Economics at Georgia State University and a Graduate Research Assistant at Georgia Policy Labs. He is an applied microeconomist working on topics related to health and education, with focuses on the intergenerational health effects of education, the effects of universal pre-K, and the effects of the Affordable Care Act. His most recent publication addresses the impact of the Affordable Care Act on insurance coverage disparities between different groups.

Paul A. Fishman, PhD

Dr. Fishman is an economist whose research has focused on improved payment models for public and private health insurance programs and health care delivery models to improve population health. He is a Professor in the University of Washington's School of Public Health and Associate Director for Research within the school's graduate programs in health service administration. Before joining the faculty at the University of Washington, Dr. Fishman spent 20 years conducting research with Group Health Cooperative (now Kaiser Permanente Washington).

Colleen M. Grogan, PhD

Dr. Grogan is a Professor at the University of Chicago in the School of Social Service Administration. Her research interests include health policy, health politics, and the American welfare state. She has written extensively on the history and current politics of the US Medicaid program. She is also completing a book manuscript titled *The Rise of America's Conservative Health Care State*, which examines the historical development of political strategies and motivations behind hiding the role of government in the US health care system. She is co-Associate Editor for the health policy section of the *American Journal of Public Health*.

Aaron B. Katz, CPH

Mr. Katz is a health policy practitioner, scholar, and teacher at the University of Washington School of Public Health in Seattle, Washington. Over more than 40 years, he has conducted research and provided support to public policy makers on issues from the HIV epidemic to the role of safety net providers to state-based health system reform, both in the U.S. and in low- and middle-income countries.

Madonna Harrington Meyer, PhD

Dr. Harrington Meyer is University Professor at Syracuse University. She is a professor of sociology at the Maxwell School of Public Affairs, the Laura J. and L. Douglas Meredith Professor of Teaching Excellence, a senior research associate at the Center for Policy Research, and a faculty affiliate at the Aging Studies Institute. Her most recent book, co-authored with Ynesse Abdul-Malak, is *Grandparenting Children with Disabilities* (forthcoming).

Samantha J. Harris, MPA

Ms. Harris is a doctoral candidate at the University of Georgia's School of Public and International Affairs in the Department of Public Administration and Policy. Her work focuses on health policy and health services related to substance use disorder treatment. Her most recent publications examine opioid use disorder medication treatment access among the publicly insured.

Pamela Herd, PhD

Dr. Herd is a professor of Public Policy at Georgetown University. Her research focuses on inequality and how it intersects with health, aging, and policy. She is an expert in survey research and biodemographic methods. She is currently the Chair of the Board of Overseers for the General Social Survey, a member of the Board of Overseers for the Panel Study of Income Dynamics, a board member for the Population Association of America, and a standing member of a National Institutes for Health review panel for the Social and Population Sciences. She has received grant awards for her work from the National Institutes for Health, National Institute on Aging, among others.

James Marton, PhD

Dr. Marton is a professor of economics at the Andrew Young School of Policy Studies at Georgia State University. His work focuses on the financing and impacts of public transfer programs. His most recent publications address the impact of the Affordable Care Act on a wide variety of outcomes, the relationship between the Medicaid program and the Supplemental Nutrition Assistance Program, as well as different delivery modes for services in state Medicaid programs.

Donald P. Moynihan, PhD

Dr. Moynihan is the inaugural McCourt Chair at the McCourt School of Public Policy at Georgetown University. His research examines how to improve how government works. He examines the behavioral effects of efforts to improve public sector outcomes through government reform, as well as the administrative burdens people encounter in their interactions with government. He is past president of the Public Management Research Association and a member of the National Academy of Public Administration.

Jill Quadagno, PhD

Dr. Quadagno is Emeritus Professor and Research Associate in the Pepper Institute on Aging and Public Policy at Florida State University. She is the author of 12 books and more than 70 articles on social welfare, aging, and health care. She is past President of the American Sociological Association and a member of the National Academy of Medicine.

Philip Rocco, PhD

Dr. Rocco is an Assistant Professor of Political Science at Marquette University. He specializes in American politics, with a focus on federalism, public policy, and the political economy of policy knowledge. He is the co-author of *Obamacare Wars: Federalism, State Politics, and the Affordable Care Act* (University Press of Kansas, 2016) and co-editor of *American Political Development and the Trump Presidency* (University of Pennsylvania Press, 2020). His work has appeared in journals such as *Political Science Quarterly*, *Journal of Health Politics, Policy, and Law*, *Health Affairs*, and the *Journal of Public Policy*.

Bikki Tran Smith, MA, MSW

Ms. Tran Smith is a doctoral candidate in the School of Social Service Administration at the University of Chicago. Her research focuses on the intersection of behavioral health services, health policy, race, and place. Her current work examines the moderating impact of area deprivation on the relationship between state substance use disorder treatment coverage and funding and outpatient addiction treatment service availability.

Carolin Spice, MS

Ms. Spice is a healthcare quality professional, clinical informaticist, researcher, and teacher whose research and work has been at the intersection of digitizing healthcare quality metrics to improve population health for over 20 years. She teaches health informatics at the University of Washington's School of Public Health. As a practitioner in healthcare quality, she has worked with integrated healthcare organizations to transform their delivery models.

J. Dalton Stevens, MA

Mr. Stevens is a PhD candidate in sociology at Syracuse University, and he is a research assistant at the Syracuse University Aging Studies Institute. His most recent publication, "Stuck in transition with you: Variable pathways to in(ter)dependence for emerging adult men with mobility impairments" appears in *Research in Social Science and Disability*.

Benjamin Ukert, PhD

Dr. Ukert is an assistant professor of Health Policy and Management at the School of Public Health at Texas A&M. His work focuses on the Affordable Care Act, insurance markets, and the delivery of care. His most recent publications address the impact of the Affordable Care Act on access to care and self-reported health, the impact of medical marijuana laws on health, and the effectiveness of provider driven care management programs on the health of the elderly.

Melissa A. Westlake, MSW

Mrs. Westlake is a doctoral candidate at the University of South Carolina's College of Social Work. Her research focus is on the impact of regulatory policy and environmental conditions on access to and quality of substance use disorder treatment. Specifically, Westlake is interested in evaluating the performance of the specialty substance use disorder treatment sector in meeting evidence-based standards for high quality treatment and determining the regulatory and environmental conditions that best predict successful quality performance.

Bill J. Wright, PhD

Dr. Wright is the director of the Center for Outcomes Research and Education at Providence Health & Services. Dr. Wright is a sociologist with a principal focus on survey design, and he specializes in longitudinal research with low-income and vulnerable populations. His research focuses on the intersection between health policy, health systems design, and the social determinants of health.

Aaron Yelowitz, PhD

Dr. Yelowitz is a professor of economics at the University of Kentucky. He is also a joint faculty member in the Martin School of Public Policy and Administration at the University of Kentucky and a senior fellow with the Cato Institute. His work focuses on the Affordable Care Act, insurance markets, and the COVID-19 pandemic. His most recent publications address the impact of government-imposed social distancing measures during the pandemic, the determinants of improper Medicaid enrollment, and the role of occupational licensing on the entry of health care professionals.

Bomy Yun, MHIHIM, MSN, ARNP

Ms. Yun is a clinical informaticist and family practice clinician at Neighborcare Health in Seattle, Washington. She has years of experience in clinical and health IT leadership. As a practicing clinician, she has provided primary health care services to underserved populations at a federally qualified health center. As an informaticist, she has led work on practice transformation and population health management through the use of informatics.

Daniela Zapata, PhD

Dr. Zapata is a Senior Research Economist at IMPAQ International. Her main areas of expertise are the design and implementation of quasi-experimental approaches to evaluate policy interventions. She has conducted impact evaluations of alternative payment models, initiatives to increase the healthcare workforce, and demonstrations to reduce the number of medical appeals. Her most recent publications focus on the effects of the Affordable Care Act on a wide variety of outcomes.

INDEX

A

access to care, xiii, 17, 60, 182, 205, 262, 281, 283, 284, 326, 374
accessibility, xvi, 283, 301, 303, 330, 358, 367
addiction, 269, 279, 303, 305, 310, 314, 326, 332, 335, 368, 373
administrative burden(s), xii, xiii, 81, 82, 83, 84, 85, 86, 87, 90, 95, 96, 97, 99, 103, 104, 105, 106, 111, 205, 262, 277, 278, 279, 281, 285, 288, 372
advocacy, 119, 130, 134, 186
Affordable Care Act, v, vi, xvi, xvii, 1, 22, 44, 49, 50, 51, 53, 54, 56, 83, 97, 102, 106, 115, 116, 132, 133, 135, 145, 174, 176, 183, 211, 212, 213, 250, 251, 252, 254, 266, 294, 302, 332, 335, 348, 361, 362, 365, 369, 372, 373, 374, 375, 376
agencies, xiv, 5, 45, 59, 72, 88, 89, 94, 99, 130, 187, 189, 196, 203, 204, 205
aging population, 353, 355, 357
alcohol (use/abuse), 314
and enrollment, 117, 202, 203, 205, 308
and health care, 4, 190, 262, 370, 372
assessment, 98, 279, 304, 323, 350
assessment of Medicaid websites, 304
assets, 133, 266, 274, 287, 299, 341, 342, 361
assisted living facilities, 338, 345
awareness, 182, 197, 198, 205

B

behavioral health, 60, 63, 65, 70, 132, 268, 269, 283, 284, 302, 303, 306, 308, 309, 310, 311, 312, 313, 314, 315, 316, 317, 319, 320, 321, 322, 323, 324, 325, 326, 327, 328, 329, 330, 331, 335, 350, 373
behavioral health benefits information, 302, 312, 331
behavioral health treatment benefits information, 315, 321
benefits, x, xi, xii, xiii, xv, xvi, 5, 16, 56, 81, 82, 83, 84, 86, 87, 88, 89, 93, 96, 100, 103, 104, 105, 112, 119, 130, 143, 144, 145, 146, 147, 155, 169, 182, 183, 192, 193, 201, 247, 261, 262, 267, 269, 280, 286, 287, 302, 303, 304, 305, 307, 308, 309, 311, 312, 313, 314, 315, 316, 319, 320, 321, 322, 323, 324, 325, 327, 328,

329, 330, 331, 332, 335, 340, 342, 350, 354, 355, 356, 362
bias, xiii, 112, 115, 116, 128, 136, 268, 273, 275, 351
buprenorphine, 136, 306, 314, 326, 331
Bureau of Labor Statistics, 28, 154

C

campaigns, 88, 147, 205, 266
caregivers, 278, 351, 352, 358, 359, 362
caregiving, 362
carved out, 322, 323, 324
carve-in, 307, 308, 323
carve-out(s), 307, 308, 314, 324, 325
census, 26, 74, 154, 156, 157, 218, 253, 254, 255, 256, 264, 265, 332
citizenship, 28, 90, 108, 215, 233, 240, 241, 242, 243, 245, 248, 311, 315
community-based services, xvi, 338
compensation, 187, 188
compliance, 81, 82, 83, 88, 89, 91, 92, 93, 98, 102, 113, 205
compliance costs, 82, 83, 88, 91, 92, 93, 98, 102, 103
consensus, 191, 206, 311, 332
consumers, xv, 203, 205, 207, 218, 247, 263, 302, 307, 308, 309, 312, 313, 317, 321, 323, 324, 325, 327, 328, 329, 330, 331
content analysis, 311, 317, 319, 320
cost of living, 154
cost saving, 183, 201, 349
counseling, 190, 203, 267, 270, 314, 346

D

daily living, 268, 279, 338, 348
dependent variable, 158, 164, 240, 241, 242, 243, 245
depression, 4, 5, 10, 15, 16, 19, 107, 280
detox, 314
disability, vi, xv, 27, 101, 217, 233, 235, 236, 240, 241, 242, 243, 245, 261, 262, 263, 264, 265, 266, 267, 268, 269, 270, 271, 272, 273, 274, 275, 276, 277, 278, 279, 280, 281, 282, 283, 284, 285, 286, 287, 288, 289, 290, 291, 292, 294, 295, 297, 298, 299, 300, 333, 338, 342, 349, 350, 374
disorder, xv, 65, 136, 264, 279, 301, 302, 303, 310, 326, 334, 367, 368, 371, 373, 374
disparities in insurance coverage, 22, 44
dolophine, 314
drug (use/abuse), 314
drug interaction, 61, 63

E

effective tax rates, 212, 215, 254, 257
elders, 348, 351, 356, 358
election, 45, 91, 97, 98, 106
eligibility, xiv, xv, 10, 49, 54, 57, 60, 82, 84, 86, 89, 90, 91, 92, 93, 94, 95, 96, 104, 107, 111, 112, 113, 131, 134, 136, 145, 169, 181, 183, 184, 190, 192, 196, 198, 202, 206, 208, 209, 215, 217, 219, 220, 235, 236, 237, 238, 247, 248, 249, 250, 252, 253, 255, 256, 257, 261, 262, 266, 270, 271, 272, 273, 276, 278, 279, 284, 287, 288, 292, 293, 296, 298, 302, 303, 311, 315, 316, 319, 320, 327, 339, 340, 341, 342, 347, 350, 355, 356, 359, 361
eligibility criteria, 96, 181, 278, 284, 315, 316, 355, 356
emergency, xi, 4, 5, 10, 11, 12, 13, 14, 15, 17, 61, 63, 325, 367
enrollment, xv, xvi, 46, 49, 58, 74, 76, 88, 90, 91, 92, 94, 95, 97, 103, 104, 106, 115, 117, 118, 119, 122, 125, 127, 128,

129, 136, 182, 185, 189, 194, 195, 196, 197, 198, 199, 200, 201, 202, 203, 204, 205, 206, 211, 213, 214, 216, 217, 221, 222, 227, 236, 238, 239, 246, 247, 248, 249, 252, 253, 257, 266, 267, 274, 275, 285, 288, 293, 296, 302, 303, 308, 311, 316, 319, 320, 323, 327, 333, 335, 355, 375
epidemic, 297, 303, 305, 308, 309, 331, 334, 370
ethnic politics, 142, 169, 365
ethnicity, 22, 25, 28, 41, 47, 149, 151, 167, 233, 240, 241, 242, 243, 245
expenditures, 5, 117, 142, 143, 153, 154, 158, 159, 164, 166, 182, 192, 266, 268, 275, 276, 285, 347, 353, 356

F

families, 3, 55, 87, 88, 91, 100, 145, 219, 238, 243, 263, 266, 274, 275, 276, 279, 288, 356, 357
family income, 183, 270
family members, 286, 338, 358
family planning, 181, 182, 183, 184, 185, 186, 187, 189, 190, 191, 192, 193, 194, 197, 199, 200, 201, 203, 205, 206, 207, 210
federal funds, 195, 350
federal government, ix, x, 83, 90, 97, 102, 104, 111, 113, 118, 119, 144, 146, 153, 154, 182, 183, 201, 308, 329, 336, 343, 356, 357
federal law, 276
federal mandate, 288
federal regulations, 118, 123, 128
federally qualified health centers, 54, 89
financial, 4, 5, 6, 7, 14, 15, 17, 18, 82, 91, 105, 207, 286, 295, 296, 344, 345, 367
financial incentives, 91, 105, 345
fiscal year, 72, 73, 195, 215, 333
Flesch Reading Ease score, 311, 315
Flesch-Kincaid grade level, 311, 315
focus groups, 186, 187, 196, 200, 201, 205
formulary, 309, 314
fraud, 86, 95, 343
funding, 54, 55, 56, 71, 88, 90, 93, 96, 97, 182, 187, 192, 195, 203, 204, 207, 209, 266, 269, 288, 305, 337, 344, 345, 346, 347, 349, 350, 351, 353, 355, 356, 369, 373
funds, 87, 88, 91, 144, 153, 192, 195, 204, 305, 339, 341, 347, 349, 350, 352, 353, 356

G

government spending, 72
governments, 86, 104, 112, 114, 115, 116, 117, 146
grants, 18, 94, 347, 367
growth, 39, 45, 57, 58, 60, 68, 143, 145, 146, 147, 148, 169, 170, 174, 222, 266, 288, 302, 305, 308, 340, 343, 351
guidance, 113, 187, 206, 294, 296, 360
guidelines, x, 86, 91, 92, 188, 194, 204, 206, 273, 274, 327, 332

H

health care costs, 144, 151, 341
health care finance, 22, 212
health care system, 7, 170, 347, 370
health condition, 17, 263, 268, 269, 278, 287
health information, xii, 65, 71, 308, 310, 324, 329
health insurance, ix, xii, xiv, 4, 10, 14, 15, 16, 22, 27, 81, 83, 84, 87, 88, 90, 92, 97, 100, 103, 104, 105, 147, 157, 165, 212, 214, 216, 218, 219, 220, 221, 227, 235,

237, 248, 268, 270, 274, 281, 284, 303, 308, 331, 367, 370
health literacy, 207, 302
health problems, 100, 357
health services, x, 55, 60, 68, 132, 185, 197, 268, 269, 284, 307, 315, 323, 324, 325, 371, 373
healthcare access, 82
HITECH Act, 54
home care services, 353
home-and-community based services, 337, 338
homes, 6, 338, 339, 340, 343, 344, 346, 347, 348, 350, 352, 353, 355, 356, 362, 368
hospice, 284, 353
household income, x, 28, 55, 95, 151, 154, 157, 216, 275
housing, 171, 267, 270, 276, 337, 347, 348, 351, 353

I

impairments, 263, 288, 374
improvements, xi, 4, 12, 56, 208, 301, 303, 329, 330
income distribution, 40, 211, 213, 214, 233, 235
increased access, 3, 4, 59, 182, 183, 185
independent living, 264
individual characteristics, 236, 240, 241, 242, 243, 245
inflation, 154, 287
information availability, 312
information on eligibility, 308
institutions, xii, 263, 274, 345, 350
Intellectual Disability, 297, 298
interest groups, 129, 131, 134, 145, 147
intergovernmental relations, 112, 116
issues, xiv, xvii, 108, 198, 215, 239, 247, 248, 282, 284, 296, 327, 343, 349, 358, 370

L

labor force, 28, 46, 100
labor force participation, 28, 46, 100
labor market, 4, 7, 46, 100, 103, 352
learning, 17, 65, 81, 82, 88, 89, 91, 92, 93, 97, 98, 102, 264
learning costs, 82, 89, 93, 97, 98, 102, 103
learning disabilities, 264
legislation, 59, 128, 130, 207, 261, 266, 285, 339
literacy, 102, 207, 302, 327, 330, 331
living arrangements, 340, 342
loan guarantees, 56
loans, 339
lobbying, 157, 173, 192, 193, 356
local community, 89, 358
local government, 91, 97
long term care, 156, 337, 338, 339, 340, 342, 343, 350, 352, 353, 354, 355, 356, 357, 358
longevity, 145
long-term services and supports, 267

M

marital status, 22, 23, 24, 25, 43, 45, 46, 233, 240, 241, 242, 243, 245
MCO Benefits Information, 320
MCO websites, 302, 309, 312, 316, 328, 329, 330, 331
media, 75, 94, 131, 144, 172, 177, 290, 295
Medicaid MCO coverage information, 304
Medicaid websites, 302, 304, 308, 309, 311, 312, 315, 317, 319, 327, 328, 331
medical assistance, 90, 93, 96, 100
medical care, 112, 267, 276, 283, 340
medication, 5, 9, 19, 304, 305, 306, 313, 314, 326, 328, 331, 349, 371
medicine, 17, 108, 112, 147, 161, 163, 165, 284

mental health, 3, 15, 16, 70, 263, 267, 268, 269, 273, 283, 285, 294, 307, 309, 314, 315, 322, 325, 326, 346, 348
mental illness, 269, 310
methadone, 304, 314, 326, 331
methadone diskets, 314
middle class, 142, 145, 169, 178, 340, 345, 358
minorities, xiii, 43, 142, 143, 146, 149, 151, 154, 155, 159, 164, 166, 167, 168, 169, 170, 174, 344
mortality, 100, 189, 207

N

naltrexone, 306, 314, 326, 331
needy, 242, 268, 272, 290, 293, 307, 340, 341, 356, 361
nursing, ix, 267, 268, 269, 279, 281, 337, 338, 339, 340, 341, 343, 344, 345, 346, 347, 348, 349, 350, 351, 352, 353, 355, 356, 357, 362
nursing care, 267, 268, 343
nursing home(s), 268, 279, 337, 338, 339, 340, 341, 343, 344, 345, 346, 347, 348, 349, 350, 351, 352, 353, 355, 356, 357
nutrition, 346, 349

O

Obama Administration, 98
Obama, President Barack, xvii, 91, 150, 178
occupational therapy, 269, 346
officials, 86, 88, 94, 111, 112, 115, 130, 131, 191, 344
online information, 104, 327
opiate, 314
opioid, 67, 136, 270, 297, 303, 305, 308, 309, 314, 326, 331, 332, 333, 334, 335, 371
opioid treatment, 314
Oregon Health Insurance Experiment, xvii, 3, 4, 5, 7, 11, 12, 14, 15, 17, 19
outpatient, 7, 304, 307, 314, 322, 323, 325, 373
outreach, 29, 60, 61, 63, 88, 89, 91, 93, 94, 97, 98, 102, 104, 187, 188, 190, 194, 196, 197, 198, 202, 203, 205, 216, 266

P

pain management, 326, 331
parents, 88, 93, 96, 100, 107, 114, 217, 278, 280, 331, 352
participants, xv, 3, 6, 8, 84, 86, 87, 88, 89, 94, 100, 117, 146, 169, 186, 187, 191, 192, 193, 196, 198, 199, 200, 203, 275, 280, 346, 347, 349
pharmaceutical(s), 56, 157, 161, 163, 165
physical health, 4, 7, 15, 307, 348
physicians, 56, 278, 279, 283, 286, 349
policy implementation, 82, 182, 185, 204
policy legacy, 142, 158, 159, 160, 162, 165, 337, 351, 358
policymakers, xi, xiii, 25, 99, 115, 143, 184, 288, 331, 337, 356, 358
political power, 84, 358
politics, ix, x, xiii, 84, 85, 104, 108, 135, 141, 142, 148, 157, 168, 169, 171, 358, 359, 365, 370, 373
poverty line, x, 95, 96, 145, 169, 226, 232, 265, 270, 272, 273, 274, 275, 280, 281
preferred drug list, 304, 309, 312, 314, 326
prescription drugs, 5, 269, 284, 346
prescription/medication, 314
prevention, 184, 190, 349
private sector, 82, 103, 345
protection, 137, 342, 356
psychiatric, 270, 278, 310, 314, 325, 335
psychological costs, 81, 82, 88, 89, 93, 98
psychological distress, 101

public assistance, 87, 95, 97, 235, 236, 240, 241, 242, 243, 245
public health, xiii, 63, 87, 88, 187, 189, 191, 194, 196, 197, 200, 206, 221, 368
Public Health Service Act, 54, 55
public opinion, 142, 143, 145, 149, 150, 151, 158, 159, 167, 170, 171, 172, 173, 174
public policy, 174, 206, 370, 373
public support, 111, 143, 145, 146, 148, 150, 166, 169, 170, 171

Q

quality assurance, 55
quality improvement, 65, 68
quality of life, 268, 275, 289, 350

R

race, 22, 23, 25, 28, 39, 40, 44, 149, 151, 153, 167, 233, 240, 241, 242, 243, 245, 262, 265, 280, 298, 373
racial differences, 148, 155
racial minorities, 168
racial politics, 142, 171
readability, 302, 311, 315, 327, 333, 335, 336
reform(s), 22, 23, 37, 38, 49, 51, 57, 71, 72, 75, 87, 104, 105, 108, 122, 134, 136, 137, 138, 145, 147, 173, 174, 176, 177, 178, 213, 217, 220, 235, 266, 291, 293, 301, 303, 308, 334, 336, 361, 370, 372
regulations, 33, 85, 117, 118, 206, 247, 305, 317, 341, 343, 344
rehabilitation, 11, 100, 353
residential treatment, 306, 314, 325
resources, 84, 100, 157, 185, 186, 187, 204, 206, 255, 276, 278, 281, 283, 329, 339, 341, 343, 349, 350, 351
restrictions, 112, 145, 146, 174, 302, 303, 313, 339, 344
retirement, 240, 241, 242, 243, 245
Revia, 314

S

Section 1115, 107, 111, 112, 114, 115, 116, 117, 118, 120, 122, 123, 127, 128, 131, 134, 135, 136, 138, 139, 181, 182, 183, 184, 190, 191, 194, 206, 219, 293
self-reported health, xi, 4, 5, 15, 374
social policy, 116, 143, 145, 150, 168, 172, 173, 368
social programs, xiii, 83, 85, 99, 145
social security, x, 18, 91, 102, 112, 146, 235, 236, 240, 241, 242, 243, 245, 274, 275, 299, 332, 339, 340, 342, 363
Social Security Administration (SSA), 18, 91, 145, 274, 275, 299, 332, 342, 363
Social Security Disability Insurance, 274
social services, 72, 113, 190
social welfare, 280, 372
stakeholder politics, 142, 148
stressful life events, 348
Suboxone, 314, 326
substance abuse, 70, 263, 279
Substance Abuse and Mental Health Services Administration (SAMHSA), 305, 336
substance use, xv, 65, 269, 285, 301, 302, 310, 314, 334, 367, 368, 371, 373, 374
substance use disorder coverage, 302
substance use disorders (SUD), xv, 122, 138, 269, 285, 301, 302, 303, 304, 305, 306, 307, 309, 312, 313, 315, 317, 322, 323, 324, 325, 326, 328, 329, 330, 331
Subutex, 314
SUD treatment coverage, 303, 304, 305, 313, 328, 330

Supplemental Nutrition Assistance Program, 372

T

target population, 89, 135, 346
technical language, 325, 328
testing, 10, 141, 150, 200, 201

U

unemployment rate, 28, 48
uninsured, x, xii, 4, 5, 6, 7, 8, 9, 10, 11, 12, 13, 15, 16, 22, 23, 24, 26, 27, 29, 30, 31, 32, 33, 34, 35, 36, 37, 38, 39, 40, 41, 42, 43, 44, 47, 48, 54, 55, 56, 58, 68, 92, 94, 107, 178, 183, 184, 185, 201, 205, 213, 216, 217, 221, 223, 224, 225, 226, 229, 230,231, 232, 261, 262, 266, 270, 293, 327, 335, 349, 361

V

Vivitrol, 314, 326

W

waiver(s), xiii, 83, 85, 86, 87, 88, 90, 95, 96, 99, 100, 103, 104, 105, 107, 111, 112, 114, 115, 116, 117, 118, 119, 120, 122, 123, 124, 125, 126, 127, 128, 129, 130, 131, 134, 136, 137, 138, 139, 147, 153, 181, 182, 183, 184, 190, 191, 192, 193, 194, 195, 196, 203, 204, 205, 206, 207, 219, 252, 268, 271, 273, 275, 285, 286, 288, 293, 296, 299, 345, 346, 347, 355, 356
webpages, 310, 316
websites, xv, 123, 196, 302, 304, 308, 309, 310, 311, 312, 315, 316, 317, 319, 322, 323, 325, 327, 328, 329, 330, 331
welfare, vi, 86, 87, 89, 93, 95, 100, 107, 112, 141, 142, 143, 144, 145, 146, 147, 148, 149, 151, 153, 154, 155, 156, 157, 164, 166, 167, 168, 169, 171, 172, 173, 174, 175, 176, 177, 178, 198, 215, 236, 247, 251, 257, 261, 262, 266, 276, 277, 280, 290, 291, 294, 299, 300, 370, 372
welfare policy, 262
welfare reform, 87, 100
welfare state, 145, 266, 370
work requirements, xiii, xv, 46, 81, 83, 84, 98, 99, 100, 101, 103, 104, 108, 111, 112, 113, 114, 115, 118, 119, 120, 125, 127, 128, 129, 130, 131, 219, 285
workforce, 100, 101, 137, 367, 376